EDUCATION AND RESEARCH CENTRE
Wythenshawe Hospital
Tel: 0161 291 57⁻⁻

This book should be returned by ·
previously recalled. Fines wiⁱⁱ ·

5ᵐ

THE EVIDENCE FOR VASCULAR SURGERY

Edited by

Jonothan J. Earnshaw and
John A. Murie

t*f*m Publishing Limited

JVRG

Publication details

Published by:-

t*f*m Publishing Limited
Brimstree View
Kemberton
Nr. Shifnal
Shropshire
TF11 9LL

Tel: 01952 586408
Fax: 01952 587654
E-mail: nikki@tfmpub.freeserve.co.uk

Design and layout: Nikki Bramhill
Cartoons: Barry Foley

First Edition   November 1999

ISBN 0 9530052 5 9

Printed by Frontier Print and Design Limited
Pickwick House
Chosen View Road
Cheltenham
Gloucestershire
GL51 9LT

Tel: 01242 573863
Fax: 01242 511643

Contents

Contents

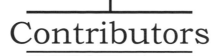

Contributors

S Ashley MS FRCS, Consultant Vascular Surgeon. *Derriford Hospital, Plymouth.*

AAB Barros D'Sa MD FRCS FRCSEd, Consultant Vascular Surgeon. *The Royal Victoria Hospital, Belfast, Northern Ireland.*

JD Beard ChM FRCS, Consultant Vascular Surgeon; **J Robinson** FRCS, Surgical Research Fellow. *Northern General Hospital, Sheffield.*

AW Bradbury BSc MD FRCSEd, Consultant Surgeon and Senior Lecturer; **RK MacKenzie** FRCSEd, Research Fellow. *Royal Infirmary of Edinburgh, Edinburgh.*

WB Campbell MS FRCP FRCS, Consultant Surgeon. *Royal Devon and Exeter Hospital, Exeter.*

J Collin MA MD FRCS, Consultant Surgeon and Reader in Surgery. *The John Radcliffe Hospital, Oxford.*

SG Darke MS FRCS, Consultant Surgeon. *Royal Bournemouth Hospital, Bournemouth.*

JJ Earnshaw DM FRCS, Consultant Surgeon. *Gloucestershire Royal Hospital, Gloucester.*

PA Gaines MRCP FRCR, Consultant Vascular Radiologist. *Northern General Hospital, Sheffield.*

RB Galland MD FRCS, Consultant Surgeon; **JMT Perkins** MD FRCS, Specialist Registrar. *Royal Berkshire Hospital, Reading.*

GL Gilling-Smith MS FRCS, Consultant Vascular Surgeon. *Royal Liverpool University Hospital, Liverpool.*

MJ Gough ChM FRCS, Consultant Surgeon; **P Tan** FRCS, Specialist Registrar; **G Maritati** MB BS, Visiting Fellow. *The General Infirmary at Leeds, Leeds.*

G Hamilton FRCS, Consultant Vascular Surgeon; **M Davis** FRCS, Specialist Registrar. *Royal Free Hospital, London.*

PL Harris MD FRCS, Consultant Vascular Surgeon; **RK Fisher** FRCS, Research Fellow. *Royal Liverpool University Hospital, Liverpool..*

BP Heather MS FRCS, Consultant Surgeon. *Gloucestershire Royal Hospital, Gloucester.*

PM Lamont MD FRCS, Consultant Vascular Surgeon and Honorary Senior Clinical Lecturer. *Bristol Royal Infirmary, Bristol.*

NJM London MB ChB MRCP FRCS MD FRCP(Edin), Professor of Surgery; **A Nasim** MD FRCS, Specialist Registrar. *Leicester Royal Infirmary, Leicester.*

PT McCollum MCh FRCSI FRCSEd, Professor of Vascular Surgery; **LD Wijesinghe** FRCS, Specialist Registrar. *Hull Royal Infirmary, Hull.*

JA Murie MA BSc MD FRCSEd FRCSG, Consultant Vascular Surgeon and Honorary Senior Lecturer. *Royal Infirmary of Edinburgh, Edinburgh.*

AR Naylor MD FRCS, Consultant Vascular Surgeon and Honorary Senior Lecturer. *Leicester Royal Infirmary, Leicester.*

SD Parvin MD FRCS, Consultant Vascular Surgeon; **A Cowan** FRCS, Specialist Registrar. *Royal Bournemouth Hospital, Bournemouth.*

DA Ratliff MD MRCP FRCS, Consultant Vascular Surgeon. *Northampton General Hospital, Northampton.*

CV Ruckley MBChM FRCS, Professor of Vascular Surgery; **AA Milne** MD FRCS, Specialist Registrar. *Royal Infirmary of Edinburgh, Edinburgh.*

DJA Scott MD FRCS, Consultant Vascular Surgeon. *St. James's University Hospital, Leeds.*

CP Shearman BSc (Hons) MS FRCS, Consultant Vascular Surgeon and Honorary Senior Lecturer; **A Chulakadabba** BA MD FRCS FRCSEd, Vascular Research Fellow. *Southampton University Hospital, Southampton.*

FCT Smith FRCS, Consultant Vascular Surgeon and Senior Lecturer. *Bristol Royal Infirmary, Bristol.*

G Stansby MChir FRCS, Honorary Consultant Surgeon and Senior Lecturer; **K Delis** MD MSc, Senior Vascular Fellow. *St. Mary's Hospital, London.*

PR Taylor MA MChir FRCS, Consultant Vascular Surgeon. *Guy's Hospital, London.*

JF Thompson MS FRCSEd FRCS, Consultant Surgeon. *Royal Devon and Exeter Hospital, Exeter.*

DC Wilkins MD FRCS, Consultant Surgeon. *Derriford Hospital, Plymouth.*

JHN Wolfe MS FRCS, Consultant Vascular Surgeon; **MJ Brooks** FRCS, Research Fellow. *St. Mary's Hospital, London.*

MG Wyatt MSc MD FRCS, Consultant Vascular Surgeon; **J Rose** FRCP FRCR, Consultant Radiologist. *Freeman Hospital, Newcastle upon Tyne.*

Foreword

The ability to pause and reflect critically on their activities is a mark of maturity in professionals and their organisations. Such reflection is particularly relevant in areas such as vascular surgery, whose exponents wield such a powerful tool. It is to the credit of vascular surgeons in general that they have been at the forefront of data collection, randomised controlled trials and clinical audit. Theirs is a young specialty, but youthful enthusiasm is now being tempered by mature reflection. It was in this spirit that in June 1999 a meeting was held in Gloucester, the theme of which was the evidence base of vascular surgery. Many leading surgeons gave of their time to present their concepts of where daily surgical practice now stands in relation to clinical science; most were (and are) members of the Joint Vascular Research Group (q.v. Appendix).

The topics considered ranged over the whole spectrum of vascular disease and its management. Carotid endarterectomy, inevitably, played a part; the initial criteria for surgery that were derived from the European Carotid Surgery Trial may have to be altered in a direction that will reduce the number of patients likely to benefit from operation. An effect will also be felt from the introduction of carotid balloon angioplasty and stenting; but this should be in the future as the evidence base of the technique is, at present, paltry. The UK Small Aneurysm Trial too has tended to reduce the numbers likely to come to surgery, with its message that it is no longer reasonable to contemplate aortic replacement for most lesions less than 55mm in diameter. Here too new technology may reduce the number of classic open procedures; endoluminal stent graft insertion proceeds with mature caution. Many other areas were considered, including some that may hitherto have been neglected, such as non-surgical factors which influence surgical outcome, and medico-legal matters. These two topics are of particular relevance in an era when hospital is being compared with hospital and surgeon with surgeon.

Those who contributed to the meeting were asked to prepare a chapter for this book 'The Evidence for Vascular Surgery'. It did not surprise the editors that the quality was uniformly high and that a thoughtful and even handed approach was the hallmark throughout. This is a book examining evidence; it has no room for the blinkered over-enthusiast ploughing his or her favourite furrow.

John A. Murie MA BSc MD FRCSG FRCSEd
Consultant Surgeon
Royal Infirmary of Edinburgh

Jonothan J. Earnshaw DM FRCS
Consultant Surgeon
Gloucestershire Royal Hospital

Chapter 1

Indications for carotid endarterectomy: lessons learned from randomised trials

JMT Perkins
Specialist Registrar
RB Galland
Consultant Surgeon

DEPARTMENT OF VASCULAR SURGERY,
ROYAL BERKSHIRE HOSPITAL, READING

Introduction

Carotid surgery as we know it today was developed in the 1950s. A number of different procedures were described for treating atheromatous stenoses of carotid arteries. These included resection of the stenosis and replacement with a homograft or saphenous vein graft. These have been largely abandoned and carotid endarterectomy has become the operation of choice. Since then, indications for carotid endarterectomy, as well as technical aspects of the operation, have been subjected to constant evaluation.

The number of carotid endarterectomies performed per annum in the United States rose from 15,000 in 1971 to 107,000 in 1985 [1] at a cost in excess of one billion dollars [2]. The rationale for this increase arose from the findings of the Joint Study Of Extracranial Arterial Occlusion, which showed that approximately 45% of the 500,000 Americans who suffered a stroke each year had a surgically accessible carotid artery stenosis [3].

However, the causes of stroke are multifactorial, and the link between asymptomatic carotid lesions or minor degrees of carotid stenosis and stroke had not been investigated or elucidated. Towards the end of the 1980s considerable uncertainty arose concerning the value of carotid endarterectomy [4]. Improvements in medical management were set against considerable geographical variation in the number of carotid endarterectomies performed [5], and striking differences in the rates of postoperative disabling stroke and death. Indications for operation were thought to be inappropriate in one-third of patients, and equivocal in a further third [6].

There was clearly a need for large scale, randomised trials to examine the relationship between degree of carotid stenosis and medical or surgical treatment for both symptomatic and asymptomatic patients.

Symptomatic carotid artery disease

The European Carotid Surgery Trial (ECST) and the North American Symptomatic Carotid Endarterectomy Trial (NASCET) published their interim results in 1991 [7,8]. Patients who had suffered a non-disabling stroke, hemispheric (carotid territory) transient ischaemic attack (TIA), or an episode of fleeting monocular blindness (amaurosis fugax) were included in the trials. Randomisation was either to carotid endarterectomy or best medical management. The degree of internal carotid artery stenosis in both trials was measured by carotid angiography. ECST stratified patients into three groups: mild stenosis (0-29%), moderate stenosis (30-69%) or severe stenosis (70-99%). NASCET randomised only those with moderate or severe stenosis, using the same percentage categories as ECST.

JVRG

Severe (70-99%) internal carotid artery stenosis

Both trials showed a clear benefit in avoiding any ipsilateral stroke, or ipsilateral disabling or fatal strokes in patients with a severe stenosis who had carotid endarterectomy.

The incidence of any peri-operative stroke or death was 7.5% in ECST and 5.8 % in NASCET. In ECST there was an additional 2.8% risk of postoperative ipsilateral stroke at 3 years after surgery compared with 16.8% after medical management (control group). The most important events to prevent are disabling or fatal strokes, and in ECST the rate of ipsilateral fatal or disabling stroke was 3.7% after surgery, with an additional 1.1% risk over 3 years. This compared with 8.4% in the control group at 3 years. The risk of fatal or disabling stroke in the medically managed patients was greatest in the first year after the onset of symptoms, and therefore if operation was delayed the benefits of carotid endarterectomy might be lost. Factors influencing the peri-operative stroke rate were not formally examined, but appeared to be greatest in those having rapid operations (<1 hour duration) or with a systolic blood pressure >160 mmHg.

The results of NASCET were similar with a 9% incidence (including peri-operative strokes) of any ipsilateral stroke at 2 years in the surgery group compared with 26% in the control group. The corresponding figures for fatal or disabling ipsilateral stroke were 2.5% (surgery) and 13.1% (medical). The yearly incidence of ipsilateral stroke in the medically treated groups was approximately 6 % in ECST, and 10% in NASCET, although the rate of stroke appeared to plateau after 3 years.

The final results from ECST were published in 1998 including longer follow-up (mean 6.1 years) [9]. This report has changed the indications for carotid endarterectomy outlined in the interim ECST report of 1991. Stroke risk and years of stroke-free survival were statistically modelled taking into account age, sex and degree of carotid stenosis. This narrowed the range of carotid stenosis over which carotid endarterectomy could be considered beneficial. Carotid endarterectomy could be expected to benefit men with a symptomatic carotid stenosis >80%, and women with a stenosis >90%. The authors conceded that there still remain areas of uncertainty, and some groups of patients contained only small numbers of patients - for example women age 55 with greater than 90% stenosis.

Long-term results from NASCET have confirmed the continuing benefit for surgery in patients with a severe (>70%) carotid stenosis [10]. At eight years follow-up, the incidence of any ipsilateral stroke was approximately 14% after surgery compared with 27% in the medical group. NASCET did not attempt to perform post hoc analysis of subgroups according to deciles of carotid stenosis as the ECST investigators have done.

Pooling of data from NASCET and ECST may make subgroup analysis more powerful, and allow confirmation of the age, sex and stenosis risk estimates outlined in the final report of ECST [9]. When considering this issue, it should be remembered that a 70% NASCET stenosis corresponds to a stenosis of >80% measured by the methods used in ECST. The continuing benefit from carotid endarterectomy seen in the long-term follow-up of NASCET may therefore correspond to the benefit shown for operation in ECST for stenoses greater than 80%.

Moderate (30-69%)stenosis

Surgery cannot be justified in symptomatic patients with moderate internal carotid artery stenosis. Whilst some benefit could not be ruled out in the very long-term, no benefit from carotid endarterectomy would be gained within 4-5 years for stenoses of 50-69%, and within 6-7 years for stenoses of 30-49% [10]. NASCET, reporting in patients with a moderate stenosis, split the results into stenoses of <50% and stenoses from 50-69% [10]. Operation was clearly not beneficial for patients with a carotid stenosis <50%. Marginal benefit from carotid endarterectomy was reported in patients with stenoses from 50-69%. The 5 year rate of any ipsilateral stroke was 15.7% in the surgery group compared with 22.2% in the medical group (p=0.045). This means that 15 patients would have to undergo carotid endarterectomy to prevent one stroke in 5 years. This degree of stenosis corresponds to an ECST stenosis of 70-80%, and the marginal benefit of surgery reported reflects the similar benefit shown for 70-79% stenoses in the final ECST results [9].

Mild (0-29%) stenosis

Surgery cannot be justified in symptomatic patients with mild internal carotid artery stenosis. Only ECST randomised patients with this degree of stenosis. The risk of ipsilateral stroke in the medical group was negligible and therefore surgery could only prove to be detrimental due to the early peri-operative mortality and morbidity [7].

Conclusions from ECST and NASCET

For the first time these two large, randomised trials clarified the indications for carotid endarterectomy in symptomatic patients, and quantified the expected benefit or lack of benefit for surgery depending on the degree of carotid stenosis. For patients with a severe (>70%) stenosis, six patients need to undergo carotid endarterectomy to prevent one stroke. Carotid endarterectomy prevents strokes in patients with severe carotid stenosis. Interim results suggested that surgery was beneficial for stenoses greater than 70%, but the final results of ECST suggest that this threshold should be 80% for men and 90% for women. This subgroup analysis requires confirmation by pooling NASCET and ECST data to make the conclusion more robust.

Results of the studies only apply to patients with the symptoms specified in the trial inclusion criteria, and without specific exclusion criteria. The results cannot be extrapolated to patients with vertebrobasilar ischaemia, non-hemispheric symptoms or other uncommon cerebrovascular complaints such as pulsatile tinnitus. Although reports have documented relief of these symptoms following carotid endarterectomy, they involve small numbers of non-randomised patients in retrospective reviews with historical controls. These reports offer no rationale for patient selection to ensure successful relief of symptoms, and non-hemispheric symptoms remain a minor and unorthodox indication for carotid endarterectomy.

Applying the results of studies to clinical practice

Trials are inevitably conducted under artificial constraints, and individual doctors have to decide the relevance of trial cohorts, methods and results to their own patient population. NASCET established entry criteria for participating centres (a review of the last 50 carotid endarterectomies within the preceding 24 months had to demonstrate a peri-operative stroke and death rate of less than 6%). NASCET excluded patients older than 79 years and those with significant cardiac, pulmonary, renal or hepatic disease likely to cause death within 5 years. ECST randomised patients where clinicians were 'substantially uncertain' if carotid surgery was indicated, and specific exclusion criteria were not given, nor were entry criteria for participating centres established. This probably means that the results of ECST are more applicable to clinical practice than NASCET.

NASCET and ECST used different methods of measurement to assess the degree of carotid stenosis from biplanar angiography. ECST compared the minimum diameter of the internal carotid artery (ICA) with the estimated diameter of the carotid bulb, whereas NASCET compared the minimum ICA diameter with the lumen of the normal ICA distal to the stenosis. The ECST method overestimates the degree of stenosis compared with the NASCET method. NASCET excluded patients with distal internal carotid artery disease (distal to the C2 vertebral body) more severe than the surgically accessible lesion.

Duplex ultrasonography is now widely used to assess carotid stenosis and angiograms are performed infrequently. Duplex images do not always detect distal internal carotid artery disease. Duplex criteria for classifying stenoses vary, and individual vascular laboratories need to perform their own validation exercise to compare duplex and angiography. Individuals will have to choose which method of angiographic measurement they prefer, and apply the results to their own individual practice. Our own recent survey of methods of carotid duplex imaging in the United Kingdom has shown little standardisation of duplex criteria. Half of the units questioned adopted literature standards, with only 50% attempting to verify their own practice against angiography (unpublished data).

Recent work has used ECST data to validate patient and angiographic factors that predict peri-operative stroke or death [12]. Prognostic risk factors and a scoring system have been derived from the data for the 0-69% stenosis group in ECST [13]. The prognostic scoring system had been validated and tested on patients with 70-99% stenoses from ECST.

These risk factors identify high risk medical patients, and also contain operative factors that predict a high rate of peri-operative stroke or death. The medical factors predicting a high probability of stroke without intervention were cerebral rather than ocular events, plaque surface irregularity, events within 2 months, and the degree of carotid stenosis (70-79, 80-89, 90-99%). Surgical risk factors were female sex, peripheral vascular disease, and systolic blood pressure >180mmHg. From these factors an overall score was derived that balanced the risk of stroke without operation against any increased peri-operative risk of stoke or death. These data allow the stoke and death risk for each patient to be assessed, rather than applying the data from ECST universally.

It should also be noted that the aspirin dose prescribed in NASCET was 1300 mg/day. This is far in excess of the doses generally prescribed to both medical and surgical patients in the United Kingdom. The risk of preoperative stroke in the moderate stenosis group of NASCET was doubled in patients taking less than 650mg of aspirin daily [10]. This dose of aspirin was also associated with greater long-term benefit after operation [10]. The dose of aspirin used in ECST was not specified.

The optimum dose of aspirin has recently been studied in the ASA and Carotid Endarterectomy Trial (ACE) [14]. This study randomised patients undergoing carotid endarterectomy to receive four different doses of aspirin:- 81mg, 325mg, 650mg, or 1300mg. Overall the combined rate of any stroke, myocardial infarction or death at 30 days and 3 months after operation was significantly reduced for the two combined low dose aspirin groups compared with the two high dose groups.

The results of this randomised trial conflict with the results on aspirin dose noted in the NASCET trial. It should be pointed out that the data from ACE demonstrate only short term differences at 3 months, and longer term results may differ. The differences observed between the groups were largely the result of a greater incidence in myocardial infarction in the high dose groups. Overall stroke rate was similar for the 81mg, 650mg and 1300mg dose groups, and was only reduced in the 350mg group. This is hard to explain in view of the equal stroke incidence in the lower (81mg) group compared with the two higher dose groups. The incidence of haemorrhagic stroke was not significantly different between the four groups.

Non-surgical patients were not included in this study, but these data do seem to suggest that for patients after carotid endarterectomy a lower dose of aspirin (81mg or 325mg per day) offers greater overall short-term protection against stroke, myocardial infarction or death than higher daily doses of aspirin (650mg or 1300mg).

Chapter 1

Asymptomatic carotid artery stenosis

Population studies have shown the prevalence of carotid stenosis greater than 50% (almost all asymptomatic) to rise from 0.5% in people in their 50's to about 10% in those over 80 years of age [15,16]. The risk of stroke in subjects with asymptomatic internal carotid artery stenosis is about 2% per year, significantly less than those with symptomatic disease [17,18]. Under these circumstances the balance between benefit and harm from prophylactic surgery is much finer. Conclusive evidence of the benefit of carotid endarterectomy would be required before prophylactic operation in an asymptomatic subject could be recommended.

Asymptomatic carotid surgery trials

Two American randomised trials were too small to provide any useful information on outcome [19,20]. One of these studies was also stopped prematurely because of the high incidence of myocardial infarction in the surgical group, who were not prescribed aspirin [20].

The CASANOVA study [21] (Carotid Artery Stenosis with Asymptomatic Narrowing: Operation versus Aspirin) randomised subjects with a carotid stenosis between 50-90%. No difference was found in the rates of stroke or death in the surgical and medical groups. However, the study design was unusual in that subjects with a stenosis greater than 90% were thought to require operation and were excluded from randomisation. Subjects in the non-surgery group also had a carotid endarterectomy if a stenosis progressed to greater than 90%, if bilateral stenoses >50% developed (operation on the more severe side), or if the patient suffered a TIA with a >50% stenosis on the side of symptoms. In total, 118 endarterectomies were performed on the 204 subjects randomised to the medical arm. Data from this study are consequently largely discredited.

The Veterans Affairs Cooperative Study Group trial did show a significant difference in the rate of ipsilateral neurological events (TIA, amaurosis fugax, or stroke) between the medical and surgical groups (8.0% surgery versus 20.6% medical at a mean follow-up of 47.9 months) [22]. However, the overall incidence of ipsilateral stroke, and the combined incidence of all strokes and death was the same in both groups. Half of the deaths in each group were attributable to cardiac events, reflecting the elderly male population studied. In the presence of such a high mortality rate from other causes, it would be difficult for the effect of less frequent events, such as strokes, to be detected. The higher incidence of TIAs in the medical group was largely irrelevant as these patients could be offered surgery as they become symptomatic, when the benefits of surgery are more clearly defined [7,8].

The value of carotid endarterectomy in reducing the risk of stroke has been demonstrated by both the Asymptomatic Carotid Atherosclerosis Study (ACAS) [18] and a subsequent meta-analysis of data from all available randomised trials [23]. ACAS randomised subjects with an asymptomatic carotid stenosis greater than 60% on angiography (equivalent to about 75% stenosis measured by the 'European' method). After a median follow-up of 2.7 years the trial was stopped. Actuarial estimated 5 year risk of stroke was 5.1% after surgery versus 11.0% in the medical group. This represented an absolute risk reduction of 5.9% or a relative risk reduction of 53%.

The Asymptomatic Carotid Surgery Trial (ACST) is a multicentre, randomised, European trial comparing carotid endarerectomy and best medical treatment for asymptomatic carotid disease. The trial is still recruiting and the results are awaited.

Meta-analysis has confirmed a definite benefit of carotid endarterectomy in preventing ipsilateral ischaemic stroke and stroke in any location [23]. The benefit is small, corresponding to an absolute risk reduction of 2% over an interval of 3.1 years.

Applying the data on asymptomatic patients to clinical practice

The benefit of carotid endarterectomy in asymptomatic subjects is extremely small, as shown by the meta-analysis referenced above. Data from the meta-analysis indicate that 50 subjects would have to have a carotid endarterectomy to prevent one stroke over a 3 year interval. If the risk of stroke in the group who did not have surgery continues beyond 3 years, then the benefit of surgery could accrue for more than 3 years and the number needed to treat might be less [24].

The data from ACAS (as used for the American guidelines on carotid surgery [25]) with an absolute risk reduction of 5.9%, pose significant problems in terms of their application to clinical practice. Centres participating in ACAS were rigorously selected to control peri-operative stroke and death rates. If the angiographic stroke rate (1.2%) were largely avoided by the use of duplex ultrasonography, then the overall peri-operative stroke and death rate in the surgical group was 1.1%. Subjects were carefully selected and about 25 were screened for every one entered into the trial [26]. Non-whites represented only 5% of the subjects enrolled. Data from the trial were projected from 2.7 years of follow-up to 5 years by actuarial analysis.

These points should be borne in mind when considering the available data on carotid endarterectomy for asymptomatic stenosis. Undoubtedly there are asymptomatic patients who would benefit from carotid endarterectomy either because they are at low risk of peri-operative stroke, or more probably because they are at high risk of stroke without operation. Unfortunately there are insufficient data at present, and until high risk subgroups can be identified, carotid endarterectomy for asymptomatic patients cannot be recommended.

Combined carotid and cardiac surgery

Carotid and coronary artery disease occur concurrently in many patients. Two to eighteen per cent of patients undergoing coronary artery bypass grafting (CABG) are estimated to have severe carotid disease, although most are asymptomatic. Forty per cent of carotid endarterectomy patients have significant coronary artery disease. The risk of stroke after CABG is increased with carotid artery disease [27]; 3.8% of patients with a unilateral carotid stenosis >50% suffer a hemispheric stroke. In patients with bilateral carotid stenoses of 80-99% the hemispheric stroke rate was 8.3% [27]. These data, showing an increased risk of stroke with significant asymtomatic carotid disease, are the rationale for performing carotid endarterectomy either prior to CABG or as a combined procedure. The results of the ACAS study [18] lend further support to the arguments of operating on asymtomatic carotid lesions. The American guidelines support the practice of carotid endarterectomy for asymptomatic stenoses >60% prior to CABG [25].

However, there is no evidence from randomised trials to guide clinicians as to whether carotid endarterectomy and coronary artery bypass grafting should be performed as a combined procedure or separately. It is suggested that where both lesions are symptomatic a combined operation is appropriate [28]. Combined procedures may be advocated for symptomatic cardiac disease with severe asymptomatic carotid stenosis, but the situation for symptomatic carotid disease with asymptomatic cardiac lesions is not clear [29].

Conclusions

There is strong evidence that carotid endarterectomy prevents strokes in patients with symptomatic internal carotid artery stenosis greater than 80%. This threshold has been revised from the original recommendation of 70% in the light of longer follow-up from ECST. Appropriate symptoms are amaurosis fugax, retinal infarction, carotid territory TIAs and non-disabling stroke. Final data from NASCET are awaited to confirm the revised thresholds for carotid endarterectomy, based on age, sex and degree of stenosis, that have arisen from the final ECST results. Symptomatic patients with mild (0-29%) or moderate (30-69%) stenoses should not undergo carotid endarterectomy. Asymptomatic patients with stenoses from 50-99% benefit from carotid endarterectomy, but the benefit is too marginal for carotid surgery to be recommended for all asymptomatic patients in this group.

Further data are required before firm conclusions can be drawn in a number of areas. No data from randomised trials exist to evaluate the role of carotid endarterectomy for other cerebral symptoms such as vertebrobasilar ischaemia, non-hemispheric symptoms and eye signs other than amaurosis fugax. Existing data from trials of carotid endarterectomy for asymptomatic disease are too few to allow identification of high-risk subgroups in whom carotid surgery could be indicated. There are no data from randomised trials to support combined carotid endarterectomy and coronary artery bypass grafting for symptomatic cardiac and carotid disease. Meta-analysis suggests that a combined operation can be performed without excess risk.

Indications for carotid endarterectomy

Sound evidence

- Patients with symptomatic ipsilateral carotid stenosis > 80% benefit from carotid endarterectomy (6 operations will prevent one stroke).

- There is no advantage from surgery over best medical therapy in patients with symptomatic ipsilateral carotid stenosis < 70%.

- Patients with asymptomatic carotid stenosis > 75% have reduced risk of stroke after carotid endarterectomy, but the advantage is marginal (50 operations will prevent one stroke).

Evidence needed

- The role of carotid endarterectomy for non-hemispheric symptoms.

- The value and timing of carotid surgery in patients undergoing coronary bypass grafting.

- The value of a search for high risk asymptomatic carotid stenosis.

Chapter 1

References (randomised trials in bold)

1. Pokras R, Dyken M. Dramatic changes in the performance of endarterectomy for diseases of the extracranial arteries of the head. *Stroke* 1988; 19: 1289-90.
2. Dyken M. Carotid endarterectomy studies: a glimmering of science. *Stroke* 1986; 17: 355-58.
3. Fields W, Maslenikov V, Meyer J, et al. Joint study of extracranial arterial occlusion. *JAMA* 1970; 211: 1993-2003.
4. Warlow C. Carotid endarterectomy: does it work? *Stroke* 1984; 15: 1068-76.
5. Chassin M, Brook R, Park R, et al. Variations in the use of medical and surgical services by the Medicare population. *N Eng J Med* 1986; 314: 285-90.
6. Winslow C, Solomon D, Chassin M, et al. The appropriateness of carotid endarterectomy. *N Eng J Med* 1988; 318: 721-26.
7. **European Carotid Surgery Trialists Group. MRC European Carotid Surgery Trial: Interim results for symptomatic patients with severe (70-99%) or with mild (0-29%) carotid stenosis. *Lancet* 1991; 337: 1235-43.**
8. **North American Symptomatic Carotid Endarterectomy Trial Collaborators. Beneficial effect of carotid endarterectomy in symptomatic patients with high-grade stenosis. *N Eng J Med* 1991; 325: 445-53.**
9. **European Carotid Surgery Trialists' Collaborative Group. Randomised trial of endarterectomy for recently symptomatic carotid stenosis: final results of the MRC European Carotid Surgery Trial. *Lancet* 1998; 351: 1379-87.**
10. **North American Symptomatic Carotid Endarterectomy Trial Collaborators. Benefit of carotid endarterectomy in patients with symptomatic moderate or severe stenosis. *N Eng J Med* 1998; 339: 1415-25.**
11. **European Carotid Surgery Trialists' Collaborative Group. Endarterectomy for moderate symptomatic carotid stenosis: interim results of the MRC European Carotid Surgery Trial. *Lancet* 1996; 347: 1591-93.**
12. Rothwell PM, Slattery J, Warlow CP. Clinical and angiographic predictors of stroke and death from carotid endarterectomy: systematic review. *Br Med J* 1997; 315: 1571-77.
13. Rothwell PM, Warlow CP. Prediction of benefit from carotid endarterectomy in individual patients: a risk-modelling study. *Lancet* 1999; 353: 2105-10.
14. **Taylor DW, Barnett HJM, Haynes RB, et al, for the ASA and Carotid Endarterectomy (ACE) Trial Collaborators. Low-dose and high-dose acetylsalicylic acid for patients undergoing carotid endarterectomy: a randomised controlled trial. *Lancet* 1999; 353: 2179-84.**
15. O'Leary DH, Polak JF, Kronm RA, et al. Distribution and correlates of sonographically detected carotid artery disease in the Cardiovascular Health Study. *Stroke* 1992; 23: 1752-60.
16. Prati P, Vanuzzo D, Casaroli M, et al. Prevalence and determinants of carotid atherosclerosis in a general population. *Stroke* 1992; 23: 1705-11.
17. European Carotid Surgery Trialists' Collaborative Group. Risk of stroke in the distribution of an asymptomatic carotid stenosis. *Lancet* 1995; 345: 209-12.
18. **Executive Committee for the Asymptomatic Carotid Atherosclerosis Study. Endarterectomy for asymptomatic carotid artery stenosis. *JAMA* 1995; 273: 1421-28.**
19. **Clagett GP, Youkey JR, Brigham RA, et al. Asymptomatic cervical bruit and abnormal ocular pneumoplethysmography: A prospective study comparing two approaches to management. *Surgery* 1984; 96: 823-29.**
20. **Mayo Asymptomatic Carotid Endarterectomy Study Group. Results of a randomised controlled trial of carotid endarterectomy for asymptomatic carotid stenosis. *Mayo Clin Proc* 1992; 67: 513-18.**
21. **CASANOVA Study Group. Carotid surgery versus medical therapy in asymptomatic carotid stenosis. *Stroke* 1991; 22: 1229-35.**
22. **Hobson R, Weiss D, Fields W, et al for the Veterans Affairs Cooperative Study Group. Efficacy of carotid endarterectomy for asymptomatic carotid stenosis. *N Eng J Med* 1993; 328: 221-7.**
23. Benavente O, Moher D, Pham B. Carotid endarterectomy for asymptomatic carotid stenosis: a meta-analysis. *Br Med J* 1998; 317: 1477-80.
24. Warlow CP. Carotid endarterectomy for asymptomatic carotid stenosis. *Br Med J* 1998; 317: 1468.
25. Biller J, Feinberg WM, Castaldo JE, et al. Guidelines for healthcare professionals from a special writing group of the Stroke Council, American Heart Association. *Stroke* 1998; 29: 554-62.
26. Mayberg MR, Winn HR. Endarterectomy for asymptomatic carotid artery stenosis. *JAMA* 1995; 273: 1459-61.
27. Schwartz LB, Bridgman AH, Kieffer RW, et al. Asymptomatic carotid artery stenosis and stroke in patients undergoing cardiopulmonary bypass. *J Vasc Surg* 1995; 21: 146-53.
28. Hertzer NR. Basic data concerning associated coronary artery disease in peripheral vascular patients. *Ann Vasc Surg* 1987; 1: 616-20.
29. Renton S, Hornick P, Taylor KM, Grace PA. Rational approach to combined carotid and ischaemic heart disease. *Br J Surg* 1997; 84: 1503-10.

Chapter 2

Improving the results of carotid endarterectomy

MJ Gough
Consultant Surgeon
P Tan
Specialist Registrar
G Maritati
Visiting Fellow

VASCULAR SURGICAL UNIT,
THE GENERAL INFIRMARY AT LEEDS, LEEDS

The aim of carotid endarterectomy (CEA) is the sustained abolition of neurological sequelae attributable to the ipsilateral carotid artery without either neurological or cardiopulmonary complications. Published results indicate that 30 day combined stroke/mortality rates after surgery vary from 1.6-9.9% [1,2] suggesting scope for improving the outcome in some centres.

Cardiac mortality

Severe, correctable, but often silent, coronary artery disease (CAD) may be present in a third of patients with carotid atherosclerosis resulting in an annual cardiac-related mortality of 6.5% in patients with >75% carotid stenosis [3]. Although CEA is not associated with the volume-dependent haemodynamic disturbances that accompany aortic surgery, changes in cardiac rhythm and blood pressure may occur and precipitate myocardial ischaemia. Thus, myocardial infarction or cardiac dysrrhythmia remain the principal cause of mortality following CEA [4], particularly in patients with pre-existing cardiac disease or in those requiring perioperative vasopressor drugs. Careful cardiac assessment is therefore essential prior to CEA.

Ideally, all patients should be screened with a dipyridamole-thallium scan or exercise ECG to identify occult CAD. However, most institutions do not have the resources for this and the overall benefit of preoperative screening is still debated. Most surgeons rely on a careful history and examination, resting ECG and chest X-ray to exclude CAD or to select patients who require coronary angiography. This leaves an intermediate group for whom screening may be justified. A small group of patients with co-existing severe CAD and carotid disease will be identified who may benefit from synchronous CEA and coronary revascularisation [5].

Anaesthetic technique

CEA may be performed under either general (GA) or locoregional (LA) anaesthesia and there is evidence that the cardiac risk of surgery is reduced with the latter [6] despite greater blood pressure instability and higher catecholamine levels that might be expected to increase the cardiac risk. Although it has been suggested that perioperative ß-adrenergic blockade may protect the myocardium, this view has not been widely accepted. Other criticisms of LA surgery include the potential for hurried and technically inadequate surgery, patient and surgeon stress and an unsatisfactory environment for training junior surgeons. Experience with the technique indicates that none of these is true.

An ideal anaesthetic will allow maintenance of normal P_aO_2 and P_aCO_2 tensions, control of arterial pressure, and preservation of cerebral autoregulation. Previous work indicates that anaesthetic agents can have both adverse and beneficial effects on cerebral perfusion and

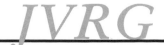

oxygenation. Thus, barbiturates reduce cerebral metabolic rate and cerebral oedema whilst propofol may protect against certain biochemical effects of reperfusion and offer greater haemodynamic stability on emergence from anaesthesia. The widely used volatile anaesthetic agents (halothane, isoflurane) may increase cerebral blood flow but suppress cerebral autoregulation and increase cerebral lactate concentration, whilst all volatile agents and nitrous oxide may increase intracranial pressure. Thus, the overall effect of many GA agents upon cerebral metabolism is unpredictable despite allowing control of P_aO_2, P_aCO_2 and blood pressure. Finally alterations in P_aCO_2 that may influence vasomotor tone do not appear to enhance cerebral blood flow.

In contrast, LA (superficial and deep cervical plexus block) preserves autoregulation and improves cerebral oxygenation during carotid clamping which induces a reflex rise in systemic blood pressure [7]. This may explain the findings of a recent meta-analysis suggesting that neurological complications, cardiac events and death following CEA are reduced by at least 50% when LA is used [6]. Intensive care unit and hospital stay may also be less. These end-points are being evaluated in a randomised trial (GALA Trial). Finally, LA allows continuous and highly reliable intraoperative monitoring (awake testing) of the need for a shunt, which advocates of selective shunting may perceive as an advantage.

Superficial and deep cervical plexus blockade, with additional intra-operative infiltration, is safe and effective. It also provides a period of postoperative analgesia. It is preferred to cervical epidural anaesthesia, which is unfamiliar to most anaesthetists and may be associated with cardiovascular complications. Some patients may be unsuitable for locoregional anaesthesia (previous stroke with dysphasia or hemiplegia or marked anxiety) and for these GA is preferred.

Surgical technique

Although specific factors that may influence the outcome of CEA are discussed below, certain aspects of general technique should be considered. Whilst not subjected to critical assessment, the authors believe them to be important. They include:

- careful positioning of the patient on the operating table - excessive rotation or extension of the neck may compromise cerebral blood flow during carotid clamping,
- minimal manipulation of the carotid arteries ('no-touch' technique) during dissection to reduce the risk of embolism,
- the use of magnifying loupes for endarterectomy and removal of residual fragments and strands, and for vessel repair,

- the use of sharp bent-on-flat scissors for clean transection of the proximal endarterectomy site and appropriate use of proximal and distal tacking sutures,
- careful flushing of debris or air with heparinised saline and continuous back-bleeding of the internal carotid artery (ICA) during final closure of the arteriotomy, followed by initial reperfusion of the external carotid artery (ECA).

Endarterectomy technique and patching

Endarterectomy technique

Three techniques have been described for CEA of which standard endarterectomy via a longitudinal arteriotomy (sCEA) is most widely used. Whilst eversion endarterectomy (eCEA) has gained in popularity, interposition grafting should be reserved for revisional carotid surgery. Data from both prospective randomised trials and retrospective studies have failed to show a difference in early ICA thrombosis and 30 day combined stroke and mortality rates, or in the frequency of cranial nerve injury and myocardial infarction, between sCEA and eCEA [8,9].

Inappropriate eCEA, particularly if the atheromatous disease extends >3cm into the ICA, may lead to difficulties with assessment and tacking of the distal endarterectomy site. Similarly, shunt insertion and retention is not easy during eCEA. Despite this, the only prospective randomised trial of eCEA versus sCEA, in which 96% of patients underwent completion angiography, angioscopy or duplex ultrasound, showed no difference in the incidence of technical defects (8% v 9%) or the need for surgical revision (4% v 3%) [8]. However, the duration of carotid clamping was shorter and recurrent ICA stenoses less common (non-significant trend) after eCEA. Patch closure is not required after eCEA.

Patching

Patch angioplasty following sCEA may reduce the rate of early ICA thrombosis (reduced thrombogenicity of the endarterectomy site, improved ICA diameter) and late restenosis (neointimal hyperplasia) and thus improve both early and long-term stroke rates. However, patching increases the carotid clamp time and the risk of patch related complications (rupture, false aneurysm, sepsis), and so the role of patching remains uncertain.

At least six randomised trials of obligatory patching or obligatory primary repair have been performed and the Cochrane Stroke Review Group has subjected the results to a meta-analysis [10]. All trials found that patching reduced the incidence of ipsilateral perioperative stroke and the meta-analysis indicated a 66% reduction in the relative odds, in the setting of an overall stroke rate of 2.7% for the two groups. This was highly significant. Similarly there was an 83% reduction in the odds of perioperative ICA occlusion together with a trend suggesting that 30 day combined stroke and death rates were reduced. Of equal importance was the finding that patching was associated with significant reductions in ipsilateral stroke or combined stroke and death during long-term follow-up. There were also fewer ICA occlusions or re-stenoses of >50%. If these differences are real, given the shortcomings of both meta-analysis and the trials examined (small numbers of events, losses to follow-up, poor methodology, reporting bias) it appears that patching could prevent 30 ipsilateral strokes and 24 deaths/1000 operations within 30 days of surgery. Furthermore, an additional 28 strokes and 75 deaths may be prevented in the subsequent 3 years. It is therefore clear that the issue of patching is important and should be investigated in a large multicentre, randomised trial. This would need to enrol at least 3000 patients to confirm a 50% reduction in stroke or death rates.

A further prospective randomised trial of 399 patients that was not included in the meta-analysis reported 30 day stroke rates of 4.4% for primary closure and 0.4% for patch repair. In addition, duplex ultrasound indicated that >50% narrowing of the ICA at 1 month was much commoner in patients with no patch. These findings were highly significant [11]. It is important to note that patients with an ICA diameter of <4mm were excluded from the study and received a patch.

Surprisingly, support for patching is not universal and one report indicates that recurrent stenosis was more common after vein patch closure. It is claimed that other factors that may influence the incidence of late re-stenosis (smoking, elevated serum lipid level, female sex) were not taken into account in previous studies [12]. These criticisms are not relevant to the early benefits of patching.

Currently most surgeons favour selective patching based on data that suggest that complications following direct repair are greater when the diameter of the ICA is 5mm or less, particularly in women, in whom the mean diameter of the ICA (4.9±0.6 mm) is 8-15 % less than in men (5.3±0.7 mm) [13,14]. With this protocol, approximately 50% of patients will need a patch. There is no randomised trial to support this view although a non-randomised study reported a lower incidence of residual/recurrent ICA stenosis when selective patching was applied in this way [15].

Further uncertainty remains regarding which patch material should be used. Autologous long saphenous vein (LSV), Dacron, polytetrafluoroethylene (PTFE) and autologous cervical vein (facial, internal and external jugular) have been proposed as suitable. Cervical vein has not been used widely but may be preferred to LSV when CEA is performed under LA. If selected, the vein should be invaginated to expose the intima and a double wall thickness used to compensate for its thin structure.

For the three materials most widely used (LSV, Dacron, PTFE) there are insufficient data upon which to make firm conclusions as to the best choice. In the meta-analysis described above, the outcomes for PTFE and vein were similar [10]. An alternative analysis of six studies (two randomised trials, one prospective audit, three retrospective reviews) indicated a trend to reduced perioperative stroke rate when vein was preferred to Dacron or PTFE. When the combined data for all synthetic patches were compared to LSV, there was no difference in the incidence of early postoperative ICA occlusion or the development of a >50% stenosis within 1 year [13].

The putative advantages of vein patches include low thrombogenicity, better handling characteristics, good haemostasis and superior resistance to infection. However, early vein patch rupture or suture line disruption with haemorrhage or false aneurysm formation may occur (0-4%), particularly when the external jugular vein or LSV from the ankle are used. Patch rupture carries a high mortality.

Proponents of synthetic patches highlight their easy availability, mechanical integrity and higher resistance to aneurysm formation. However, risks of patch sepsis are increased and heparin reversal with protamine is usually required for PTFE patches. This may also influence the outcome of surgery (see below).

In summary, available evidence favours patch angioplasty after sCEA, although debate continues as to which type of patch to use. It remains uncertain whether a patch should be used routinely, or only in patients with an ICA diameter of 5mm or less. If these questions are subjected to a randomised trial one treatment arm should include eCEA if all uncertainties are to be answered. Such a study would require 3000-6000 patients.

Cranial and cervical nerve injury

Several cranial and cervical nerves are at risk during CEA and postoperative nerve dysfunction may occur in 3-27% of patients. The majority recover after 12 months although 7% are permanent. Even when temporary, such injuries may cause disability, particularly when the recurrent laryngeal or XII nerves are involved. Such lesions assume greater importance when proceeding to contralateral CEA since bilateral palsies of either nerve may result in upper airway obstruction, and difficulties with speech and swallowing.

Neck haematoma, re-exploration for bleeding, shunting, patch closure, a trainee surgeon and high carotid lesions all increase the risk of nerve palsy. Whilst more important considerations dictate the use of shunts and patches, the integrity of cranial/cervical nerves following CEA is largely surgeon-dependent.

Nerve transection should be rare given sound anatomical knowledge, although neuropraxia may result from stretching or retraction. Thus, adequate exposure of the carotid arteries, careful deployment of self-retaining retractors and circumspect use of diathermy are important. Key points of anatomy and methods of minimising nerve injury are shown in Figure 1 and Table 1.

Shunting and intraoperative monitoring

Shunt use during CEA has attracted considerable debate with three approaches to surgery evolving. Some surgeons use a shunt for all patients, believing that the risk of intraoperative ischaemic stroke is reduced and that additional time is available, particularly when a patch is required or if a trainee is performing surgery. Conversely, others never use shunts, suggesting that they cause platelet and air emboli, intimal damage, late restenosis and arterial dissection. In addition shunts may kink, dislodge and reduce access to the operative field. Finally,

Table 1. Prevention of injury to cranial nerves during carotid endarterectomy.

Nerve	Anatomy	Mode of Injury	Avoidance	Incidence
Recurrent laryngeal (RLN)	Tracheoesophageal groove. A non-RLN may leave vagus at level of bifurcation or distal CCA and cross medially, posterior to the CCA to enter the larynx.	Retraction Clamping Dissection	Minimise circumferential dissection CCA, ICA, ECA. Be aware of a non-RLN. Direct laryngoscopy prior to staged contralateral CEA.	1-25%
Superior laryngeal	Vertical in the carotid sheath behind ICA and ECA close to superior thyroid artery where it divides into internal (sensory) and external (motor) branches.	Stretch Retraction Clamping	As for RLN and control superior thyroid artery at junction with CCA (external branch). Care with clamps on ECA	Not known
Vagus	Posterolateral to CCA/ICA in carotid sheath. May occupy anteromedial position.	Clamping Dissection	Care with clamping CCA/ICA, close dissection of CCA.	Not known
Hypoglossal	Crosses ICA and ECA 2-4 cm above bifurcation. Tethered by the descendens hypoglossi/ansa and sternomastoid artery and vein. Can be as low as bifurcation and adherent to posterior surface of the anterior facial vein.	Stretch Retraction Ligation	Careful mobilisation of nerve with division of tethering structures. Do not separate fused vagus and hypoglossal.	1-13.5 %
Marginal mandibular branch of facial nerve	Lies inferior and parallel to the ramus of the mandible deep to the platysma.	Incision Stretch Retraction	Avoid excessive hyperextension of the neck (nerve is pulled down closer to the operative field). Curve superior extent of skin incision posteriorly. Avoid retracting onto mandible.	0.5-15 %
Greater auricular and transverse cervical nerves	Greater auricular nerve (GAN) crosses the uppermost portion of transverse incision. Transverse cervical nerve (TCN) crosses lower end of the standard neck incision.	Incision	Properly placed skin incision if possible though many patients complain of numbness over ear lobe/angle of jaw (GAN) or in submental or submandibular area (TCN).	1.1-60 %

CCA - common carotid artery
ECA - external carotid artery
ICA - internal carotid artery

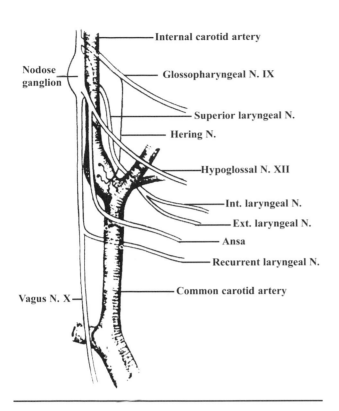

Internal carotid artery

Glossopharyngeal N. IX

Superior laryngeal N.

Hering N.

Hypoglossal N. XII

Int. laryngeal N.

Ext. laryngeal N.

Ansa

Recurrent laryngeal N.

Common carotid artery

Nodose ganglion

Vagus N. X

Figure 1. Anatomy of operative field during carotid endarterectomy.

some surgeons deploy shunts selectively when intraoperative monitoring demonstrates evidence of cerebral ischaemia following carotid clamping.

Counsell et al have reviewed the trials of routine shunting versus no shunting [16]. These demonstrate trends suggesting fewer strokes and stroke-related deaths and lower 30-day mortality in patients who have a shunt. However, the number of outcome events was small and the trials varied in randomisation methods, risk stratification, surgical technique and the frequency of patching. Thus there is no conclusive evidence to support either routine shunting or non-shunting. Counsell further suggested that a multicentre prospective randomised trial to provide a definitive answer to this question would require some 5000 patients, provided that the methodological criticisms of previous studies were eliminated.

The logical approach to safe CEA is reliable detection of intraoperative cerebral ischaemia, which occurs in up to a third of patients, and then selective use of a shunt. The search for a suitable method of monitoring has been difficult; many techniques have been examined. These include physiological tests reflecting cerebral perfusion (electroencephalography, measurement of somatosensory

Chapter 2

Table 2. Methods of cerebral monitoring and criteria for selective shunt insertion.

Technique	Suggested Criteria	Comments	False +ve	False -ve
Stump pressure	<50 mm Hg (other criteria 'established' during LA CEA not reliable).	Cheap, universally available. No continuous monitoring. Changes in BP, P_aCO_2, P_aO_2 may affect Circle of Willis flow during CEA.	High	0-23%
Cerebral blood flow (xenon[133] washout)	<18-20ml/100gm/min.	Limited availability, expensive, radiation hazard. Technician required.	Unknown	Unknown
Transcranial Doppler (TCD)	Variously stated as >50% - >70% decrease in middle cerebral arterial velocity.	Expensive technician required, 10% of patients do not have an acoustic window. Affected by change in P_aCO_2, BP.	Depends on cut off	Up to 17% if >70% fall used as criterion
Near infra-red spectroscopy	Decrease in cerebral O_2 saturation of >10%.	Expensive, research tool, Uncertain contribution of extracranial perfusion.	50%	4%
Local anaesthesia (awake testing)	Altered neurological function.	Cheap, reliable and continuous monitoring.	0%	0%
Electroencephalography (EEG)	Decreased amplitude, slowing, loss of fast activity.	Continuous. Technician required. Assesses superficial cortex > deeper tissue, affected by diathermy, some types of GA, P_aCO_2 and previous stroke.	8-13%	5-50%
Somatosensory evoked potentials (SSEP)	>50% decrease in amplitude of SSEP complex or >1ms increase in central conduction time following median nerve stimulation.	Moderate cost. Easier than EEG. Technician required. Influenced by some types of GA and analgesics. Assesses internal capsule viability (unlike EEG).	0-17%	1-17% (<1% in most studies)

evoked potentials (SSEP)), direct assessments of cerebral blood flow (stump pressure, transcranial Doppler (TCD), cerebral oximetry) or direct neurological examination (awake testing during LA surgery). The relative merits of these are summarised in Table 2. With the exception of awake neurological testing which should be regarded as the gold standard, none is perfect.

Monitoring techniques with a high false positive rate will result in unnecessary shunt deployment diminishing the benefit of selective shunting. Conversely, techniques with a significant false negative rate increase the risk of ischaemic stroke. Thus methods of monitoring require verification to establish their sensitivity and specificity. This is almost impossible to achieve when CEA is performed under GA, although it has been suggested that different techniques could be calibrated against the need for a shunt in patients having LA surgery. This concept is flawed because, whilst LA preserves cerebral autoregulation, this is lost under GA. Thus physiological indicators of cerebral ischaemia cannot be extrapolated from LA to GA [7].

From present data it is clear that awake testing is the only technique that accurately identifies patients for selective shunting. Of the others, measurement of SSEP is perhaps the most promising since it is continuous, relatively easy to perform, and applicable to all patients.

Anticoagulation and heparin reversal during CEA

Whilst anticoagulation with heparin during CEA is universally practised, the dose administered varies considerably; some surgeons use up to 15,000 units. There is no evidence to suggest that dose variations influence stroke or death rates, although two reports indicate that heparin reversal with protamine increases perioperative stroke rates [17,18]. In these studies there were no strokes in non-reversed patients compared to rates of 2.6% (5/193) and 6.5% (2/31) in those given protamine. If real, this effect may be due to increased platelet adhesiveness and thrombosis at the endarterectomy site, although heparin has other actions that may reduce stroke susceptibility after CEA [18]. This possible benefit was achieved at the expense of more frequent re-exploration for haematoma and increased drainage volumes following surgery. A third study has shown that protamine reduces the risk of wound haematoma without increasing the risk of stroke [19].

The value of these reports is uncertain since only one study was randomised [17], and variations in shunt use and patch angioplasty in all three studies may have influenced the results. Indeed, in one report all strokes occurred in non-patched patients [18], whilst in another the frequency of primary closure was 50% higher in the group given

protamine [17]. Given these variables the true impact of heparin reversal in the pathogenesis of post-CEA stroke is almost impossible to elucidate.

Other factors that may influence the outcome of CEA

A number of other factors may affect the results of CEA but have not been tested in a randomised trial. They include:

- ## *hospital and surgeon clinical volume*

Studies from the USA have shown that the risk of stroke and death after CEA is highest when surgery is undertaken by surgeons who perform five or fewer procedures/year, or in institutions carrying out <100 endarterectomies each year [20,21]. This suggests that CEA is more likely to have a satisfactory outcome in specialist units.

- ## *adjuvant pharmacological therapy*

Pharmacological neuroprotection is an attractive concept although little explored. It is reported that administration of sodium thiopentone prior to carotid clamping, in doses sufficient to suppress EEG burst activity, allows surgery to be undertaken without a shunt, with a combined stroke and death rate of 0-1.4% [22]. Whilst of interest, EEG monitoring is mandatory to confirm that the desired effect is achieved and recovery from anaesthesia is prolonged with patients often requiring postoperative ventilation.

A number of authors have reported that some 5% of patients monitored with TCD during the first few hours following CEA experience multiple middle cerebral artery emboli (>50/hr) of whom 60% progress to acute carotid thrombosis and stroke [23,24]. This phenomenon may represent a technical error during arteriotomy closure or enhanced thrombogenicity of the endarterectomised vessel or patch. One approach to these emboli would be re-exploration of the carotid vessels, although this is unlikely to be useful if there is no correctable abnormality. The Leicester group, who have a rigorous policy of quality assessment on completion of CEA, investigated the role of administering incremental doses of dextran 40 (20-40 ml/hr), an anti-platelet agent, to patients who developed multiple emboli postoperatively but in whom technical problems had been excluded. Embolic events ceased in all patients (5/100 CEA) and no strokes occurred [23]. This protocol requires corroboration but may have promise, provided that TCD monitoring during the first 6hr after CEA is available.

Finally, preoperative colloid volume expansion with 500-1000ml 6% hetastarch has been shown to reduce the frequency of ischaemic EEG changes following application of the carotid clamps by some 40-60%, although there is no work to assess its impact on stroke and death rates [25].

- ### *quality control methods*

TCD can be used during surgery to monitor shunt performance and detect release of emboli during vascular dissection. This may be useful to both experienced surgeons and trainees. Following CEA, angioscopy, completion angiography and duplex imaging have all been described as methods of examining the adequacy of surgical repair. However, apparent defects are detected more often than the anticipated stroke rate if no assessment were performed. Gaunt et al found abnormalities requiring further intervention in 12/100 patients undergoing angioscopy [26]. The risk of embolic complications or vessel damage following angiography or angioscopy should also be considered.

Of the techniques available, duplex imaging is perhaps the most attractive. It is non-invasive and can identify residual stenoses, intimal flaps and intraluminal thrombus. Although Gaunt et al report technical difficulties with the technique a more recent study has confirmed its efficacy [27].

Those who are enthusiastic about quality control suggest that a lesion requiring surgical revision may be discovered in 6-12% of patients, although there are no randomised trials to confirm the benefit. Similarly there is no consensus as to which abnormalities warrant revisional surgery.

Summary

On current knowledge the gold standard for carotid endarterectomy might include:

- full preoperative cardiac assessment,
- surgery performed under local anaesthesia,
- selective shunting on the basis of awake testing,
- standard endarterectomy with patch closure,
- completion duplex imaging,
- surgery by an experienced surgeon in a specialist unit.

Measures requiring further evaluation:

- the risk/benefit of local and general anaesthesia,
- a comparison of eversion endarterectomy with patch angioplasty,
- a comparison of synthetic and venous patches,
- the use of protamine for heparin reversal,
- the benefit of intra and postoperative TCD monitoring,
- postoperative dextran therapy.

Improving the results of carotid endarterectomy

Sound evidence

- **As part of a standard carotid endarterectomy, patch angioplasty reduces perioperative ICA occlusion and postoperative restenosis.**

- **If TCD detects postoperative cerebral emboli, these can be abolished by Dextran 40.**

Evidence needed

- **Randomised trials containing thousands of patients are needed to prove the value of other perioperative interventions.**

- **The ideal method of anaesthesia for CEA is under investigation.**

Chapter 2

References (randomised trials in bold)

1. Hertzer N R, O'Hara P J, Mascha E J, et al. Early outcome assessment for 2228 consecutive carotid endarterectomy procedures: The Cleveland Clinic experience from 1989 to 1995. *J Vasc Surg* 1997; 26: 1-10.

2. **Brown MM on behalf of the CAVATAS investigators. Results of the carotid and vertebral artery transluminal angioplasty study (CAVATAS). *Br J Surg* 1999; 86: A710-11.**

3. Norris JW, Zhu CZ, Bornstein NM, Chambers BR. Vascular risks of asymptomatic carotid stenosis. *Stroke* 1991; 22: 1485-1490.

4. Riles TS, Kopelman I, Imparato AM . Myocardial infarction following carotid endarterectomy: A review of 683 operations. *Surgery* 1979; 85: 249-252.

5. Mackey WC. Carotid and coronary disease: staged or simultaneous management? *Semin Vasc Surg* 1998; 11: 36-40.

6. Tangkanakul C, Counsell C, Warlow CP. Local versus general anaesthesia in carotid endarterectomy: a systematic review of the evidence. *Eur J Vasc Surg* 1997; 13: 491-499.

7. McCleary AJ, Dearden NM, Dickson DH, Watson A, Gough MJ. The differing effects of regional and general anaesthesia on cerebral metabolism during carotid endarterectomy. *Eur J Vasc Surg* 1996; 12: 173-181.

8. **Cao P, Giordano G, De Rango P, et al, Collaborators of the EVEREST study group. A randomized study on eversion versus standard carotid endarterectomy: Study design and preliminary results: The EVEREST Trial. *J Vasc Surg* 1998; 27: 595-605.**

9. Darling RC, Paty PSK, Shah DM, Chang BB, Leather RP. Eversion endarterectomy of the internal carotid artery: technique and results in 449 procedures. *Surgery* 1996; 120: 635-640.

10. **Counsell C, Salinas R, Naylor AR, Warlow CP. A systematic review of the randomised trials of carotid patch angioplasty in carotid endarterectomy. *Eur J Vasc Surg* 1997; 13: 345-354.**

11. **Aburahma AF, Khan JH, Robinson PA, et al. Prospective randomized trial of carotid endarterectomy with primary closure and patch angioplasty with saphenous vein, jugular vein and polytetrafluoroethylene: Perioperative (30 day) results. *J Vasc Surg* 1996; 24: 998-1007.**

12. Gelabert HA, Sherif EM, Moore WS. Carotid endarterectomy with primary closure do not adversely affect the rate of recurrent stenosis. *Arch Surg* 1994; 129: 648-654.

13. Archie JP. Patching with carotid endarterectomy: when to do it and what to use. *Semin Vasc Surg* 1998; 11: 24-29.

14. Schneider JR, Droste JS, Golan JF. Carotid endarterectomy in women versus men: Patient characteristics and outcome. *J Vasc Surg 1997; 25: 890-898.*

15. Golledge J, Cuming R, Davies AH, Greenhalgh RM. Outcome of selective patching following carotid endarterectomy. *Eur J Vasc Surg* 1996; 11: 458-463.

16. **Counsell C, Salinas R, Naylor AR, Warlow CP. Routine or selective carotid artery shunting during carotid endarterectomy and the different methods of monitoring in selective shunting (Cochrane Review). *The Cochrane Library* 1998; Issue 3: 1-12.**

17. **Fearn SJ, Parry AD, Picton AJ, Mortimer AJ, McCollum CN. Should heparin be reversed after carotid endarterectomy? A randomised prospective trial. *Eur J Vasc Surg* 1997; 13: 394-397.**

18. Mauney MC, Buchanan SA, Lawrence WA, et al. Stroke rate is markedly reduced after carotid endarterectomy by avoidance of protamine. *J Vasc Surg* 1995; 22: 264-270.

19. Treiman RL, Cossman DV, Foran RF, Levin PM, Cohen JL, Wagner WH. The influence of neutralising heparin after carotid endarterectomy on postoperative stroke and haematoma formation. *J Vasc Surg* 1990; 12: 440-445.

20. Cebul RD, Snow RJ, Pine R, Hertzer NR, Norris DG. Indications, outcomes, and provider volumes for carotid endarterectomy. *JAMA* 1998; 279: 1282-1287.

21. Hannan EL, Popp AJ, Tranmer B, Fuestel P, Waldman J, Shah D. Relationship between provider volume and mortality for carotid endarterectomies in New York State. *Stroke* 1998; 29: 2292-2297.

22. Frawley JE, Hicks RG, Horton DA, Gray LJ, Niesche JW, Matheson JM. Thiopental sodium cerebral protection during carotid endarterectomy: Perioperative disease and death. *J Vasc Surg* 1994; 19: 732-738.

23. Lennard N, Smith J, Dumville J, et al. Prevention of postoperative thrombotic stroke after carotid endarterectomy: the role of transcranial Doppler ultrasound. *J Vasc Surg* 1997; 26: 579-584.

24. Levi CR, O'Malley HM, Fell G, et al. Transcranial Doppler detected cerebral microembolism following carotid endarterectomy: high microembolic signal loads predict postoperative cerebral ischaemia. *Brain* 1997; 120: 621-629.

25. Gross CE, Bednar MM, Lew SM, Florman JE, Kohut JJ. Preoperative volume expansion improves tolerance to carotid artery cross-clamping during endarterectomy. *Neurosurgery* 1998; 43: 222-228.

26. Gaunt ME, Smith JL, Ratliff DA, Bell PR, Naylor AR. A comparison of quality control methods applied to carotid endarterectomy. *Eur J Vasc Surg* 1996; 11: 4-11.

27. Walker RA, Fox AD, Magee TR, Horrocks M. Intraoperative Duplex scanning as a means of quality control during carotid endarterectomy. *Eur J Vasc Surg* 1996; 11: 364-367.

Chapter 3

Carotid angioplasty: a radiologist's perspective

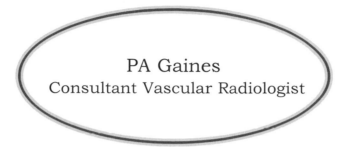

PA Gaines
Consultant Vascular Radiologist

SHEFFIELD VASCULAR INSTITUTE,
NORTHERN GENERAL HOSPITAL, SHEFFIELD

Introduction

Stroke is the third commonest cause of death in the Western World and is the principal cause of prolonged neurological morbidity [1]. In the UK 125,000 patients suffer their first stroke each year and this results in a 10% usage of NHS bed days and 5% of the annual healthcare expenditure [2,3]. Stroke principally affects older people and because of the relative increase in this part of the population, the overall incidence of stroke could increase by 30% by the year 2033 [4].

Not surprisingly, stroke prevention is important for the health of a nation. It must be both accessible to the elderly and cost effective. The major single cause of carotid territory infarction is thrombo-embolic disease, but unfortunately only 20% of major strokes are heralded by minor neurological embolic symptoms (transient ischaemic attack (TIA), amaurosis fugax, recovered stroke). Pure haemodynamic changes account for only 1-2% of all strokes [5]. Patients who suffer a TIA increase their risk of stroke by seven times over the next 7 years. The actuarial risk of stroke is approximately 11.6% during the first year after a TIA and approximately 5.9% per year in each of the subsequent 5 years. With increasing stenosis of the ipsilateral internal carotid artery the risk may increase by up to 36 % over 2 years [6]. Medical therapy has been directed towards limiting thromboembolism from an unstable carotid plaque, principally using anti-platelet agents, but the risk of stroke remains high.

Following the publication of two large trials [6,7] surgery combined with best medical therapy is now considered the treatment of choice for symptomatic high grade carotid stenosis. The role of carotid endarterectomy as the mainstay of treatment has been challenged by the introduction of minimally invasive endovascular techniques (angioplasty and stenting) to treat these stenoses.

The potential of endovascular therapy

The value of carotid endarterectomy relies on the balance between the eventual stroke prophylaxis and the major events surrounding surgery. In two large randomised studies, the European Carotid Surgery Trial (ECST) and the North American Symptomatic Carotid Endarterectomy Trial (NASCET), symptomatic patients with a high grade internal carotid artery stenosis were randomised to best medical therapy or carotid endarterectomy [6,7]. Patients with >70% carotid stenosis had a 3.7% risk of disabling stroke or death within 30 days of surgery in ECST. This rose to 7.5% if all strokes of more than 7 days were included. Similarly, within NASCET there was a 2.1% risk of major stroke or death related to surgery and a 5.8% risk of all peri-operative stroke or death. Clearly carotid endarterectomy, even in these highly selected patients and centres, is not without problems. A recent systematic review of published trials

JVRG

indicated the risk of stroke and/or death following surgery was 5.6% (95% CI 4.4-6.9%) [8]. In addition NASCET detailed further surgical complications, including cranial nerve injury (7.6%), wound haematoma (5.5%), wound infection (3.4%), myocardial infarction (0.9%), congestive heart failure (0.6%) and other cardiovascular problems (1.2%).

The combination of evolving clinical practice and a close collaboration with commercial expertise in providing outstanding miniaturisation and safety of endovascular devices, has resulted in the use of balloon dilatation and stent placement to manage carotid artery stenoses. If it can be shown to be as safe as endarterectomy, either in all patients or in those identified as being at high risk from surgery, then endovascular therapy may become attractive, particularly as it does not have the non-cerebral complications associated with conventional therapy and if it is confirmed as a cost effective day-case procedure (Figure 1).

Current data on endovascular techniques

A Cochrane review is available and includes all the early, small series of carotid angioplasty [9]. However, the majority of data have emerged since 1996. Gil-Peralta and colleagues [10] treated 87 patients with high grade (>70%) symptomatic internal carotid artery disease with simple balloon dilatation. A 4.9% death and disabling stroke rate was recorded, with 3.7% of patients suffering a TIA. They failed to cross the lesion in 5% of patients. At 4 years over 95% of their patients were free from ipsilateral disabling stroke. The Alabama group [11] has published a series of 107 patients with 126 carotid arteries treated by primary stenting (using a variety of devices) and without cerebral protection. All treatments were completed successfully reducing the mean stenosis from 78% (range 53 to 100%) to 20% (range -10 to 25%). The procedural complications included 4.7% minor stroke, 0.8% major stroke and no deaths. At 30 days

there was a further major stroke in one patient, one minor stroke and one death. Overall they reported a 30 day major stroke and death rate of 2.4% from 126 carotid stent procedures. Some 64% of their patients were symptomatic and all but two minor strokes occurred in this group. At short term follow-up there were no further strokes. Eckert and colleagues [12] treated 58 patients with symptomatic internal carotid artery stenoses of >70% according to the NASCET criteria. They had an 81% success rate, with no deaths and only one major stroke (2%). At a mean of 16 months follow-up there was one stroke death and a further stroke following restenosis.

At the Sheffield Vascular Institute there has been endovascular carotid intervention in 207 patients [13]. Some 189 carotid interventions occurred in 182 patients with atherosclerotic disease. All were symptomatic apart from two who underwent carotid stenting prior to coronary artery by-pass surgery. The carotid artery had a low grade stenosis (NASCET scoring method) in 19 patients (50-69%), a high grade stenosis in 121 (70-95%), and was pre-occlusive in 49 (greater than 95%). The contralateral internal carotid artery was significantly diseased (greater than 70%) in 55 patients. In the total group of 189 interventions there were three deaths (1.6%); 2.6% patients had a disabling major stroke and 2.6% a non-disabling stroke. The overall death and disabling major stroke rate was therefore 4.2%; the death and major stroke rate (i.e. including disabling and non-disabling major strokes) was 6.9%. There were, in addition, 2.1% minor strokes, 13% TIAs and 1.5% branch retinal artery occlusions.

These 30 day results from endovascular treatment of carotid stenosis are within the 95% CIs reported by Rothwell et al [8] and include a large number of patients who would have been considered high risk for endarterectomy using the NASCET criteria.

The data relating to the long term success of endovascular techniques as stroke prophylaxis are limited. The data from Gil-Peralta et al [10] are shown in Table 1. These 4-year data can be compared against

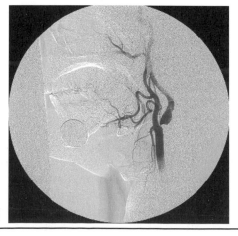
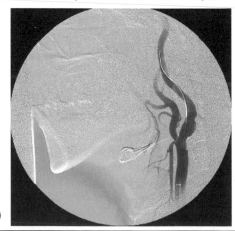

Figure 1. A 90% stenosis at the origin of the internal carotid artery is demonstrated on a subtraction angiogram (a). An excellent result following the placement of a Cordis carotid stent (b).

Table 1. Data from Gil-Peralta et al [10] and the Alabama Group[11].

	%
Gil-Peralta et al:	
Freedom from ipsilateral disabling ischaemic stroke at 4 years	95
Freedom from ipsilateral disabling stroke or vascular death at 4 years	91.5
Freedom from any ipsilateral stroke or death at 4 years	87
University of Alabama, Birmingham, USA:	
Freedom from any stroke or neurological death at 1 year	94±2
Freedom from any stroke or neurological death at 2 years	91±3

surgery; in the NASCET study freedom from major or fatal ipsilateral stroke at 2 years was 96.3% and freedom from any ipsilateral ischaemic stroke was 91%. Within ECST, freedom from any stroke lasting greater than 7 days at 3 years was 97.2%.

For comparison against the Alabama Group results [11] (Table 1), 2 year data from NASCET and ECST were again chosen. In NASCET, freedom from any major or fatal stroke was 96.3%, any stroke or death 84.2%, and any major stroke or death 81.9%. In ECST freedom from any stroke lasting greater than 7 days or surgical death was 89%; freedom from any disabling or fatal stroke or surgical death was 95%.

Any historical comparisons will necessarily be crude but the outcome data between surgery and endovascular treatments of carotid stenosis do appear to be comparable.

The Carotid and Vertebral Artery Transluminal Angioplasty Study (CAVATAS)[14]

This study is the only randomised trial investigating the safety and long term efficacy of endovascular techniques in the management of symptomatic carotid disease. Twenty four centres from around the world randomised 560 patients to two limbs of the trial to compare endovascular therapy against surgery (if patients were fit for surgery) or endovascular therapy against best medical therapy (if patients were unfit for surgery). As with ECST, patients were only randomised if they were suitable for

both forms of treatment and if there was doubt as to the best management. The best medical therapy limb of the trial, however, recruited too few patients for any conclusions to be drawn.

Five hundred and four patients with significant, symptomatic carotid stenosis were randomised between endovascular treatment and conventional surgery. Demographics, presenting symptoms and risk factors were similar. The 30 day adverse event rates following treatment were:
a) disabling stroke and death
- surgery 5.9%
- endovascular 6.4%
b) all stroke (>7days) and death
- surgery 9.9%
- endovascular 10.0%

The non-cerebral complications were also similar in both groups except for significantly more cranial nerve palsies after surgery (not surprisingly there were none after endovascular treatment). At follow-up, there was identical freedom from all stroke and death, and ipsilateral stroke and death, for both treatments up to 3 years.

In summary in CAVATAS there was identical safety, as judged by major indices, and stroke prevention, between the two treatment strategies. Concern has been raised regarding the number of 30 day strokes following surgery. Well conducted randomised trials tend to show a higher complication rate than single centre retrospective audits; it should be noted that many of the patients in this study would have been excluded from NASCET because of co-morbid risk factors.

Chapter 3

The future

The current status of carotid endarterectomy has taken 44 years to achieve. There is little to indicate that this operation will change greatly in the future. Performing carotid endarterectomy under local anaesthesia may remove some of the risks of surgery, but as yet data do not exist to substantiate this claim.

By contrast, the endovascular management of carotid disease began in 1983 and has developed only in earnest over the last 4-5 years. The future is exciting. Pharmaceutical cover surrounding the procedure can be optimised. A great deal of time and money is currently being invested in cerebral protection systems designed to limit embolisation. One such device, based on Therons' original concept of balloon occlusion, already has a CE mark and is undergoing extensive investigation around the world. Other systems designed to limit embolisation by filtration are already developed and entering clinical trials. Dedicated stents will have low profile delivery systems, small interstices, and a coating to limit embolisation and restenosis. Already, in this unit and others, the treatment is being undertaken as a day-case procedure and the cost benefits of this will surely be realised.

I predict that in future large studies will confirm the benefits of endovascular management of symptomatic carotid disease. The future is bright, but not surgical!

References (randomised trials in bold)

1. Warlow CP. Disorders of the cerebral circulation. In: Walton J (Ed). *Brains diseases of the nervous system*. Oxford: Oxford University Press, 1993: 197-210.
2. Bamford J, Sandercock P, Dennid M, Burn J, Warlow CP. A prospective study of acute cerebrovascular disease in the community. The Oxfordshire Community Stroke Project 1981-1986. *J Neurol Neurosurg Psychiatry* 1988; 51: 1373.
3. Dunbabin D, Sandercock P. Stroke prevention. *Hospital Update* 1992; July: 540-5.
4. Malmgren R, Bamford J, Warlow CP, Sandercosk PAG, Slettery JM. Projecting the number of patients with first ever strokes and patients newly handicapped by stroke in England and Wales. *Br Med J* 1989; 298: 656-60.
5. Ringlestein EB, Sievers C, Echer S, Schneider PA, Otis SM. Non-invasive assessment of CO_2 induced cerebral vasomotor response in the normal individual and patients with internal carotid artery occlusions. *Stroke* 1988; 19: 963-9.
6. **North American Symptomatic Carotid Endarterectomy Trial Collaborators. Beneficial effect of carotid endarterectomy in symptomatic patients with high-grade carotid stenoses. *N Eng J Med* 1991; 325: 445-453.**
7. **European Carotid Surgery Trialists Collaborative Group. MRC European Carotid Surgery Trial: interim results for symptomatic patients with severe (70-99%) or with mild (0-29%) carotid stenosis. *Lancet* 1991; 337: 1235-1241.**
8. Rothwell PM, Slattery J, Warlow CP. A systematic review of the risks of stroke and death due to endarterectomy for symptomatic carotid stenosis. *Stroke*. 1996; 27: 260-265.
9. Crawley F, Brown MM. Percutaneous transluminal angioplasty and stenting for carotid artery stenosis (Cochrane Review). In: *The Cochrane Library*, Issue 1, 1999. Oxford: Update Software.
10. Gil-Peralta A, Mayol A, Marcos JRG, et al. Percutaneous transluminal angioplasty of the symptomatic atherosclerotic carotid arteries: results, complications and follow-up. *Stroke*. 1996; 27: 2271-2273.
11. Yadav JS, Roubin GS, Iyer S, et al. Elective stenting of the Extracranial Carotid Arteries. *Circulation*. 1997; 95: 376-381.
12. Eckert B, Zanella FE, Thie A, Steinmetz J, Zeumer H. Angioplasty of the internal carotid artery: results, complications and follow-up in 61 cases. *Cerebrovasc Dis* 1996; 6:97-105.
13. Gaines P, Cleveland T, Beard JD, Venables G. Endovascular carotid intervention - a single centre audit. *JVIR (suppl)*. 1999; 10; 213.
14. **Brown MM for the CAVATAS investigators. Results of the Carotid and Vertebral Artery Transluminal Angioplasty Study (CAVATAS). *Cerebrovasc Dis* 1998; 8(suppl 4): 21.**

Chapter 4

Carotid angioplasty: a surgical perspective

AR Naylor
Consultant Vascular Surgeon and
Honorary Senior Lecturer

DEPARTMENT OF SURGERY,
LEICESTER ROYAL INFIRMARY, LEICESTER

Rationale

Ischaemic stroke secondary to carotid artery disease is an embolic phenomenon and the rationale underlying carotid endarterectomy (CEA) is primarily the removal of the source of embolism. Because pure haemodynamic failure is a relatively rare cause of stroke, the removal of a flow limiting stenosis is of secondary importance. The rationale underlying carotid angioplasty (CA) is to dilate the stenosis and somehow favourably alter the physical and rheological characteristics of the plaque [1]. Procedural embolisation still remains a significant risk [2].

Thus from the outset, there is a subtle difference in therapeutic emphasis compared with CEA, although CA could confer other potential advantages such as avoidance of wound complications, cranial nerve injury and the potential for day case intervention.

Feasibility

CEA has been an accepted means of preventing ischaemic stroke for 45 years but only achieved level I evidence of benefit in 1991 [3,4]. Conversely, CA is a relatively new treatment modality and has not been subject to the same scrutiny. However, an overview of all published series in 1992 [5] showed that it was both feasible and a potential alternative to CEA. The current situation is therefore analogous to that which faced clinicians before the introduction of peripheral angioplasty in the 1970s and coronary angioplasty in the 1980s. The latter has now assumed an accepted role in the management of patients with ischaemic heart disease, albeit with occasional grumbles from cardiac surgeons; most vascular surgeons would now concede that without peripheral angioplasty they would not be able to cope with their increasing workload.

Evolution of carotid angioplasty

The internal carotid artery (ICA) is one of the last major vessels to be considered for angioplasty, primarily because of concerns about the adverse effects of procedural embolisation. Prior to 1992, a number of authors published their preliminary experience and the fears about embolisation appeared to be unfounded. In an overview of the published results in 123 patients (Table 1), Brown observed that CA was associated with a procedural risk of <1% [5]. These results thereafter became a catalyst for the rapid development and proliferation of CA. However, instead of developing a consensus as to how CEA and/or CA may benefit patients in the future, much of the current debate has focussed on interdisciplinary 'turf wars' between vascular surgeons, interventionists and latterly cardiologists.

In the current era of evidence-based practice, vascular surgeons may be forgiven for criticising the atmosphere

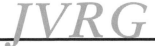

Chapter 4

surrounding the evolution of CA (which appears to be driven by industry and the media rather than by science), while interventionists perceive vascular surgeons to be protectionist and driven by dogma and surgical paranoia.

Interpreting the published results of carotid angioplasty

Irrespective of the criticisms of earlier published series, it remains an indisputable fact that the beneficial effect of CEA has been proven in level I trials [3,4]. However, the results of these trials have also forced surgeons to face some unpalatable truths. There is increasing evidence that the current results following CEA may not match those published in the international trials. Hsai audited outcome in all Medicare beneficiaries undergoing CEA while NASCET was recruiting and showed that the operative mortality was five times higher [6]. When the audit was repeated in 1996, the operative mortality was still almost 2% [7]. Wennberg [8] observed that by 1998 NASCET centres comprised only 3% of institutions performing CEA in the United States (performing only 7% of all CEAs) and that operative mortality was directly related to surgeon experience and annual operative volume [9]. Similarly, the surgical arm of the Carotid And Vertebral Artery Transluminal Angioplasty Study (CAVATAS) reported procedural risks that were significantly worse than those of the ECST in 1991 [3,10].

Even the Asymptomatic Atherosclerosis Study reported a 1.2% stroke rate after angiography in asymptomatic individuals [13].

By 1998, in excess of 2000 CAs had been reported with a very creditable stroke/death rate of 3.74%. However if the data are analysed more closely, it is observed that seven series (1201 patients) reported a death/any stroke rate of 1.16%, while thirteen series (857 patients) reported a 7.5% procedural risk [14]. The tendency to encounter adverse results in more recently published series tends to be dismissed by advocates of CA as simply reflecting the learning curve, or poor technique. Even if this were partially true, it does suggest that CA (like CEA) may not be generalisable to future clinical practice, as any learning curve will not only have to be absorbed by current interventionists but by all trainees in the future. To date, the inclusion of procedural risk associated with angioplasty by trainees has never been considered, while this has been standard practice in carotid surgical centres for some time.

In reality, it is perverse and altogether too simplistic to ascribe 'inevitable learning curve difficulties or poor technique' to those encountering adverse outcomes following carotid angioplasty. A simple review of Table 1 suggests that the pioneers of CA developed the optimal angioplasty technique from the outset, none encountered any learning curve (despite the fact that four series contained fewer than ten patients and eight fewer than

Table 1. Overview of published results of carotid angioplasty prior to 1992 (adapted from Brown [5]).

Author	year	number	death	major stroke	minor stroke
Wiggli	1983	2	0	0	0
Brockenheimer	1983	3	0	0	0
Tsai	1986	6	0	0	0
Theron	1987	5	0	0	0
Freitag	1987	11	0	0	0
Mathias	1987	15	0	0	0
Kachel	1987	24	0	0	0
Brown	1990	12	0	0	0
Theron	1990	13	0	0	0
Porta	1991	32	0	0	1
TOTAL		123	0	0	1

Death and disabling stroke = 0.00%
Death and any stroke   = 0.81%

Thus concerns about the generalisability of CEA appear to have predominated, while the very real potential that a similar problem might face CA has largely been ignored. In the original overview by Brown (Table 1), CA was associated with no deaths, no major strokes and only one non-disabling stroke in 123 patients [5]. These results were remarkable, even better than the published risks of diagnostic carotid angiography alone which is generally accepted to be 1-2% in symptomatic patients [11,12].

20). It is probable that these excellent results were obtained by performing CA in highly selected, low risk patients, but this does no more than prove that CA is feasible. A similar phenomenon was encountered in the Leicester carotid angioplasty trial. Here the radiologist encountered no complications in a series of highly selected individuals but when 'routine CEA' patients were randomised in the trial, the ensuing stroke rate following angioplasty was unacceptably high [15].

Whether CA is better than CEA can only be answered by further randomised, controlled trials. To date, many proponents of angioplasty have been reluctant to participate in such trials, usually on the grounds that 'now is not the time' or because 'future advances in catheter technology will render any trials obsolete'. The argument regarding timing could be used *ad infinitum*. It should be borne in mind that, were CA shown to have a beneficial role (even in selected patients), it is vital that this information is obtained quickly. The argument regarding future improvements in catheter technology is a poor excuse for not performing a randomised trial. Carotid surgeons could similarly argue that advances in monitoring, quality control and operative technique have reduced the procedural risk to 2% [16].

To date, only two randomised trials have been performed. Neither has shown that CA confers any benefit over CEA. CAVATAS recorded a 10% angioplasty stroke risk [10], while the Leicester trial had to be abandoned because of a significant excess of strokes in the angioplasty arm of the trial [15]. Until further trials have been performed and the issue of generalisability addressed, there remains no scientific evidence that CA is safer than CEA.

Predicting high risk patients

A significant proportion of CA series currently include a preponderance of asymptomatic patients. This might be justified, by some, on the basis of the Asymptomatic Carotid Artery Study findings, but just as there have been concerns regarding the role of CEA in asymptomatic patients, the same criticisms will inevitably face practitioners of CA. Even if CA achieved a procedural stroke risk of 2-3% (including the diagnostic angiogram risk), CA could only ever confer an actual risk reduction of late stroke of 1% per annum and reliance on angioplasty would only ever prevent about 3% of all strokes [17]. This author believes that, just as the surgical indications for operating on asymptomatic individuals will reduce in the future, the same will apply to CA. Both treatment modalities are unlikely ever to achieve the combination of generalisability, clinical effectiveness and cost-effectiveness.

It seems inevitable that the indications for intervention on symptomatic patients will become stricter. At present, 70-80% of patients with symptomatic 70-99% stenoses undergoing CEA would otherwise have remained stroke free had they received best medical therapy; there is no evidence to suggest that the overall risk:benefit ratio will be any different following CA. In the future, there will be legitimate calls to limit CEA or CA to the subgroup of patients who are at highest risk of late stroke. Evidence suggests that a combination of clinical features (women versus men, ocular versus non-ocular symptoms, peripheral vascular disease, systolic hypertension) and angiographic criteria (degree of stenosis, surface irregularity/thrombus) can contribute towards a scoring system that could identify patients with a >40% risk of stroke during follow-up [18]. In this way, up to 80% of otherwise low risk patients would not need to undergo surgery (or CA) with the net effect that treatment would become more clinically beneficial and cost-effective and 80% of patients might not be subjected to an unnecessary (and occasionally risky) procedure.

Paradoxically, however, were such a policy to be introduced, the same data suggest that peri-operative risks would also increase significantly, i.e. surgeons could find themselves operating on a smaller number of patients with a higher risk of procedural stroke [18]. Should that become the case, any patient considered for either CEA or CA will be highly likely to have overlying plaque thrombus which could severely limit the ability of interventionists to undertake a safe angioplasty procedure. Moreover, for some interventionists who rely on angiography to identify high risk patients with luminal thrombus (as was the case in CAVATAS) in order to exclude them from CA, but the latest ECST data suggest that this is unreliable. Up to 58% of patients with an angiographically smooth stenosis will have ulceration at operation and 25% will have unsuspected surface thrombus [19]. The presence or absence of luminal thrombus is never a contra-indication to CEA.

What of the future?

It is inevitable that CA will have a role in the management of selected patients with carotid artery disease but appropriate selection criteria will only ever evolve from properly conducted randomised trials where inclusion and exclusion criteria are clearly stipulated. Until this is done, the results will never be generalisable. The problem will remain the ability reliably to predict the high risk carotid plaque. Figure 1 illustrates two pre-angioplasty stenoses and their completion films. Both patients presented with a TIA and the stenoses look very similar, yet one of the patients (case 2) suffered a procedural stroke. Similarly, amid the haste to pioneer aids and technological advancements to make both CEA and CA safer, it should not be forgotten that only high risk patients require intervention. Surgeons and radiologists cannot justify intervening in low risk patients in order to ensure optimal procedural outcomes.

In the future, it seems inevitable that both surgeons and interventionists will become subject to increased independent audit and accountability. Those who quote the results of other trials or centres to justify individual practice face the daunting prospect of medicolegal action. It also seems likely that the volume of symptomatic patients being referred for CEA or CA will be greatly reduced in the future, thereby paving the way for centralisation of carotid surgery and/or angioplasty into larger centres. Such a trend would serve to optimise outcomes, training, multi-disciplinary team input, cost and audit/research. The question as to whether CA will be able to meet these increasing demands in the future remains to be seen. At present there is no evidence that, even with future technological advances, CA will be any more generalisable or safer than CEA.

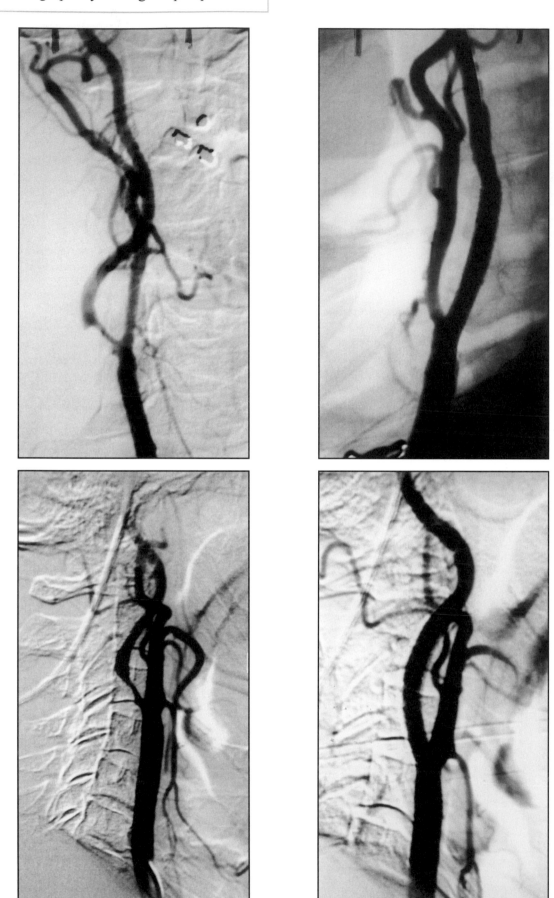

Figure 1. Spot the difference? Pre-angioplasty and completion angiograms in two patients with similar symptomatic carotid stenoses. Patient 1 (top left and right) proceeded uneventfully. Patient 2 (bottom left and right) suffered a procedural stroke. The problem for the interventionist is the ability to predict reliably the high risk plaque.

References (randomised trials in bold)

1. Ferguson RDG, Ferguson JG, Lee LI. Endovascular revascularization therapy in cerebral athero-occlusive disease. *Neurosurg Clin North Am* 1994; 5: 511-527.
2. Goldsmith MF. Cerebral percutaneous angioplasty in second year of trials. *JAMA* 1992; 268: 3039-3040.
3. **European Carotid Surgery Trialists' Collaborative Group. Randomised trial of endarterectomy for recently symptomatic carotid stenosis: final results of the MRC European Carotid Surgery Trial (ECST). *Lancet* 1998; 351: 1379-1387.**
4. **Barnett HJM, Taylor DW, Eliasziw M, et al. Benefit of carotid endarterectomy in patients with symptomatic moderate or severe stenosis. *N Engl J Med* 1998; 339: 1415-1425.**
5. Brown MM. Balloon angioplasty for cerebrovascular disease. *Neurol Res* 1992; 14(suppl); 159-163.
6. Hsai DC, Krushat WM, Moscoe LM. Epidemiology of carotid endarterectomy among Medicare beneficiaries. *J Vasc Surg* 1992; 16: 201-208.
7. Hsai DC, Krushat WM, Moscoe LM. Epidemiology of carotid endarterectomy among Medicare beneficiaries: 1985 - 1996 update. *Stroke* 1998; 29: 346-350.
8. Wennberg DE, Lucas FL, Birkmeyer JD, Bredenberg CE, Fisher ES. Variation in carotid endarterectomy mortality in the Medicare population. *JAMA* 1998; 279: 1278-1281.
9. Karp HR, Flanders D, Shipp CC, Taylor B, Martin D. Carotid endarterectomy among Medicare beneficiaries: a statewide evaluation of appropriateness and outcome. *Stroke* 1998; 29: 46-52.
10. **Brown MM on behalf of the CAVATAS Investigators. Results of the Carotid and Vertebral Artery Transluminal Angioplasty Study (CAVATAS). *Br J Surg* 1999; 86: A710-11.**
11. Hankey GJ, Warlow CP, Sellar RJ. Cerebral angiographic risk in mild cerebrovascular disease. *Stroke* 1990; 21: 209-222.
12. Davies KN, Humphrey PR. Complications of cerebral angiography in patients with symptomatic carotid territory ischaemia screened by carotid ultrasound. *J Neurol Neurosurg Psych* 1993; 56: 967-972.
13. Executive Committee for the Asymptomatic Carotid Atherosclerosis Study. Endarterectomy for asymptomatic carotid artery stenosis. *JAMA* 1995; 273: 1421-1461.
14. Naylor AR. Carotid artery disease. In: *Vascular Surgery Highlights* 1998-1999. Ed: Davies AH. Health Press, Oxford 1999; 56-63.
15. **Naylor AR, Bolia A, Abbott RJ, et al. Randomised trial of carotid endarterectomy versus carotid angioplasty: a stopped trial. *J Vasc Surg* 1998; 28: 326-334.**
16. Naylor AR, Hayes PD, Allroggen H, et al. Reducing the risk of carotid surgery: a seven year audit of the role of monitoring and quality control assessment. *Stroke* (in press).
17. Hankey GJ. Asymptomatic carotid stenosis: how should it be managed? *Med J Aust* 1995; 163: 197-200.
18. Rothwell PM, Warlow CP, on behalf of the European Carotid Surgery Trialists' Collaborative Group. Prediction of benefit from carotid endarterectomy in individual patients: a risk modelling study. *Lancet* 1999; 353: 2105-10.
19. Rothwell PM, Villagra R, Gibson R, Donders R, Warlow CP on behalf of the European Carotid Surgery Trialists' Collaborative Group. Evidence for a chronic systemic cause of irregularity and rupture of atherosclerotic plaques. *Lancet* (in press).

Chapter 4

Carotid angioplasty: a surgical perspective

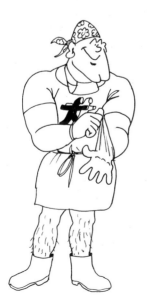

Chapter 5

The value of risk factor management in patients with peripheral arterial disease

CP Shearman
Consultant Vascular Surgeon and
Honorary Senior Lecturer
A Chulakadabba
Vascular Research Fellow

DEPARTMENT OF VASCULAR SURGERY,
SOUTHAMPTON UNIVERSITY HOSPITAL, SOUTHAMPTON

Introduction

Peripheral arterial occlusive disease in the leg (PAOD), is a significant health care problem. The disease may remain asymptomatic or manifest as intermittent claudication (IC) or critical limb ischaemia (CLI). The Edinburgh Artery Study found in a survey of a population of subjects aged between 55 to 74 years that 4.5% had symptomatic claudication, 8% had major asymptomatic disease and a further 16.6% had abnormal haemodynamic variables indicative of PAOD. Over the following 5 years the majority of patients subsequently presenting with IC were those who had previously been found to have asymptomatic PAOD [1]. In elderly men, IC is even more prevalent; as many as one in five suffer claudication. CLI is an equally daunting problem with an annual incidence of between 500-1000 patients per million of the population [2].

At least 70% of patients with IC have ischaemic heart disease and their 10 year mortality from cardiovascular disease, largely due to myocardial infarction and stroke, is approximately 50%, or 3.8 times greater than patients without PAOD [3]. The outlook for a patient with CLI is even more gloomy. One in five will be dead from cardiovascular disease within a year of diagnosis [4]. There is little to suggest that treatment of POAD by revascularisation has any influence on the progression and outcome of local or systemic atherosclerotic disease, possibly other than by selection of the fitter patients for intervention.

It is apparent that atheroma is not a slowly progressive disease, but can undergo periods of intense biological activity resulting in intra-plaque haemorrhage or rupture. These sudden changes either occlude a vessel or expose the highly thrombogenic subintimal surface, promoting platelet adherence and activation. This process is termed atherothrombosis and it seems that most clinical events (such as myocardial infarction) are associated with such acute changes in the plaque [5].

Based on the above observations, a major component of treatment of patients with PAOD should include measures to reduce the progression of arteriosclerosis. The potential benefits include reduction of cardiovascular mortality and morbidity, preventing deterioration of the local disease as well as improving the long-term benefit of revascularisation procedures. However, lack of direct evidence of benefit and problems with patient compliance, coupled with concerns about cost effectiveness, have limited the widespread application of such an approach. This chapter examines the current evidence for the role of identification and treatment of cardiovascular risk factors in patients with PAOD. A number of factors that increase the risk of cardiovascular morbidity and mortality or local disease are well established, while other life-style changes or adjunctive medication may be of value (Table 1).

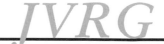

Table 1. Risk factors associated with cardiovascular disease. They are closely interrelated. An asterisk denotes that evidence of benefit from correction of the factor is unproven.

FIXED	MODIFIABLE	LIFE STYLE
Age	Smoking	Exercise
Sex	Cholesterol	Anti-platelet drugs
Family history	Hypertension	Vitamins and anti-oxidant*
Diabetes	Obesity	
	Homocysteine*	
	Oestrogen*	

Chapter 5

Smoking

Cigarette smoking is the leading cause of preventable death in the Western World; one in five of all deaths are attributable to cigarettes [6]. It is also the single most important risk factor for PAOD, associated with a three-fold increased risk of developing the disease [7]. Clinically significant disease progression is also more likely in persistent smokers and subsequent intervention less likely to succeed. Amputation is more common in smokers than non-smokers [8].

Both nicotine and carbon monoxide in cigarette smoke appear to cause harm in a number of ways including affecting other risk factors. Smoking increases blood pressure and total serum cholesterol, reduces oxygen carriage, increases vascular resistance and vasospasm (which may cause plaque rupture), and adversely affects vascular endothelium, platelets and thrombotic mechanisms [9].

There are short term and long-term benefits of stopping smoking. Nicotine levels fall by half within 8 hours and carbon monoxide levels return to normal in 24-48 hours, while oxygen carriage and blood pressure take longer to normalise. Evidence of the benefit of stopping smoking has never been established in a randomised controlled trial, but several large cohort studies have clearly shown that stopping smoking carries cardiovascular benefit [10]. The excess cardiovascular risk is halved within one year and is the same as non-smokers within 5-15 years. After surgical intervention the benefit of stopping smoking is still apparent. In the Coronary Artery Surgery Study (CASS) patients who had undergone coronary artery bypass surgery and given up smoking had significantly better survival rates at 10 years (84% v 68%) and less re-interventions than those who continued to smoke [11]. Several observational studies have identified an improvement in walking distance in patients with IC and less risk of amputation in those who give up cigarettes.

Persuading patients to stop smoking is notoriously difficult with success rates as low as 2% reported. However, the rate can be improved to 27% with support such as nicotine patches, counselling and behaviour modification [12]. The large benefit of stopping smoking and the large numbers of people at risk mean that even a modest reduction in the number of smokers will have a big impact on overall outcome for patients with PAOD.

Diabetes

Patients with Type 2 (non-insulin dependent) diabetes have a 3-5 fold increased risk of developing PAOD compared to non-diabetics. Intensive blood glucose control appears to reduce the risk of microvascular diabetic complications but has little impact on macrovascular disease and amputation. However, control of other risk factors in Type 2 diabetics, such as hypertension and hyperlipidaemia, will reduce the risk of cardiovascular events [13,14,15]. Similarly, in Type 1 diabetics good blood glucose control reduces the risk of microvascular disease, but although this should reduce cardiovascular mortality and morbidity, this has not been established clearly.

Cholesterol

The observation that elevated cholesterol levels increase the risk of ischaemic heart disease in a linear manner is well established [16]. Although the relationship is more complex in PAOD, there remains a strong association [17]. Dietary attempts to reduce cholesterol levels have been disappointing, achieving only modest reductions of 5-10% and requiring considerable patient encouragement to achieve even this. The statin class of drugs (HMG-CoA reductase inhibitors) produce reductions in serum cholesterol of around 25-30% and appear safe. Several large, prospective primary intervention studies (West of Scotland Coronary Prevention Study [18], Air Force/Texas Coronary Atherosclerosis Prevention Study [19]) and secondary intervention studies (Scandinavian Simvastatin Survival Study [20], Cholesterol and Recurrent Events Study [21]) have demonstrated a significant reduction in cardiovascular events associated with cholesterol lowering therapy using the statin drugs. Cholesterol tended to be lowered after intervention by around 25% and the risk reduction was approximately 30%. The benefits then, were greatest in subjects with the greatest risk of cardiovascular events, that is those with established ischaemic heart disease and elevated serum cholesterol; in this group approximately 13 patients will require treatment for 5 years to prevent one cardiovascular event. In studies of subjects with elevated cholesterol, without established arterial disease the benefit is less and around 40 patients require treatment to prevent one event [22]. In light of this evidence it has been accepted that subjects with elevated cholesterol following myocardial infarction should be treated with statins. Although patients with symptomatic PAOD have similar risks of cardiac events, and so should gain at least the same benefit, the case for treatment has not been widely proven [23]. This is partly due to the lack of direct evidence in patients with PAOD and concerns that the above results do not apply to patients over 65 years of age, although recent analysis suggests that they probably do. There is no evidence to support concerns that there is increased mortality from cholesterol lowering therapy [24]. The debate therefore must focus on the cost of treating these relatively elderly patients against any potential benefit they may gain.

It would be appealing if lipid-lowering therapy also had an effect on the atheroma in the lower limb arteries. This might prevent disease progression. More recently the possibility of encouraging plaque stability has been suggested. Several small studies have examined this in the femoral and carotid arteries where plaque size was assessed using ultrasound imaging. Any positive changes were small. Although encouraging, there is currently no good evidence to support the suggestion that lipid lowering therapy arrests or causes regression of peripheral artery atheroma, let alone affects symptoms.

Hypertension

Elevated blood pressure is very common and it has been estimated that up to 24% of the adult population may be hypertensive. It is also a strong independent predictor of cardiovascular disease, especially stroke and ischaemic heart disease, but also increases the risk of PAOD approximately three-fold. Clear benefit in treating hypertension has been demonstrated in a number of studies. Stroke rate can be reduced by 38%, cardiovascular deaths by 14% and other cardiovascular events by 26%; these effects are also apparent in elderly subjects. Some evidence has been produced to support the suggestion that lowering systemic blood pressure may adversely affect PAOD, but this is probably of little clinical significance in relation to the systemic benefits gained from blood pressure control. Also of some interest is the observation that despite theoretical concerns about ß-blockers in patients with PAOD, there is no evidence to suggest that they do in fact have an adverse effect.

Exercise

A sedentary life-style is a major risk factor for cardiovascular disease. People who undertake even a moderate amount of exercise on a regular basis, such as 30 minutes walking per day, have half the cardiovascular mortality rate of those who rarely exercise. Increasing physical activity in previously inactive adults is beneficial but the effect is lost if the individual returns to their previous inactive life-style. The relationship of obesity and cardiovascular disease is less clear, but exercise

combined with weight loss is associated with a reduction in cholesterol and blood pressure and a number of small observational studies suggest clinical benefits.

Exercise may also improve the walking ability of patients with PAOD and a recent meta-analysis of 21 studies suggested an improvement in distance walked of 124%. Although none of the studies was large enough to be conclusive in its own right, the weight of evidence seems to suggest that this is a real finding [25]. In these studies walking for 30 minutes a day, three times a week for 6 months had the most benefit. Although some form of walking seems best, the optimal method and frequency of exercise therapy or whether it needs to be supervised has not been clearly established. Numerous mechanisms have been proposed for this improvement including muscle fibre type transformation, metabolic adaptation, increased muscle capillary blood flow, reduction in blood viscosity or simply using non-ischaemic muscles. On balance, exercise is essential for patients with PAOD. It may not only improve the primary problem with the leg, but may also reduce the cardiovascular risk. It is surprising that more attention has not been paid to exercise therapy.

Antiplatelet agents

In patients with PAOD platelets show evidence of increased activation. Atheromatous plaque rupture may lead to further platelet activation and aggregation at the site of disruption. This can cause occlusion of the vessel or sudden increase in plaque volume, resulting in a clinical event. Aspirin irreversibly blocks platelet cyclo-oxygenase-mediated production of thromboxane A_2, a powerful promoter of platelet aggregation. Experimentally, low doses of 40 to 80 mg aspirin seem to be effective at blocking cyclo-oxgenase for the 10-day life span of the platelet, while higher doses may have an adverse effect on cyclo-oxygenase in the vascular endothelium.

The Antiplatelet Trialists' Collaboration analysed 145 placebo-controlled, randomised studies and found that aspirin in doses ranging from 75-1500mg per day reduced the risk of death, myocardial infarction, and stroke by 25% in patients with established arteriosclerosis [26]. Other antiplatelet agents examined did not have any advantage over aspirin. Up to 20% of patients cannot tolerate aspirin; gastro-intestinal side effects occur in up to 5% and are dose-related. A recent study compared a new antiplatelet agent, clopidogrel, to aspirin in patients following recent stroke, myocardial infarction or established claudication [27]. There was a significant reduction in cardiovascular events in both treatment groups compared to what would have been expected if the patients had received no treatment. Clopidogrel was found to be more effective, with a reduction in relative risk of 8.7%, than aspirin. From these data it was estimated that 1000 patients with arterial disease who did not receive aspirin would suffer 77 cardiovascular events in 1 year. Treatment with aspirin would reduce this by 19 events, but clopidogrel could reduce it by 24 events. On subgroup analysis, patients with PAOD gained more benefit than the patients who had myocardial infarction or stroke, with a relative risk reduction of 23.8%. Clopidogrel is at least as safe as aspirin but more expensive, so use as a first line antiplatelet agent will be determined by cost effectiveness. Currently it offers a powerful alternative for those patients unable to tolerate aspirin.

Homocysteine

There have been several reports of the strong relationship between elevated serum homocysteine and PAOD. In particular, elevated homocysteine is strongly associated with early onset atheroma. The mechanism of homocysteine-induced atheroma is multifactorial but may involve impaired endothelial production of nitric oxide, proliferation of smooth muscle cells and thrombosis. Plasma homocysteine can be lowered with folate and vitamins B_{12} and B_6 dietary supplementation. There have been no randomised, controlled studies of this treatment, but there are preliminary claims that therapy can slow atherosclerotic plaque progression

Antioxidants and vitamins

Oxidative damage seems to play a significant role in the genesis and progression of arteriosclerosis. Patients with claudication have less antioxidant capacity, supporting the hypothesis that it has been mopped up by continued oxidant activity. It is possible then that antioxidants such as vitamins C and E, ß carotene and selenium could be used to reduce the risk of cardiovascular disease. Although appealing, and probably safe, there is no evidence to support the use of these vitamins as a protection against atherosclerosis.

Oestrogen

Cardiovascular disease is the commonest cause of death in post-menopausal women. Several observational studies have suggested a reduction in cardiovascular death in women on hormone replacement therapy, prompting the suggestion that oestrogen may be cardioprotective. However, a recent study which randomised women following myocardial infarction to placebo or oestrogen therapy failed to show any benefit from hormone replacement therapy [28].

Conclusions

When considering the role of risk factor identification and reduction, the potential benefit to a patient has to be weighed against the risk of intervention and the cost of identifying and treating the risk factor. There is overwhelming evidence to suggest that active risk factor intervention significantly reduces cardiovascular mortality in patients with PAOD. In general, most of the interventions discussed above are safe, or at least low risk. Some, such as statin therapy for hypercholesterolaemia, are relatively expensive; others are very economical so it is surprising that they are not more widely applied. It has been shown that up to 20% of patients with proven atherosclerotic arterial disease are not taking aspirin. The cost of rehabilitating a patient following a stroke or myocardial infarction is so high that anything which makes even a modest impact on this problem is worthwhile.

In the United Kingdom most patients with PAOD will be treated either by a vascular surgeon or general practitioner. The responsibility then must lie with these two clinicians to take on the challenge of risk factor management. Although largely falling into a medical sphere, the essence of risk factor management lies in having well developed protocols and good relationships with other medical teams, such as diabetic physicians. The real challenge lies in devising a way of encouraging patients with PAOD to comply with such protocols. To date, the most successful programmes have encompassed intervention at a number of different levels and tend to be part of a community-based health awareness campaign. Although not easy, tackling some of the reversible causes of PAOD could have as much impact on patient survival and quality of life as any revascularisation procedure.

The value of risk factor management in patients with peripheral arterial disease

Sound evidence

- Patients with peripheral arterial disease should stop smoking, take aspirin (or similar), exercise and have high blood pressure and high cholesterol treated as this reduces the chance of subsequent adverse cardiovascular events.

Evidence needed

- Whether any of the above affects the natural history of peripheral arterial insufficiency.

References (randomised trials in bold)

1. Leng GC, Lee AJ, Fowkes FGR, et al. Incidence, natural history and cardiovascular events in symptomatic and asymptomatic peripheral arterial disease in the general population. *Int J Epidemiol* 1996; 25: 1172-1181.

2. European Consensus on critical limb ischaemia. *Lancet* 1989; I: 737-738.

3. Bainton D, Sweetnam P, Baker I, Elwood P. Peripheral vascular disease: consequence for survival and association with risk factors in the Speedwell prospective heart disease study. *Br Heart J* 1994; 72: 128-132.

4. Norgren L. Life expectancy for critical limb ischaemia. In: Greenhalgh RM, Ed. *The durability of vascular and endovascular interventions.* London: WB Saunders, 1999; 163-173.

5. Libby P, Geng YJ, Aikawa M, et al. Macrophages and atherosclerotic plaque stability *Curr Opin Lipidol* 1996; 7: 330-335.

6. Centers for disease control and prevention. Cigarette smoking - attributable mortality and years of potential life lost - United States,1990. *Morb Mort Wkly Rep* 1993; 42: 645-649.

7. Hiatt WR, Hoag S, Hamman RF. Effect of diagnostic criteria on the prevalence of peripheral arterial disease. The San Luis Valley Diabetes Study. *Circulation* 1995; 91: 1472-1479.

8. Hirsch AT, Treat-Jacobsfn D, Lando HA, Hatsukami DK. The role of tobacco cessation, antiplatelet and lipid lowering therapies in the treatment of peripheral arterial disease. *Vasc Med* 1997; 2: 243-251.

9. Jonas MA, Oates JA, Ockene JK, Hennekens CH. Statement on smoking and cardiovascular disease for health professionals. AHA Medical/Scientific Statement. *Circulation* 1992; 86: 1664-1669.

10. Doll R, Peto R, Wheatley K, Gray R, Sutherland I. Mortality in relation to smoking: 40 years' observations on male British doctors. *Br Med J* 1994; 309: 901-911.

11. **Cavender JB, Rogers WJ, Fisher LD, Bush BJ, Coggin CJ, Meyers WO. Effects of smoking on survival and morbidity in patients randomized to medical or surgical therapy in the Coronary Artery Surgery Study (CASS): 10-year follow-up. *J Am Coll Cardiol* 1992; 20: 287-294.**

12. Joseph AM, Norman SM, Ferry LH, et al. The safety of transdermal nicotine as an aid to smoking cessation in patients with cardiac disease. *N Eng J Med* 1996; 335: 1792-1798.

13. **UK Prospective Diabetes Study Group. Tight blood pressure control and risk of macrovascular and microvascular complications in type 2 diabetics. UKPDS 38. *Br Med J* 1998; 317: 703-713.**

14. Pyorala K, Pedersen TR, Kjekshus J, Faergeman O, Olsson AG, Thorgeirsson G. Cholesterol lowering with simvastatin improves prognosis of diabetic patients with coronary heart disease. A subgroup analysis of the Scandinavian Simvastatin Survival Study (4S). *Diabetes Care* 1997; 20: 614-620.

15. **UK Prospective Diabetes Study (UKPDS) Group. Intensive blood-glucose control with sulphonureas or insulin compared with conventional treatment and risk of complications in patients with type 2 diabetes (UKPDS 33). *Lancet* 1998; 352: 837-853.**

16. Consensus Conference from the Office of Medical Applications of Research, National Institutes of Health, Bethesda, Md. Lowering blood cholesterol to prevent heart disease. *JAMA* 1985; 253: 2080-2086.

17. Murabito JM, D'Agostino RB, Silbershatz H, Wilson WF. Intermittent claudication. A risk profile from the Framingham Heart Study. *Circulation* 1997; 96: 44-49.

18. **Shepherd J, Cobbe SM, Ford I, et al, for the West of Scotland Coronary Prevention Study Group. Prevention of coronary heart disease with pravastatin in men with hypercholesterolemia. *N Engl J Med* 1996; 333: 1301-1307.**

19. **Downs JR, Clearfield M, Weis S, et al. Primary prevention of acute coronary events with lovastatin in men and women with average cholesterol levels. *JAMA* 1998; 279: 1615-1622.**

20. **Scandinavian Simvastatin Survival Study Group. Randomised trial of cholesterol lowering in 4444 patients with coronary heart disease: the Scandinavian Simvastatain Survival Study (4S). *Lancet* 1994; 344: 1383-1389.**

21. **Sacks FM, Pfeffer MA, Moye LA, et al, for the Cholesterol and Recurrent Events Trial Investigators. The effect of pravasatin on coronary events after myocardial infarction in patients with average cholesterol levels. *N Eng J Med* 1996; 335: 1001-1009.**

22. Haq IU, Ramsay LE, Pickin DM, Yeo WW, Jackson PR, Payne JN. Lipid-lowering for prevention of coronary heart disease: what policy now? *Clin Sci* 1996; 91: 399-413.

23. Haq IU, Yeo WW, Jackson PR, Ramsay LE. The case for cholesterol reduction in peripheral arterial disease. *Critical Ischaemia* 1997; 7: 15-22.

24. Gaziano JM, Castelli WP. Cholesterol Reduction. In: Hennekens CH, Ed. *Clinical Trials in Cardiovascular Disease.* Philadelphia: WB Saunders, 1999; 327-340.

25. Leng GC, Fowler B, Ernst E. Exercise for intermittent claudication. (Cochrane Review) In: *The Cochrane Library*, Issue 2. Oxford: Update Software; 1998.

26. **Antiplatelet Trialists' Collaboration. Collaborative overview of randomised trials of antiplatelet therapy - I: Prevention of death, myocardial infarction and stroke by prolonged antiplatelet therapy in various categories of patients. *Br Med J* 1994; 308: 81-106.**

27. **Caprie Steering Committee. A randomised, blinded, trial of clopidogrel versus aspirin in patients at risk of ischaemic events (CAPRIE). *Lancet* 1996; 348: 1329-1339.**

28. **Hulley S, Grady D, Bush T, et al. Randomized trial of estrogen plus progestin for secondary prevention of coronary heart disease in post menopausal women. Heart Estrogen-progestin Replacement Study Research Group. *JAMA* 1998; 280: 605-613.**

Chapter 5

The value of risk factor management in
patients with peripheral arterial disease

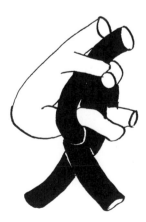

Chapter 6

Management of intermittent claudication

PM Lamont
Consultant Vascular Surgeon and
Honorary Senior Clinical Lecturer

DEPARTMENT OF VASCULAR SURGERY,
BRISTOL ROYAL INFIRMARY, BRISTOL

Introduction

The management of intermittent claudication remains one of the most controversial areas in vascular surgery. Scientific studies are confounded by the natural tendency of claudication symptoms to improve spontaneously. Clear guidelines are lacking and only a few good randomised studies in selected patient populations are available. The clinician can choose from masterly inactivity, through drug treatment, to exercise training, to balloon angioplasty or even bypass surgery without serious fear of criticism. Evidence in favour of any one of these therapies can be produced by judicious review of the literature, although consensus on which is the most appropriate can be more difficult to elicit. Little wonder that the public health physicians who guard the public purse on health expenditure are astounded by the lack of agreement on the correct way to manage claudication.

Claudication is, in itself, a relatively benign condition that need not produce major disability if patients are happy to accept the limitations imposed on their lifestyle. The first step in managing claudication is to decide whether it needs management at all, other than modification of risk factors (see previous chapter). Many patients present for treatment in the fear that their claudication is a harbinger of imminent gangrene and subsequent amputation. Often simple reassurance about the natural history of claudication is all that is required. In a prospective study of nearly 2,000 patients with untreated claudication followed for 1 year reported by Dormandy in 1991, symptoms deteriorated to the extent of needing intervention in only 111 patients (5.5%) and 32 (1.6%) required a major amputation [1]. In the longer term, McAllister's study showed over 6 years that a patient with claudication had a 50% chance of improving spontaneously, a 30% chance of remaining unchanged and a 20% chance of deterioration; only 7 of 100 patients studied lost their leg (six of whom had severe diabetes) [2].

At what stage should the clinician consider active treatment for claudication? Assessment of walking distance alone is a poor guide. The patient's own assessment is notoriously unreliable and a treadmill test does not simulate a patient's normal walking pace. The patient's perception of disability may have little to do with actual walking distance. Compare the 55 year old sedentary working man, happy to continue with 50 metre claudication because he is never far from his car, to the 82 year old lady devastated by 300 metre claudication because she can no longer take her dog for a walk in the park. Some assessment of the patient's quality of life in relation to their walking distance is clearly required. Another catch is a patient with other smoking related disease, who can only walk 20 metres because of claudication but previously only walked 25 metres because of angina or shortness of breath. Treating claudication under these conditions is unlikely to improve walking distance or quality of life.

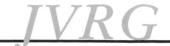

Sufficient time, usually 2 to 3 months, must have passed from the onset of claudication to ensure that the need for treatment will not be pre-empted by spontaneous improvement. If no improvement occurs, both clinician and patient should come to a view about the effect of the claudication on quality of life. What exactly is the patient unable to do and can their lifestyle be modified to reduce disability. No self-respecting golfer would ever contemplate giving up the game, but what about playing with only a seven iron so that the ball is never hit further than the claudication distance. Can the employer reassign working practice to lie within the limits of the claudication? Is the quality of life so bad that the patient is willing to lose their leg should an interventional treatment go horribly wrong? If the patient remains keen for treatment after examining these issues, which treatment is most appropriate?

Exercise training

Simple advice to exercise and walk at least a mile a day is all very laudable, but has little effect on the quality of life as measured by an SF-36 questionnaire [3]. To this extent, Dr. Housley's treatment of claudication in five words 'Stop smoking and keep walking' [4] is unlikely to improve symptoms on its own. In order to have an impact on walking distance and quality of life, exercise programmes need to be well structured, supervised initially and continued at home indefinitely [5].

Insufficient research exists to specify the ideal exercise programme, but it is clear that some form of supervision in an exercise class is important initially to motivate the patient. After a period of supervision the patient may well become self-motivated as the resulting improvement in walking distance becomes evident. Out of a cohort of 22 patients in Southampton, randomised to supervised exercise classes once a week for 1 month and then left to perform daily exercise sessions at home, the reported compliance 1 year later was 4.9 sessions per week out of a potential maximum of seven [5].

In a meta-analysis of exercise rehabilitation programmes for claudication, Gardner and Poehlman analysed those factors producing the greatest improvements in pain-free walking distance [6]. These factors included exercise continued for more than 30 minutes per session, at least three exercise sessions per week, walking used as the mode of exercise, near maximal pain during training used as the claudication end point and a programme lasting at least 6 months.

Systematic review of randomised trials on the effects of exercise on claudication comes up with remarkably consistent results [7]. All ten of those good quality trials identified in the review demonstrated an unequivocal improvement in pain-free and maximum walking distance/time, ranging from 28% - 210% (mean 105%, SD 56%). Five of these trials had an untreated control group and in all five studies the exercise training programme showed superior results to untreated controls.

There seems little doubt that supervised exercise has a place in the management of intermittent claudication. Despite a wealth of evidence, dating back over the past 30 years [8,9,10,11], few UK vascular centres offer supervised exercise training to their patients, including some who have advocated such programmes in the literature. The reasons for this poor provision are not clear but may include difficulty in persuading patients to take part and patient demands for interventional treatment (many have seen balloon angioplasty on television). The presence of co-morbidity may also limit adequate exercise. Perhaps there is reluctance by some vascular surgeons to consider non-interventional therapy. Even though angioplasty or surgery may offer an apparent 'quick fix', there is often a lengthy wait between outpatient clinic and intervention. This interval might readily be occupied by a supervised exercise class that may may obviate the need for further intervention.

Drug therapy

Poor study design of drug trials and the natural history of spontaneous improvement in patients with claudication make the value of drug treatment difficult to assess. In a meta-analysis of drug therapy for claudication, 75 different trials of 33 different pharmacological agents were analysed and deficiencies were found in 57 of 75 (76%) [12]. The most frequently studied drug was oxpentifylline, which in seven placebo-controlled trials showed an average improvement of 65% in claudication distance. A significant inverse relationship between sample size and response in these studies suggested a bias produced by non-publication of negative results. The authors concluded that the information available did not establish convincingly that any drug consistently improved exercise performance in claudicants.

Current guidelines in the British National Formulary suggest that oxpentifylline, along with cinnarizine, prazosin and thymoxamine, are not established as effective in the management of claudication [13]. The formulary does suggest that naftidrofuryl may alleviate symptoms and improve pain-free walking distance in moderate disease. In a meta-analysis of two French and two German placebo-controlled trials, a beneficial effect of naftidrofuryl on pain-free walking distance was found in patients with claudication [14]. The effects were most marked in non-smokers whose initial pain-free walking distance was over 150 metres before treatment commenced. After 3 months of treatment the mean improvement in walking distance of treated patients over controls was 54 metres.

Two British randomised controlled trials have failed to show any overall benefit for naftidrofuryl over placebo [15, 16]. Subset analysis in the larger of these two trials showed a significant advantage in patients over 60 years of age who took the active drug. Patients over 60 on placebo did not improve their walking distance by a significant amount, but 6 months into the study their mean walking time to onset of pain was 155 seconds, compared to 166 seconds in the drug treated group. Again the order of magnitude of the improvement with naftidrofuryl was not very marked and the cost-effectiveness of such treatment is questionable.

None of these studies has questioned whether such modest improvements in pain-free walking distance objectively influence a patients' quality of life. Certainly the evidence in favour of drug treatment remains weak. If drugs are to be used then it would seem sensible to discontinue them after 2 or 3 months to see if any improvement is dependent on drug ingestion or whether it is simply a result of spontaneous improvement. There is little sense in continuing drug therapy for more then a couple of months if symptoms are not improving.

Balloon angioplasty

Balloon angioplasty remains a popular choice in the management of intermittent claudication. Complications are low with good patient selection and an experienced radiologist. Many patients with moderate claudication between 100 and 300 metres are keen to have treatment but rightly balk when the risks of surgery are explained. Many of these patients will have a discrete stenosis or occlusion less than 10 cm long that can be dilated successfully. Technical failure to dilate the lesion is a possibility in 10% to 20% of patients, but the need for surgical intervention to salvage the situation after an angioplasty is now less than 2%, with a risk of amputation less than 0.3% and of death less than 0.17% [17].

Patients who undergo balloon angioplasty do show improvement in their quality of life scores on an SF-36 questionnaire 3 months after the procedure [3]. Although restenosis occurs in over 20% of patients, not all develop recurrent symptoms and only one in ten patients with restenosis returns with more severe symptoms than those present before the original angioplasty. Restenosis and disease progression above or below the angioplasty site cause a steady longer-term risk of recurrent symptoms, such that there is only a 60% chance of continuing clinical success 3 years after angioplasty. Likewise quality of life scores revert to pre-angioplasty levels within 2 years [5].

Comparison of angioplasty with surgical bypass procedures shows no significant differences on survival, limb loss, haemodynamic improvement or quality of life over a median follow-up of 4 years [18]. As it is a much less invasive procedure with shorter hospital stay and improved recovery, there seems little doubt that angioplasty is a better alternative than bypass surgery in the presence of a suitable lesion. The main area of current controversy remains whether such interventional treatment provides superior results to supervised exercise programmes.

A Cochrane review of angioplasty versus non-surgical management for intermittent claudication [19] has identified only two appropriate studies, one from Edinburgh [20,21] and one from Oxford [22,23]. The Edinburgh study compared the results of balloon angioplasty against simple advice to stop smoking and keep walking. After 6 months the angioplasty group had significantly improved pain-free walking distance compared to the conservative group (median 667m versus 172m) as well as an improved quality of life measured by the Nottingham Health Profile. After 2 years of follow-up the picture changed dramatically. There was now no difference in either pain-free walking distance (median 383m versus 333m) or in the quality of life between the two groups. Thus, although there was a short-term benefit from angioplasty, the effects were not sustained in the medium-term. The trial illustrates the difficulties produced by a condition with markedly heterogeneous patterns of disease distribution. In order to find 62 patients with comparable stenoses or occlusions, the authors had to screen 600 patients with claudication. This high degree of patient selection is a concern when applying the findings of the study to clinical practice, but does beg the question whether angioplasty may be less effective in the management of claudication than current clinical opinion suggests.

The Oxford study compared angioplasty to a supervised exercise programme. In the angioplasty group, maximum improvement in claudication distance had occurred by 3 months after treatment and showed no further improvement over the ensuing 15 months. In the exercise group (supervised classes twice a week for 6 months) there was a continuing and incremental improvement in claudication distance at each of the 6, 9, 12 and 15 month intervals. From 6 months onwards the claudication distances were better in the exercise group than in the angioplasty group. In the longer-term, after a median follow-up of 70 months, only a third of the patients remaining in the exercise group were still exercising more than twice a week and there was no longer any significant difference in the maximum walking distance between the two groups. The exercise group had deteriorated from a peak exercise tolerance of over 400m at 15 months, back down to the same level as the angioplasty group (around 150m) after 70 months.

The number of patients in the Oxford study was small; only 37 were available for long-term follow-up. The suggestion remains that the success of exercise training is at least equivalent to, if not better than, that of angioplasty and that serious further evaluation with bigger patient numbers and at least 2 years follow-up is now required [19].

Atherectomy, lasers and stents

Other interventional radiology methods have been used to try and improve on the success of balloon angioplasty, especially atherectomy, laser-assisted angioplasty and stenting. Atherectomy is the interventional radiology equivalent of endarterectomy and, like its surgical counterpart, has been dogged by a high rate of restenosis. One year after atherectomy, patency can be as low as 25% compared to 75% after balloon angioplasty. Atherectomy offers no significant improvement in clinical outcome with maintenance of symptom relief in 57% of patients compared to 74% of patients after angioplasty in one randomised, controlled trial [24].

Laser-assisted angioplasty also went through a period of popularity in the early 1990s, when it was thought that laser-assistance would improve recanalisation rates by aiding the passage of guide-wires and catheters through occlusions. Subsequent randomised trials sadly demonstrated no benefits of laser assistance over normal angioplasty [25,26]. Around 70-80% of occlusions in the femoropopliteal segment were recanalised with either method and 1 year patency also showed no difference at around 60%.

The latest enthusiasm is to try and maintain patency by placing an endovascular stent across the angioplasty site. The technique is mostly used in the iliac segment, where it is favoured for the primary treatment of occlusions and the secondary treatment of restenosis. In the femoral segment there is no difference in the clinical or haemodynamic outcome using stents compared to balloon angioplasty alone (1-year patency of 62% versus 74%, respectively) [27].

Even in the iliac segment the value of stent placement is controversial. Meta-analysis of six angioplasty and eight stent studies showed 4-year patencies in patients with iliac stenosis causing claudication of 65% for angioplasty and 74% for stenting [28]. In iliac occlusions the patencies were 54% for angioplasty and 61% for stenting. This small difference in favour of stenting was not confirmed in a randomised trial from the Netherlands [29]. In this study of 279 patients there were no differences in technical success, clinical outcomes or re-intervention rates after 2 years follow-up. Two-year cumulative patency rates were 71% in the stent group versus 70% in the angioplasty group. Quality of life improved significantly after intervention, regardless of the technique used. Since stent placement adds a significant cost to the procedure, there is little evidence to support the use of stents as a primary adjunct to balloon angioplasty. There

may be some value in the use of stents to maintain secondary patency, but there are no randomised trials of secondary stenting versus revisional balloon angioplasty alone to support this approach.

Surgery

Surgical reconstruction of the aorto-iliac and femoropopliteal segments can be performed with good results; the question is not so much whether surgery can offer a successful outcome for claudication but whether surgery is appropriate in the light of the risks involved, for what is essentially a benign condition. The quality of life does improve after successful surgery [3], but every vascular surgeon knows of a patient who came into hospital with the moderate disability of claudication and left hospital with the major disability of amputation after a failed bypass graft. Even if the risk of this adverse event is less than 1%, can it be justified for a condition in which the natural history for 80% of the patients is either to improve spontaneously or to have no progression of symptoms over time? [2] The pragmatic answer is that some patients have severely disabling and progressive symptoms that interfere with their work or leave them housebound. In this selected group with major disability, surgery may be offered if the patient understands and accepts the risks involved. Such surgery should always be preceded by a period of conservative management to ensure that spontaneous improvement in symptoms does not occur.

If a patient has a lesion suitable for balloon angioplasty, then that should be the preferred option to surgery. A study of 263 patients randomly assigned to surgery or balloon angioplasty showed no significant difference in outcomes during a median follow-up of 4 years [18]. The less invasive nature of angioplasty dictates its preferential use where possible. Conventional angioplasty is restricted to occlusions less than 10cm in length, but the newer technique of subintimal angioplasty has been performed with better success in infra-inguinal lesions over 10cm long. This new technique may offer an alternative to femoropopliteal bypass grafting in the future and the outcome of randomised trials comparing subintimal angioplasty and surgery in long femoropopliteal occlusions is awaited with interest (see Chapter 7).

As there is no apparent difference between exercise training and balloon angioplasty [22,23], and no difference between balloon angioplasty and surgery [18], perhaps exercise training might produce equivalent results to surgery in patients with claudication. A group from Goteborg in Sweden studied this issue in 75 patients, comparing not just surgery alone to exercise training alone, but also to surgery combined with subsequent exercise training [30]. After a 1 year follow-up all three study groups showed improvements in walking distance.

The best results were found in patients who had the combination of surgery followed by exercise training. There is a certain logic in this finding that treatment with two different modalities might be additive and beneficial. The study used small numbers of patients and the follow-up was only 1 year. Again conclusions can only be limited at the present time but this is undoubtedly an area where further studies are needed.

Conclusions

There is now a wealth of evidence to support the use of regular exercise as a lifestyle change in patients with cardiovascular disease. In the specific case of intermittent claudication, all patients should be advised to exercise regularly and vascular surgeons need encouragement to develop supervised exercise programmes. Such programmes should encourage and monitor patient compliance with (what to many will be) quite a stringent exercise regimen of walking exercises for more than 30 minutes at least three times a week. The majority of patients who comply with this regimen need never come to interventional treatment and require education that the outcomes in the medium to long-term will be just as good.

Drug treatment is not very effective for claudication, but in patients over 60 years of age with resistant claudication, a 2-3 month trial of naftidrofuryl may produce a modest improvement in walking distance.

Balloon angioplasty is an effective treatment for claudication but needs to be tempered with the knowledge that supervised exercise training may prove more cost-effective. A question mark exists over the role of adjunctive iliac stenting after angioplasty. Although it is currently popular in clinical practice, the stents are expensive and randomised trials to date do not support their use.

The role of surgery must remain restricted to the more severe and disabling claudication. Even patients thought suitable for surgery can improve with supervised exercise training, with the chance of avoiding surgery as a consequence. More use should be made of exercise before surgery and most certainly exercise is a useful adjunct afterwards should the operation take place.

Chapter 6

Management of intermittent claudication

Sound evidence

- 50% of patients improve spontaneously.

- Supervised exercise training improves claudication symptoms in the medium term and is more effective than balloon angioplasty in selected patients.

- Drug therapy is mostly ineffective or unproven in rigorous clinical trials.

- Exercise training is a useful adjunct to surgery.

Evidence needed

- Better definition of the relative indications for exercise training versus angioplasty.

- The role of exercise training as an adjunct to angioplasty

- The role of stenting in iliac angioplasty.

- Surgery versus subintimal angioplasty for infra-inguinal disease.

- Comparative trials of exercise training versus surgical management.

References (randomised trials in bold)

1. Dormandy JA, Murray GD. The fate of the claudicant - a prospective study of 1969 claudicants. *Eur J Vasc Surg* 1991; 5: 131-133.
2. McAllister FF. The fate of patients with intermittent claudication managed non-operatively. *Am J Surg* 1976; 132: 593-595.
3. Currie IC, Wilson YG, Baird RN, Lamont PM. Treatment of intermittent claudication: the impact on quality of life. *Eur J Vasc Endovasc Surg* 1995; 10: 356-36.
4. Housley E. Treating claudication in five words. *Br Med J* 1988; 296: 1483-1484.
5. Tisi P, Shearman C. The impact of treatment of intermittent claudication on subjective health of the patient. *Health Trends* 1999; 30: 109-114.
6. Gardner AW, Poehlman ET. Exercise rehabilitation programs for the treatment of claudication pain. A meta-analysis. *JAMA* 1995; 27: 975-980.
7. Robeer GG, Brandsma JW, van den Heuvel SP, Smit B, Oostendorp RA, Wittens CH. Exercise therapy for intermittent claudication: a review of the quality of randomised clinical trials and evaluation of predictive factors. *Eur J Vasc Endovasc Surg* 1998; 15: 36-43.
8. Skinner JS, Strandness DE. Exercise and intermittent claudication. II. Effect of physical training. *Circulation* 1967; 36: 23-29.
9. Larssen OA, Lassen NA. The effect of daily muscle exercise in patients with intermittent claudication. *Lancet* 1966; ii: 1093-1096.
10. Ekroth R, Dahlhöf A, Gundevall B, Holm J. Physical training of patients with intermittent claudication: indications, methods and results. *Surgery* 1978; 84: 640-643.
11. Clifford P, Davies PW, Hayne JA, Baird RN. Intermittent claudication: Is a supervised exercise class worthwhile? *Br Med J* 1980; 280: 1503-1505.
12. Cameron HA, Waller PC, Ramsey LE. Drug treatment of intermittent claudication: a critical analysis of the methods and findings of published clinical trials, 1965-1985. *Br J Clin Pharmacol* 1988; 26: 569-576.
13. British National Formulary 1999; 37: 103.
14. Lehert P, Riphagen FE, Gamand S. The effect of naftidrofuryl on intermittent claudication; A meta-analysis. *J Cardivasc Pharmacol* 1990; 16 (Suppl. 3): S81-S86.
15. **Ruckley CV, Callam MJ, Ferrington CM, Prescott RJ. Naftidrofuryl for intermittent claudication: a double blind controlled trial. *Br Med J* 1978; 1: 622.**
16. **Clyne CAC, Galland RB, Fox MJ, Gustave R, Jantet GH, Jamieson CW. A controlled trial of naftidrofuryl (Praxilene) in the treatment of intermittent claudication. *Br J Surg* 1980; 67: 347-348.**
17. Lewis DR, Bulbulia RA, Murphy P, et al. Vascular surgical intervention for complications of cardiovascular radiology; 13 years experience in a single centre. *Ann R Coll Surg Eng* 1999; 81: 23-26.
18. **Wolf GL, Wilson SE, Cross AP, Deupree RH, Stason WP. Surgery or balloon angioplasty for peripheral vascular disease; a randomised clinical trial. Principal investigators and their Associates of Veterans Administration Cooperative Study Number 199. *J Vasc Interv Radiol* 1993; 4: 639-648.**
19. Fowkes FGR, Gillespie IN. Angioplasty (versus non surgical management) for intermittent claudication (Cochrane Review). In: *The Cochrane Library* 1999; 2: Update Software.
20. **Whyman MR, Fowkes FGR, Kerracher EMG, et al. Randomised controlled trial of percutaneous transluminal angioplasty for intermittent claudication. *Eur J Vasc Endovasc Surg* 1996; 12: 167-172.**
21. **Whyman MR, Fowkes FGR, Kerracher EMG, et al. Is intermittent claudication improved by percutaneous transluminal angioplasty? A randomised controlled trial. *J Vasc Surg* 1997; 26: 551-557.**
22. **Creasy TS, McMillan PJ, Fletcher EWL, Collin J, Morris PJ. Is percutaneous transluminal angioplasty better than exercise for claudication? - preliminary results of a prospective randomised trial. *Eur J vasc Surg* 1990; 4: 135-140.**
23. **Perkins JMT, Collin J, Creasy TS, Fletcher EWL, Morris PJ. Exercise training versus angioplasty for stable claudication. Long and medium term results of a prospective randomised trial. *Eur J vasc Endovasc Surg* 1996; 11: 409-413.**
24. **Vroegindeweij D, Kemper FJM, Tielbeek AV, Buth J, Landman G. Recurrence of stenosis following balloon angioplasty and Simpson atherectomy of the femoropopliteal segment. A randomised comparative 1 year follow-up study using colour flow Duplex. *Eur J Vasc Surg* 1992; 6: 164-171.**
25. **Jeans WD, Murphy P, Hughes AO, Horrocks M, Baird RN. Randomized trial of laser-assisted passage through occluded femoro-popliteal arteries. *Br J Radiol* 1990; 63: 19-21.**
26. **Lammer J, Pilger E, Decrinis M, Quehenberger F, Klein GE, Stark G. Pulsed excimer laser versus continuous-wave Nd:YAG laser versus conventional angioplasty of peripheral arterial occlusions: prospective, controlled, randomised trial. *Lancet* 1992; 340: 1183-1188.**
27. **Vroegindeweij D, Vos LD, Tielbeek AV, Buth J, van der Bosch HC. Balloon angioplasty combined with primary stenting versus balloon angioplasty alone in femoropopliteal obstructions: A comparative randomised study. *Cardiovasc Intervent Radiol* 1997; 20: 420-425.**
28. Bosch JL, Hunink MG. Meta-analysis of the results of percutaneous transluminal angioplasty and stent placement for aortoiliac occlusive disease. *Radiology* 1997; 204: 87-96.
29. **Tetteroo E, van der Graaf Y, Bosch JL, et al. Randomised comparison of primary stent placement versus primary angioplasty followed by selective stent placement in patients with iliac artery occlusive disease. Dutch Iliac Stent Trial Study Group. *Lancet* 1998; 351: 1153-1159.**
30. **Lundgren F, Dahlhof AG, Lundholm K, Sehesten T, Volkman R. Intermittent claudication - surgical reconstruction or physical training? A prospective randomised trial of treatment efficiency. *Ann Surg* 1989; 209: 346-355.**

Chapter 7

The role of subintimal angioplasty

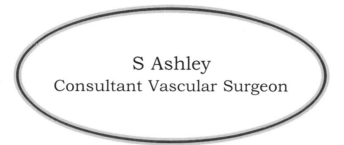

S Ashley
Consultant Vascular Surgeon

VASCULAR SURGICAL UNIT,
DERRIFORD HOSPITAL, PLYMOUTH

Introduction

Percutaneous transluminal balloon angioplasty (PTA) is an accepted and successful method of treating chronic atherosclerotic stenoses and occlusions in peripheral arteries. However, it has long been recognised that the results of PTA for treatment of long chronic femoropopliteal occlusions (greater than 10cm) are poor both in terms of ability initially to recanalise the occlusion (primary technical success) as well as subsequent vessel patency [1,2]. In the mid to late 1980s, a host of new laser and mechanical atherectomy devices emerged to assist PTA [3,4,5]. It was hoped that such devices would be superior to PTA alone in the treatment of long occlusions by removing rather than displacing atheromatous plaque, thereby enhancing primary recanalisation and patency of lesions treated successfully. Despite promising initial results, clinical studies demonstrated that such expectations were unfounded and laser devices have now largely been abandoned in favour of cheaper conventional catheter and guidewire techniques [4,6].

In pursuit of the optimal method of recanalisation using conventional PTA as well as laser angioplasty devices, it became apparent that unintentional subintimal or extraluminal dissection of the arterial wall occurs frequently but usually without sequelae, even if vessel perforation occurs [6,7]. Until recently, vessel dissection was regarded as an indication to abandon the angioplasty procedure and was a principal cause of primary recanalisation failure. However, it was observed that a successful outcome could be achieved if the false lumen created by accidental subintimal passage was pursued, with re-entry into the true lumen beyond the distal extent of the occlusion [8,9]. Subsequently, the technique of deliberate subintimal angioplasty has developed, facilitated by advances in catheter and guidewire technology.

Technique of subintimal angioplasty

The main proponent of subintimal angioplasty is Dr Bolia, a Vascular Radiologist at Leicester Royal Infirmary. His technique for recanalising femoropopliteal occlusions is well described elsewhere [10] but the essential steps are as follows (Figure 1):

An ipsilateral antegrade approach to the occlusion is made via puncture of the common femoral artery for occlusions that begin near the origin of the superficial femoral artery (only a small stump of 5mm or less is needed). Alternatively, selective puncture of the superficial femoral artery may be used for more distal occlusions. Heparin (5000 units) and tolazoline (12.5mg) are injected intra-arterially prior to crossing the lesion. Tolazoline, a vasodilator, helps to dilate the distal vessels and reduces spasm during the procedure. A straight floppy tipped 0.035 inch diameter guidewire is used to enter the occlusion. The tip of the wire is directed to the arterial wall. Sometimes this requires use of a preshaped

JVRG

Longitudinal section

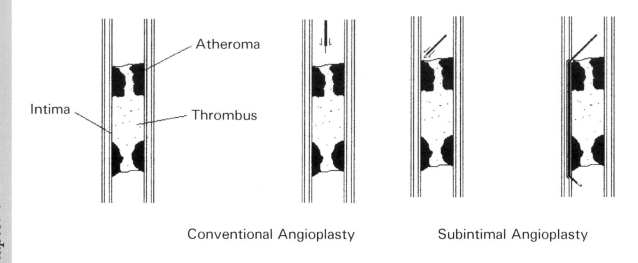

Conventional Angioplasty   Subintimal Angioplasty

Cross section

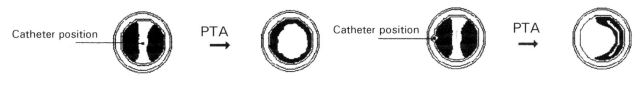

Conventional Angioplasty   Subintimal Angioplasty

Figure 1. Schematic diagram comparing conventional 'intraluminal' guidewire recanalisation with 'extraluminal' subintimal recanalisation. Cross-section shows lumen before and after balloon dilatation (PTA).

catheter (Cobra). The wire/catheter combination is then advanced in the occlusion and, in the vast majority of cases advances into the path of least resistance which is usually in a plane between the intima and the media. Patients frequently experience pain as the vessel is deliberately dissected and analgesia may be required. Entry into the subintimal space is confirmed by injection of a small volume of dilute contrast medium. Once in the subintimal space the guidewire moves freely, encountering very little resistance. The straight wire is now replaced with a 0.035 inch tapered tip J wire. The length of the occlusion is traversed using the J wire itself or by advancing the catheter with a J wire protruding from it. Digital subtraction angiography with road mapping is used to monitor the path of the guidewire and displays the exact length of the occlusion. When the catheter is 2 to 3cm from the distal end of the occlusion, it is retracted back 2 to 3cm and the J wire manipulated to form a large loop. Forward pressure on this loop enables re-entry into the true arterial lumen distally. Once the lesion has been crossed, a 5 or 6mm balloon catheter is inflated throughout the length of the subintimal passage using 10 to 12 atmospheres of pressure for 15s inflations at a time. Redilatation is carried out if there is a residual stenosis of greater than 30%. At the completion of the procedure a further dose of tolazoline (12.5mg) is given. Aspirin (150 - 300mg) is prescribed to all patients but oral anticoagulation is not used routinely.

Although in one sense, as long as the procedure is successful, it does not matter, confirmation that a subintimal recanalisation has been performed is achieved in several ways in addition to contrast injection. Easy passage of the guidewire in chronic, hard occlusions, implies the wire has taken the path of least resistance, which is a dissection. The guidewire loops and moves freely in the subintimal space. Contrast frequently fills the adjacent femoral vein due to shunting across vasa vasora. Distal re-entry beyond the end of an occlusion corroborates that the occlusion has been traversed extraluminally. Immediate postangioplasty arteriography characteristically demonstrates a smooth-walled 'spiral ribbon' appearance within the new lumen with eccentric entry and exit points (Figure 2).

A similar technique can also be used to treat tibial artery occlusions longer that 3cm. Here, an angled hydrophilic guidewire is used for recanalisation and subsequent dilatation is performed with a 3mm diameter balloon.

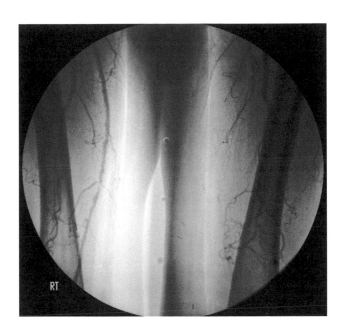

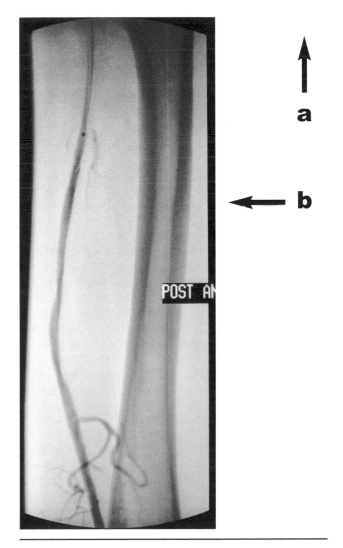

a

b

Figure 2. Arteriograms demonstrating long left superficial femoral artery occlusion (a) before and (b) after successful subintimal angioplasty.

Results

Femoropopliteal occlusions

Reekers et al [9] reported the results of intentional percutaneous extraluminal recanalisation of 40 long chronic occlusions of the femoropopliteal segment. In 30 patients with occlusions longer than 10cm, extraluminal recanalisation was used primarily. In the remaining 10 patients with shorter occlusions extraluminal recanalisation was performed after failure of conventional techniques. Eleven patients had severe intermittent claudication (27.5%) and 29 had ischaemic rest pain and/or ulceration/gangrene (72.5%). The mean length of occlusion in the superficial femoral artery (SFA) was 17cm (range 4-30cm) and in the popliteal artery was 12cm (range 5-18cm). Five patients had an SFA occlusion extending into the popliteal artery with a mean length of 28cm (range 16-45cm). All patients received intravenous heparin for 24h after the procedure and aspirin was administered prior to the procedure and subsequently. Follow-up was by clinical assessment and ankle-brachial pressure index (ABPI).

Primary technical success was achieved in 85% of angioplasties and was independent of the length, location or duration of the occlusion. All six primary failures were due to heavily calcified vessels. Complications occurred in eight patients (20%); seven had a groin haematoma, one required surgery. There was one traumatic arteriovenous fistula that closed spontaneously. There were five early reocclusions within 7 days, all without successful reintervention. Therefore, the cumulative 30-day primary patency was 72.5%. The primary and secondary cumulative patencies based on clinical follow-up and ABPI were 50% and 60% at 1 year, and 50% and 55% at 2 years respectively. In none of the patients was the option for bypass surgery compromised.

Bolia et al [11] reported the results of 200 attempted subintimal angioplasties in 176 patients over 64 months. This represented 20% of all leg angioplasties performed during the same interval and 81% of angioplasties done for femoropopliteal occlusive disease. The indication for treatment was intermittent claudication in 178 legs (89%) and critical ischaemia in 22 legs (11%). The site of occlusion was the femoral artery in 154 legs (77%) and the popliteal artery in 46 (23%). The median occlusion length was 11.5cm (range 2-37cm). All patients received aspirin but anticoagulants were not prescribed routinely. Follow-up was based on clinical symptoms and ABPI measurement.

Primary technical success was achieved in 80% (159/200) and was unrelated to the length or site of occlusion, indication for treatment or presence of diabetes. Five (3%) technically successful procedures failed within 24 hours. There were two major complications (1%) and 13 minor complications (6.5%). Major complications included one retroperitoneal haematoma and one scrotal haematoma, both required surgical evacuation. The minor complications were two groin haematomas, seven distal emboli and four vessel perforations. The groin haematomas resolved spontaneously. Two perforations required no treatment and two were managed by spring coil embolisation. Of the seven distal emboli, six were aspirated using an 8F non-tapered aspiration catheter; in addition, one required intra-arterial streptokinase for 24 hours. There were three deaths (30-day mortality 1.5%), all resulting from myocardial infarction. There were no deaths or amputations directly related to the procedure.

The cumulative primary haemodynamic patencies at 1, 12 and 36 months based on ABPI measurements for all procedures were 73, 56 and 46%, respectively. Univariate analysis was performed to identify factors affecting patency in technically successful procedures. The most significant variables influencing patency were smoking, number of run-off vessels and occlusion length.

Tibial artery occlusions

Bolia et al [12] reported the results of subintimal angioplasty to treat 32 infra-popliteal artery occlusions for 28 critically ischaemic legs in 27 patients. In three legs (11%) multiple vessels were recanalised. In 19 (68%) of the 28 legs, adjunctive angioplasty of superficial femoral or popliteal artery lesions was performed. Twenty four legs (86%) had distal tissue necrosis. Nine patients (33%) were diabetic. The median length of occlusions was 7cm (range 2-30cm). Patency after the procedure and at follow-up was determined by duplex imaging. Patients received aspirin, as before.

The immediate technical success rate was 84% (27/32) for occlusions and 82% for legs (23/28). The five failed procedures were due to vessel perforation in three cases and failure to advance the guidewire in two. Of these, two patients went on to have a femorodistal bypass and three had residual ischaemic rest pain. There were three minor complications including a groin haematoma, a vessel perforation with no consequence and one distal embolus. No surgical intervention was needed. There were no legs lost as a result of the procedure and zero mortality within 30 days. The minimum follow-up was 18 months. The cumulative primary haemodynamic patency at 1 year was 53%; the corresponding limb salvage rate was 85% and the patient survival rate was 81%.

Discussion

Published results of subintimal angioplasty are limited at present, although it is known that several centres are attempting this technique. The paucity of published results from centres other than Leicester might reflect the fact that subintimal angioplasty has a steep learning curve or could be indicative of a desire to avoid premature reporting. A weakness common to the first two studies quoted above is that long term patency was determined primarily from clinical assessment and ABPI, as opposed to duplex imaging or angiography. Therefore, patency of treated vessels could well have been overestimated in these studies. Furthermore, comparisons with conventional intraluminal angioplasty and surgical revascularisation are lacking, although it is acknowledged that patient populations undergoing these treatments are likely to be substantially different. Despite these reservations, the results of subintimal angioplasty are encouraging, particularly as the incidence of major complications appears to be low. In addition, there is no suggestion that subsequent performance of arterial bypass surgery, if necessary, is compromised by immediate or late failure of subintimal angioplasty; hence there is no harm in trying.

It remains to be determined whether the newly created extraluminal channel results in a better long term patency than an intraluminal approach. Theoretical advantages of subintimal angioplasty are that thrombogenic, crushed atheroma is displaced to one side of the new lumen, and the false lumen is smooth and wider than the true lumen permitting greater blood flow. In addition less mechanical trauma is required to recanalise in the extraluminal plane. A potential complication of subintimal angioplasty is damage to collateral or main vessels distal to the occlusion if these are included in the dissected portion. It is important, therefore, that the dissection is not extended too far distal to the occlusion. An interesting observation from arteriograms performed months or even years following successful subintimal angioplasty is that filling of branch arteries and collaterals can be observed in the previously recanalised segment.

Due to differences in case mix and the characteristics of lesions treated it is impossible to make meaningful comparisons between the results of subintimal angioplasty reported thus far and other studies of the outcome of PTA. However, the results of subintimal angioplasty appear favourable, both in terms of the rate of technically successful recanalisation and subsequent vessel patency when compared with previous studies of PTA in the treatment of long femoropopliteal occlusions. Whether centres other than those of the main proponents will be able to reproduce good outcomes following subintimal angioplasty remains to be seen. More studies using duplex imaging to determine the true haemodynamic success and long term patency of lesions treated by subintimal angioplasty are urgently required. Whether preferential use of deliberate subintimal angioplasty for recanalising short occlusions suitable for intraluminal angioplasty is justified needs to be examined by a randomised trial. Similarly, a comparison between long segment subintimal angioplasty and femoropopliteal bypass, examining clinical outcomes as well as quality of life variables is needed. Perhaps the most exciting prospect of subintimal angioplasty is the potential to offer an alternative to femorodistal grafting in elderly, frail patients with critical ischaemia. Considerably more experience from different centres is required before the role of subintimal angioplasty in this difficult group of patients becomes established.

References

1. Murray RR, Hewes RC White RI, et al. Long segment femoropopliteal stenosis: is angioplasty a boon or a bust? *Radiology* 1987; 162: 473-476.

2. Krepel VM, Van Andel GJ, Van Erp WF, et al. Percutaneous angioplasty of the femoropopliteal artery: initial and long-term results. *Radiology* 1985; 156: 325-328.

3. Sandborn TA, Cumberland DC, Greenfield AJ, et al. Percutaneous laser thermal angioplasty: initial results and 1-year follow-up in 129 femoropopliteal lesions. *Radiology* 1988; 168: 121-125.

4. Ashley S, Brooks SG, Gehani AA, et al. Percutaneous laser recanalisation of femoropopliteal occlusions using continuous wave Nd YAG laser and sapphire contact probe delivery system. *Eur J Vasc Surg* 1994; 8: 494-501.

5. Gehani A, Sheard K, Ashley S, et al. Dynamic angioplasty of total arterial occlusions *Br J Surg* 1990; 77: 1139-1141.

6. Ashley S, Kester RC. Laser angioplasty. *Br J Surg* 1993; 80: 550-551.

7. Belli AM, Proctor AE, Cumberland DC. Peripheral vascular occlusions: mechanical recanalisation with a metal laser probe after guidewire dissection. *Radiology* 1990; 176: 539-541.

8. Bolia A, Miles KA, Brennan J, Bell PRF. Percutaneous transluminal angioplasty of occlusions of the femoral and popliteal arteries by subintimal dissection. *Cardiovasc Intervent Radiol* 1990; 13: 357-63.

9. Reekers JA, Kromhout JG, Jacobs JHM. Percutaneous intentional extraluminal recanalisation of the femoropopliteal artery. *Eur J Vasc Surg* 1994; 8: 723-728.

10. Bolia A, Bell PRF. Femoropopliteal and crural artery recanalisation using subintimal angioplasty. *Sem Vasc Surg* 1995; 8: 253-264.

11. London NJM, Srinivasan R, Naylor AR, et al. Subintimal angioplasty of femoropopliteal artery occlusions: the long-term results. *Eur J Vasc Surg* 1994; 8: 148-155.

12. Nydahl S, Hatshorne T, Bell PRF, Bolia A, London NJM. Subintimal angioplasty of infrapopliteal occlusions in critically Ischaemic legs. *Eur J Vasc Endovasc Surg* 1997; 14: 212-216.

Chapter 7

The role of subintimal angioplasty

Sound evidence

- None.

Evidence needed

- Are good results reproducible in different centres?

- Patency following subintimal angioplasty assessed by duplex imaging.

- Comparison of subintimal versus intraluminal angioplasty for short (<10cm) femoropopliteal artery occlusions, and subintimal angioplasty versus femoropopliteal bypass for longer occlusions.

- The role of subintimal angioplasty for treating infrapopliteal occlusions.

The role of subintimal angioplasty

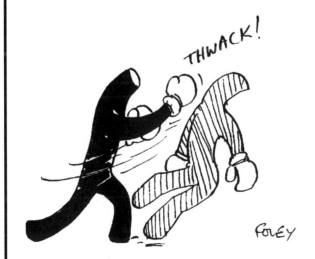

THWACK!

FOLEY

Improving the patency of femorodistal bypass

RK Fisher
Research Fellow
PL Harris
Consultant Surgeon

REGIONAL VASCULAR UNIT,
ROYAL LIVERPOOL UNIVERSITY HOSPITAL, LIVERPOOL

Introduction

Critical limb ischaemia has an incidence of 40/100,000 in the United Kingdom affecting about 20,000 patients per annum with an amputation rate approaching 25% [1]. Treatment frequently involves arterial reconstruction in the form of bypass to distal calf vessels. Although patency rates are inferior with distal bypass [2], an active approach has been justified by Cheshire et al, who showed primary and secondary reconstruction to distal vessels is cheaper than primary amputation [3]. Such policy heralded the introduction of a variety of alternative grafts and adjuvant techniques in an attempt to improve graft patency and limb salvage rates.

The bypass graft

Autologous vein vs. prosthetic material

The bypass graft is one of the most important factors determining long-term patency. Autologous vein remains the preferred choice since its introduction by Kunlin in 1949. Vein, however, is absent or of insufficient quality in up to one third of patients, necessitating the use of prosthetic material such as polytetrafluoroethylene (PTFE), Dacron or Human Umbilical Vein (HUV) [4]. A study by Kumar et al in 1995 did not demonstrate any significant difference in patency rates between PTFE and Dacron [5], but randomised trials comparing PTFE and HUV reported significant improvement in favour of HUV (Table 1) [6,7,8]. Long term follow-up, however, revealed graft dilatation and aneurysm formation in up to 30 % of HUV bypasses and its popularity diminished subsequently [8].

The preference of vein over PTFE has been established by randomised trials, Tilanus et al in 1985 reported a significant difference in long-term patency between PTFE (37%) and autologous vein (70%) (p<0.001) (Table 2) [4,5,9,10]. The data reported by Bergan et al in 1982 did not entirely corroborate this, identifying a difference between the two grafts only when taken to infrapopliteal vessels. The latter study only reported patency rates up to 30 months follow-up, whereas the benefit of using vein becomes more evident with time [10].

It is generally accepted that autologous vein achieves the optimum patency, particularly for bypass to tibial vessels performed for critical limb ischaemia, and that PTFE should be reserved for arterial reconstruction in the absence of vein.

In situ or reversed vein bypass

The potential benefit of *in situ* over reversed vein bypass has stimulated much debate. The intact vasa vasorum should maintain nutrition to the vessel,

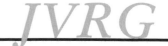

Table 1. Randomised trials comparing the patency of HUV and PTFE infrainguinal bypass grafts.

Author	distal vessel	bypass material	follow-up years	1^0 patency	2^0 patency
Eickhoff et al [6] 1987 (n=105)	Bk pop	HUV PTFE	4	--	42%* 22%
McCollum et al [7] 1991 (n=191)	Ak and Bk pop	HUV PTFE	3	57% 48%	66%* 49%
Aalders et al [8] 1992 (n=85)	Ak pop	HUV PTFE	5	65%* 32%	73%* 41%

*   statistical significance (p<0.05)
Ak pop   above knee popliteal artery
Bk pop   below knee popliteal artery

Table 2. Randomised trials comparing vein and PTFE/Dacron grafts for infrainguinal bypass.

Author	procedure/ anastomosis		number	follow-up years	1^0 patency	2^0 patency	limb salvage
Bergan et al [10] 1982	Akpop	vein PTFE	41 33		70% 72%	-- --	-- --
	Bkpop	vein PTFE	50 46	2.5	76% 62%	-- --	-- --
	Infrapop	vein PTFE	57 58		50%* 20%	-- --	-- --
Tilanus et al [4] 1985	Fempop	vein PTFE	25 24	5	-- --	70%* 37%	-- --
Veith et al [9] 1986	Akpop	vein PTFE	85 91	4	61% 38%	-- --	-- --
	Bkpop	vein PTFE	62 80	4	76%* 54%	-- --	-- --
	Combined fempop	vein PTFE	147 171	5	68%* 38%	-- --	75% 70%
	Infrapop	vein PTFE	106 98	4	49%* 12%	-- --	61% 57%
Kumar et al [5] 1995	Akpop	vein PTFE Dacron	50 49 46	4	73%* 47% 54%	90%* 47% 60%	-- -- --

*   statistically significant results (p<0.05)
Ak pop   above knee popliteal artery
Bk pop   below knee popliteal artery
Infrapop   infrapopliteal
Fempop   femoropopliteal

preserving desirable properties such as endothelial secretion of plasminogen activators, and thereby promoting lower thrombogenicity. Natural vein wall compliance may also be retained, reducing myointimal hyperplasia and early graft occlusion. The taper of the *in situ* vein affords better matching for size between graft and artery at both proximal and distal anastomoses. Proponents of this technique claim that vein too small to be reversed may successfully be used *in situ*. This may have particular relevance in femorotibial bypass.

Harris et al in 1987 reported a series of 200 femoropopliteal bypasses, randomised to *in situ* or reversed vein. There was no significant difference in 3 year cumulative patency rates between the two groups (68% vs. 77% respectively). Patency was adversely affected, however, by vein calibre of <4mm internal diameter (p<0.005), long grafts taken below, (as opposed to above) the knee (p<0.01) and poor run-off (p<0.05). No difference in patency was observed between the two bypass techniques within each of these high risk sub-groups [11].

A subsequent multicentre randomised trial reported by the same author confirmed similar results for infrapopliteal vein grafts, with secondary cumulative patency rates at 3 years of 68% and 66%, respectively, for *in situ* and reversed grafts [12]. Claims for superior patency with the *in situ* operation may be considered to be based almost entirely on credence given to the well recognised, but unproven, theoretical advantages outlined previously. They are supported only by comparison with results of non-contemporaneous series of reversed vein operations. Results from these and other randomised trials provide strong evidence that neither procedure achieves significantly better patency, irrespective of the level of distal anastomosis (Table 3) [12-16].

Superior patency rates for small diameter vein bypasses (<4mm) have been reported, when anastomosed *in situ,* as opposed to reversed. Although these do not achieve statistical significance, they may substantiate claims that an *in situ* graft is indicated when the vein is so small that the surgeon cannot perform a

Chapter 8

Table 3. Trials comparing patency and limb salvage rates for *in situ* and reversed autologous vein bypass.

Author	procedure	level of bypass	follow-up years	1⁰ patency	2⁰ patency	limb salvage
Wengerter et al* [13] 1991	in situ (n=62) reverse(n=63)	Infrapopliteal	2.5	58% 61%	69% 67%	76% 87%
Moody et al* [14] 1992	in situ (n=101) reverse(n=114)	Fempop AK/BK	5	64% 62%	-- --	-- --
Harris et al* [12] 1993	in situ (n=82) reverse(n=80)	Infrapopliteal	3	-- --	68% 66%	78% 87%
Watelet et al* [15] 1997	in situ (n=50) reverse(n=50)	Fempop AK/BK	10	42%** 65%	65% 70%	74% 74%
Lawson et al [16] 1999	in situ (n=307) reverse(n=775)	Fempop AK/BK	2	67%** 74%	85% 84%	89% 92%
	in situ (n=193) reverse(n=180)	Infrapopliteal	2	52%** 63%	74% 71%	82% 85%

*   randomised controlled trial

**   statistically significant p<0.05. Differences only identified in primary patency.

Fempop	femoropopliteal
AK	above knee
BK	below knee

reversed procedure [13]. Ultimately, a flexible approach is advocated, determined by the surgeon's clinical preference.

Alternative veins

When ipsilateral long saphenous vein is unavailable, alternative vein may be harvested, including contralateral saphenous, the cephalic and/or basilic arm vein, short saphenous or deep leg veins. If a single vein is of insufficient length, two or more segments may be spliced together forming a composite vein graft. Composite grafts combining proximal PTFE with distal vein segments are advocated by some, particularly using PTFE in the thigh and vein to cross the knee joint [17].

Contralateral long saphenous vein

It has been suggested that the contralateral saphenous vein should be used as the first alternative. In the series by Hölzenbein et al, however, contralateral long saphenous vein was only available in 38% of patients. There was a 60% probability that the vein would be required for contralateral bypass within 3 years. Hölzenbein et al therefore recommended that the contralateral limb should be left intact, preserving the vein for future contralateral bypass [18].

The deep leg veins

Superficial femoral and popliteal vein bypass was originally described as an alternative conduit in the absence of ipsilateral long saphenous vein. Schulman et al reported excellent long-term patency rates [19] and progressed to a randomised trial comparing saphenous vein (n=56) with deep leg veins (n=41) in primary femoropopliteal bypass. There were similar primary and secondary patency rates in the two groups at 3 years (60% and 63% for reversed saphenous vein versus 64% and 68% for superficial femoral vein, respectively). Schulman now recommends the use of deep leg veins as the primary conduit for femoropopliteal bypass, preserving the saphenous vein for future distal arterial reconstruction or coronary artery bypass. Although the technique is protracted and more demanding, and has the potential for postoperative swelling of the leg, Schulman did not report any long term disability in his series [20].

Despite these good results the use of deep vein remains less popular than other sources of vein, mainly due to the demanding nature of the surgery and the relatively short length of harvested vein, making it inappropriate for long femorodistal bypass.

Arm vein and composite venous grafts

Hölzenbein et al used arm veins as the primary alternative when ipsilateral saphenous vein was unavailable in 250 patients. The grafts included cephalic vein alone (50%), cephalic and basilic vein (36%) and basilic vein alone (14%). Cumulative primary and secondary patency rates at 1 year of 70.6% and 76.9% respectively were reported with a limb salvage rate of 88.2%. Cumulative primary and revised patency rates at 3 years were 49.5% and 52.8% respectively, with a limb salvage rate of 80.4%. There was no statistically significant difference between the anatomical origin of the arm vein or the type of procedure performed [18]. These results, although encouraging, represent a single retrospective case series which made no comparison with alternative techniques. Other series report less promising results. Schulman et al reported 2 and 5 year patency rates of 31% and 15% respectively for femorotibial bypasses. They also provided the first long-term data on patients up to 10 years after arm vein bypass, which revealed a pattern of graft elongation and aneurysmal dilatation [21].

The composite-PTFE and sequential graft

McCarthy et al performed 67 composite sequential bypasses using 6mm PTFE to the popliteal artery, with long or short saphenous vein extensions to tibial vessels. They reported cumulative patency rates at 1 year (72%) and 3 years (48%) with a limb salvage rate at 4 years of 70% [17]. Once again, care should be taken in drawing conclusions from this retrospective study; other centres have reported significant differences in patency rates at 5 years between autologous vein (63%) and composite-prosthetic vein grafts (28%, p=0.005) [22].

There can be little doubt that autologous vein offers the optimum graft patency rate. When ipsilateral long saphenous vein is unavailable there is evidence that single and even composite vein grafts from alternative sites may achieve acceptable patency. There have been no randomised controlled trials comparing alternative autogenous vein, composite and prosthetic grafts in femorodistal bypass, and until such evidence exists the surgeon's own preference will continue to be a major deciding factor.

Polytetrafluoroethylene grafts

In the absence of vein, expanded PTFE is commonly used, representing up to one third of all infrainguinal bypasses. The patency and limb salvage rates are significantly worse below the knee, but may approach those achieved by autologous vein when anastomosed to the above knee popliteal artery [9]. In view of this, some surgeons advocate its preferential use in femoropopliteal bypass, as a way of preserving the ipsilateral vein for subsequent, more distal procedures [23].

Poor patency in femorodistal bypass is attributed to early graft occlusion from progression of distal disease and/or the deposition of myointimal hyperplasia (MIH) at critical points within the end-to-side anastomosis. These points are situated at the graft heel, toe and recipient artery floor, all areas of flow division and separation resulting in abnormally low wall shear stress, an important factor in the development of MIH [24].

Techniques developed to improve the patency and limb salvage rates of prosthetic grafts after femorodistal bypass include the interposition of vein cuffs and patches, formation of arteriovenous fistulas and the design of a pre-cuffed graft.

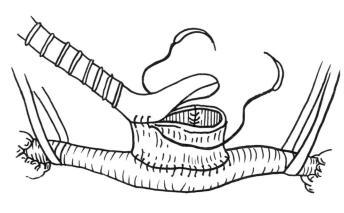

Figure 1. The Miller cuff.

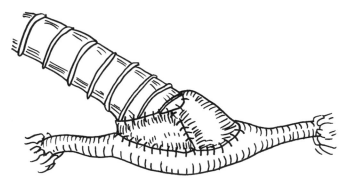

Figure 2. The St. Mary's boot.

The interposition of vein

The vein cuff

The vein cuff was first described by Siegman in 1979 as a method of anastomosing mismatched prosthetic grafts to small distal arteries. A later modification by Miller et al in 1984 was popularised and has undergone subsequent adaptation, including the St. Marys' Boot (Figures 1 and 2) [25,26]. Theoretical advantages of interposing vein between PTFE and a small distal artery include a technically less demanding distal anastomosis, possibly reducing imperfections [25]. In addition, Suggs et al, in an experimental study, showed that MIH was significantly inhibited within a distal cuffed anastomosis, initially attributed to the improved compliance of the vein [27]. Subsequent work by Sottiurai, however, indicated that changes in haemodynamic forces induced by the cuff may be the main advantage, rather than compliance improvement [24]. Da Silva et al described how the configuration adopted by the Miller cuff forms a highly stable, cohesive vortex (Figure 3), which may increase wall shear stress at critical points within the anastomosis, thereby inhibiting the accretion of MIH [28].

There are several clinical series reporting good patency rates using the Miller cuff and St. Mary's boot [25,26], but there remains only one prospective, multicentre randomised trial, by Stonebridge et al [29]. Two hundred and sixty-one PTFE bypass operations to above- and below-knee arteries were randomised to groups with and without a distal vein cuff. There was no difference in patency between the two groups after above knee bypass. Below-knee femoropopliteal grafts with a cuff had higher patency rates at 12 and 24 months (80% and 52%, respectively) than those without a cuff (65% and 29%, p=0.03). Limb salvage rates between the groups were not statistically significantly different in either above or below knee procedures.

The vein patch

In 1992 Taylor et al described the incorporation of a vein patch into the roof of a standard PTFE end-to-side anastomosis (Figure 4). Five year patency rates of 71% for femoropopliteal and 54% for infrapopliteal grafts were described in a series of 256 procedures [30]. These figures compared favorably to historical series. It was speculated that potential benefit may partly arise from increased anastomotic volume, and partly from the presence of vein at a critical point within the anastomosis known to be susceptible to MIH.

The benefits of vein interposition for distal bypass remain somewhat speculative. Larger randomised studies with longer follow-up are required before a definitive technique can be recognised. Until then personal preferences will continue to dictate clinical practice, but many surgeons now use a distal vein cuff or patch routinely for prosthetic femorodistal bypass.

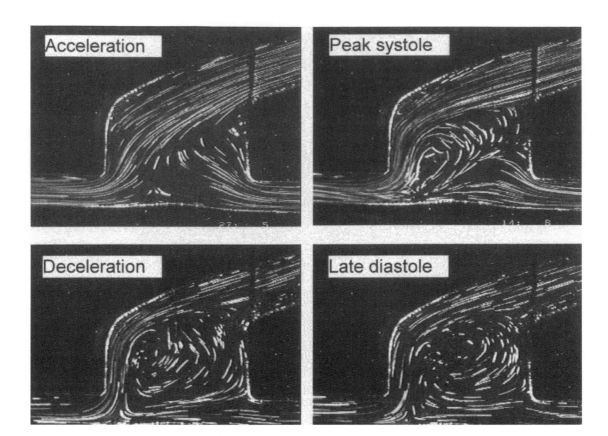

Figure 3. The cohesive vortex developing within the Miller cuff, potentially increasing wall shear stress and inhibiting myointimal hyerplasia.

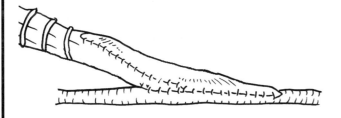

Figure 4. The Taylor patch.

The arteriovenous fistula

A complementary distal arteriovenous fistula (AVF) was proposed as a simple solution to circumvent the problems encountered when a prosthetic graft is used as a bypass to a small calibre distal vessel with a low-flow/high resistance system. The comparatively low resistance/high-flow of the venous outlet theoretically increases graft blood flow above its thrombotic threshold velocity, whilst maintaining an acceptable perfusion of the distal artery. Previous canine studies have indicated a trend for improved graft patency in bypasses with adjunctive AVF [31].

The fistula is created between the distal artery and the deep concomitant vein, and may be pre- or post-anastomotic, involve a common ostium with the artery, or incorporate the bypass graft, forming a complementary AVF with deep vein interposition (Figures 5, 6 & 7). Fistula formation is relatively safe if sufficient time and care is taken, however, there are recognised complications including venous hypertension, distension and (potentially) right sided cardiac failure due to increased preload on a myocardium with suboptimal function. A steal phenomenon by the venous system may also arise; banding of the venous outflow is recommended if the systolic graft pressure is less than 100mmHg or if the systolic pressure gradient between distal graft and radial artery exceeds 30mmHg [31]. Intraoperative graft pressure measurements, completion arteriography and/or Doppler ultrasound are recommended to exclude steal phenomena and to confirm prograde arterial flow and cephalad venous flow [32]. Subsequent graft surveillance is usually undertaken with duplex imaging, confirming patency of the AVF by colour flow and high diastolic velocity.

Adjunctive AVF formation was popularised during the 1980s, and series by Dardik et al and Ascer et al indicated satisfactory patency rates (Table 4) [31,32]. Adjunctive AVF was recommended for all prosthetic bypasses to tibial arteries; relative contraindications included very poor arterial run-off, small venae comitantes and extensive sclerosis or other sequelae of

Table 4. Results of adjuvant distal arteriovenous fistula (AVF).

Author	patient number	type of fistula	1 year patency	2 year patency	limb salvage
Dardik et al [32] 1991	69	side-side	--	44%	--
Ascer et al [31] 1996	68	AVF/VI	64.7%	57%	86%
Hamsho et al [33] 1999*					
Control	48	--	52.2%	--	54.1%
AVF	41	common ostium or preanastomotic	53.4%	--	43.2%
*	randomised controlled trial of infrapopliteal Miller cuff anastomoses, with and without AVF. No statistical difference demonstrated.				
VI	vein interposition				

deep vein thrombosis. Graft patency was found to be longer than that of the fistula and it was suggested that the graft may increase its thrombotic threshold with time, possibly due to neo-endothelialisation. Mean velocity was reported to be 74% higher in grafts with a patent AVF compared to grafts with an occluded fistula (p<0.01), confirming some of the theoretical benefits of AVF [32].

These studies were encouraging, but in a prospective randomised trial comparing graft patency and limb salvage rates after femorotibial prosthetic bypass with and without adjunctive AVF, Hamsho et al in 1999 found no significant difference [5]. Although small patient numbers (AVF n=48, control n=41) may have masked an early benefit in patency with AVF, any difference diminished after the first 6 months. It was concluded that there is no evidence of worthwhile benefit associated with routine use of an AVF in prosthetic femorotibial bypass [33].

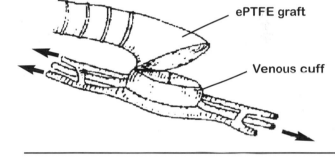

Figure 6. Common ostium arteriovenous fistula. (With permission from the European Journal of Vascular and Endovascular Surgery. Hamsho A, Nott D, Harris PL. Prospective randomized trial of distal arteriovenous fistula as an adjunct to femoro-infrapopliteal PTFE bypass. *Eur J Vasc Endovasc Surg* 1999; 17: 197-201).

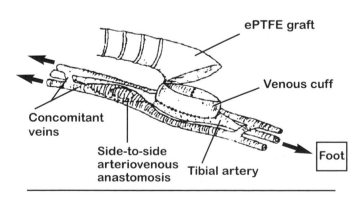

Figure 5. Pre-anastomotic arteriovenous fistula. (With permission from the European Journal of Vascular and Endovascular Surgery. Hamsho A, Nott D, Harris PL. Prospective randomized trial of distal arteriovenous fistula as an adjunct to femoro-infrapopliteal PTFE bypass. *Eur J Vasc Endovasc Surg* 1999; 17: 197-201).

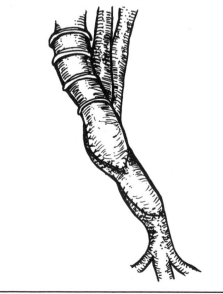

Figure 7. Arterio-venous fistula with deep vein interposition.

Chapter 8

Chapter 8

Pre-cuffed prosthetic bypass

Improving the patency of prosthetic femorotibial bypass grafts remains the focus of much attention, and research derived from da Silva's work has led to the development of a pre-cuffed PTFE graft (Figure 8). The shape of the dilated end has been designed to optimise the potentially beneficial flow patterns and haemodynamic forces observed in anastomoses, including a Miller cuff [34]. Pre-cuffed grafts have only recently been incorporated into clinical practice and randomised trials will be needed to validate the theoretical benefits.

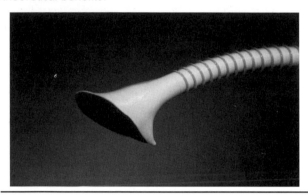

Figure 8. Pre-cuffed PTFE graft.

Intraoperative monitoring and investigation

The cause of graft failure is related to the interval since insertion. Failure after 3 months is associated with intrinsic graft or anastomotic problems, commonly myointimal hyperplasia, whilst disease progression either proximal or distal to the graft accounts for late occlusion. Failure within the first month occurs in between 10-15% of grafts and is largely attributed to technical error, inherent thrombogenicity or inadequate run-off [35]. The technical adequacy of a femorodistal bypass may be assessed by external inspection, restoration of peripheral pulses and perfusion, non-invasive Doppler ultrasound or invasive procedures such as angiography or angioscopy.

Until recently, completion angiography was almost obligatory after femorodistal bypass as a method of confirming technical success. Studies such as that by Miller et al heralded it as the 'gold standard' for intraoperative assessment based on a greater sensitivity than Doppler examination. When angiography detected defects that were subsequently corrected, early graft patency rates were excellent [36]. Noting the associated risk and expense, however, Dalman et al retrospectively compared the long term patency of grafts that had undergone completion angiography with those that had not, and found a similar likelihood of occlusion [37].

Blankenstein et al, in a prospective study of intraoperative determinants of bypass patency, reported that continuous wave Doppler (CWD) was the best indicator of technical error and concluded that intraoperative angiography was best reserved for anatomical assessment of those grafts with abnormalities identified by CWD [35].

Arteriography, although limited by an inability to provide haemodynamic information, does afford further benefits in identifying the quality of the outflow. Angioscopy has been advocated as superior to angiography for disclosing graft defects, although it remains costly and demanding, with a potential for significant complications [38]. Another recent development has been the introduction of intravascular ultrasound that images the anatomy of the bypass, detecting luminal and anastomotic irregularities, as well as inflow and outflow problems.

It has been postulated that some of these techniques may be too sensitive and result in unnecessary revision of some grafts [35]. At present there is no clear evidence identifying any one technique as superior, and policy varies between institutes, usually based on personal preference and availability of equipment. A truer reflection of the benefits associated with each method will only be revealed by undertaking randomised trials comparing the short and long term patency of each method.

Improving graft patency with drugs

With the advent of a more aggressive policy towards distal vascular reconstruction, adjuvant pharmacological intervention has been introduced to maintain patency in high risk grafts, particularly those with compromised run-off. Watson et al in 1999 reviewed the current literature to evaluate the evidence for the use of various agents [39].

Platelet inhibition

Early graft occlusion due to myointimal hyperplasia is initiated by accumulation of activated platelets at sites of endothelial denudation and subsequent release of myofibroblastic mitogens. Inhibition of platelets may therefore have some benefit in the prevention of MIH and improve graft patency.

Aspirin

Placebo-controlled randomised studies have suggested that the benefit of aspirin may be greater in preventing occlusion in prosthetic grafts; whilst a meta-analysis by The Antiplatelet Trialists' Collaboration provided evidence that aspirin afforded additional benefit by reducing the rate of incidental stroke, myocardial infarction and vascular death [40]. The use of aspirin is widely advocated after prosthetic bypass, although care is still required to avoid the adverse effects in this predominantly elderly population. Current evidence is deplete concerning optimum dosage, and inconsistent regarding combination therapy with agents such as dipyridamole, sulphinpyrazone and indobufen.

Ticlopidine

There is strong evidence from a multicentred, double blind, placebo-controlled study that ticlopidine produces a significant treatment benefit in maintaining patency of vein grafts, however, no data on other grafts or comparisons with other agents are currently available. Continued research into its benefits may reveal further applications for this agent [39].

Prostanoids

The prostacyclin analogue, Iloprost, used as a single intragraft injection on completion of a distal bypass may improve early postoperative graft patency. This is attributed to its action reducing peripheral resistance, thereby improving graft blood flow. The Iloprost Bypass International Study Group performed a multicentre, double blind, randomised controlled trial of a 3 day treatment regimen of Iloprost in 517 patients. There was a significant difference in early patency only in prosthetic grafts. There were no differences in patency or limb salvage rates in either vein or PTFE after 12 months. Although Iloprost has had some success in the treatment of critical ischaemia, its use as an adjunct to femorodistal bypass appears limited [41].

Anticoagulants

Warfarin

A study by Arfvidsson et al in 1990 failed to show significant improvements in graft patency or limb salvage in patients given coumarin after vein or prosthetic bypass [42]. However, when considering vein grafts alone, Kretschmer et al, in a series of studies, identified improved graft patency and patient survival with coumarin in both the short and the long-term [43].

A recent trial reported significantly improved patency when aspirin was combined with warfarin in high-risk vein grafts, i.e. those with poor run-off, inferior quality vein or revisional procedures [44].

Low molecular weight heparin (LMWH)

Although widely used as both a prophylactic and therapeutic anticoagulant, there are no reports of double-blind trials with LMWH, and therefore the data available do not provide sufficient evidence to draw definitive conclusions on its clinical application. This is a particular area that would benefit from further studies.

Conclusions

There is strong evidence that autologous saphenous vein has superior patency over prosthetic materials, especially in femorotibial bypass. No difference can be demonstrated, however, between in situ or reversed vein graft techniques. In the absence of saphenous vein, no convincing studies exist to suggest the preferred alternative. Patency of PTFE grafts may be improved with the interposition of vein at the distal anastomosis, but the formation of an arteriovenous fistula appears to offer no additional benefit. Intraoperative quality control may improve early patency, although none of the investigation techniques has been shown to be superior or decrease long-term occlusion rates. Aspirin is beneficial in prosthetic bypasses, whilst venous grafts may remain patent longer with oral anticoagulation.

The Second European Consensus Document on Chronic Critical Leg Ischaemia quotes 1-year patency rates for patients with critical leg ischaemia of 75% for above knee femoropopliteal, 70% for below-knee femoropopliteal and 70% for infrapopliteal grafts using autologous vein. With prosthetic grafts the respective figures were reported to be 65, 60 and 40% at 1 year [45]. Evidence that the various adjuvant techniques discussed have the potential to improve these figures remains scarce, and only through continued attention to scientific methodology will it be possible to identify those of genuine benefit.

Chapter 8

Improving the patency of femorodistal bypass

Sound evidence

- **Graft patency improved by**
  - use of autologous vein.
  - interposition of vein in below-knee femoropopliteal and femorotibial prosthetic grafts.
  - anticoagulant and antiplatelet agents may improve patency but their main benefit is to reduce the risk of other vascular thrombotic events.

Evidence needed

- **Arm vein vs composite vein vs a prosthetic graft.**
- **Interposition vein cuffs vs patches vs pre-cuffed prosthetic grafts.**
- **Ideal method of intraoperative quality control.**
- **Which anticoagulant/antiplatelet agents improve graft patency.**

References (randomised trials in bold)

1. The Vascular Surgical Society of Great Britain and Ireland. Critical limb ischaemia: management and outcome. Report of a National Survey. *Eur J Vasc Endovasc Surg* 1995; 10: 108-113.

2. Cranley JJ, Hafner CD. Revascularization of the femoropopliteal arteries using saphenous vein, polytetrafluoroethylene, and umbilical vein grafts. *Arch Surg* 1982; 117: 1543-1550.

3. Cheshire NJW, Wolfe MS, Noone MA et al. The economics of femorocrural reconstruction for critical limb ischaemia with and without autologous vein. *J Vasc Surg* 1992; 15: 167-175.

4. **Tilanus HW, Obertop H, van Urk H. Saphenous vein or PTFE for femoropopliteal bypass. A prospective randomized trial. *Ann Surg*; 202: 780-2.**

5. **Kumar KP, Crinnon JN, Ashley S, Case WG, Gough MJ. Vein, PTFE or Dacron for above knee femoropopliteal bypass? *Int Angiol* 1995; 14: 200.**

6. **Eickhof JH, Broome A, Ericson BF, et al. Four years' results of a prospective, randomised clinical trial comparing polytetrafluoroethylene and modified human umbilical vein for below-knee femoropopliteal bypass. *J Vasc Surg* 1987; 6: 506-11.**

7. **McCollum C, Kenchington G, Alexander C, Franks PJ, Greenhalgh RM. PTFE or HUV for femoropopliteal bypass: A multicentre trial. *Eur J Vasc Surg* 1991; 5: 435-443.**

8. **Aalders GJ, van Vroonhoven TJMV. Polytetrafluoroethylene versus human umbilical vein in above knee femoropopliteal bypass: six-year results of a randomized clinical trial. *J Vasc Surg* 1992; 16: 816-24.**

9. **Veith FJ, Gupta SK, Ascer E, et al. Six-year prospective multicentre randomized comparison of autologous saphenous vein and expanded polytetrafluoroethylene grafts in infrainguinal arterial constructions. *J Vasc Surg* 1986; 3: 104-14.**

10. **Bergan JJ, Veith FJ, Bernhard VM, et al. Randomization of autogenous vein and polytetrafluoroethylene grafts in femorodistal constructions. *Surgery* 1982; 92: 921-930.**

11. **Harris PL, How TV, Jones DR. Prospectively randomized clinical trial to compare *in situ* and reversed saphenous vein grafts for femoropopliteal bypass. *Br J Surg* 1987; 74: 252-255.**

12. **Harris PL, Veith FJ, Shanik GD, Nott D, Wengerter KR, Moore DJ. Prospective randomized comparison of *in situ* and reversed infrapopliteal vein grafts. *Br J Surg* 1993; 80: 173-176**

13. **Wengerter KR, Veith FJ, Gupta SK, et al. Prospective randomized multicenter comparison of *in situ* and reversed vein infrapopliteal bypasses. *J Vasc Surg* 1991; 13: 189-199.**

14. **Moody AP, Edwards PR, Harris PL. *In situ* versus reversed femoropopliteal vein grafts: long-term follow up of a prospective randomized trial. *Br J Surg* 1992; 79: 750-752.**

15. **Watelet J, Saour N, Menard J-F, et al. Femoropopliteal bypass: *in situ* or reversed vein grafts? Ten-year results of a randomized prospective study. *Ann Vasc Surg* 1997; 11: 510-519.**

16. Lawson JA, Tangelder MJD, Algra A, Eikelboom BC, on behalf of the Dutch BOA Study Group. The myth of the *in situ* graft: Superiority in infrainguinal bypass surgery? *Eur J Vasc Endovasc Surg* 1999; 18: 149-157.

17. McCarthy WJ, Pearce WH, Flinn WR, McGee GS, Wang R, Yao JS. Long-term evaluation of composite sequential bypass for limb-threatening ischaemia. *J Vasc Surg* 1992; 15: 761-770.

18. Hölzenbein TJ, Pomposelli FB, Miller A, et al. Results of a policy with arm veins used as the first alternative to an unavailable ipsilateral greater saphenous vein for infrainguinal bypass. *J Vasc Surg* 1996; 23: 130-40.

19. Schulman ML, Badhey MR, Yatco R, Pillari G. An 11-year experience with deep leg veins as femoropopliteal bypass grafts. *Arch Surg* 1986; 121: 1010-1015.

20. **Schulman ML, Badhey MR, Yatco R. Superficial femoral-popliteal reversed saphenous veins as primary femoropopliteal bypass grafts: a randomized comparative study. *J Vasc Surg* 1987; 6: 1-10.**

21. Schulman ML, Badhey MR. Late results and angiographic evaluation of arm veins as long bypass grafts. *Surgery* 1982; 96: 1032-1041.

22. Londrey GL, Ramsey DE, Hodgson KJ, Barkmeier LD, Sumner DS. Infrapopliteal bypass for severe ischaemia: comparison of autologous vein, composite, and prosthetic grafts. *J Vasc Surg* 1991; 13: 631-636.

23. Prendiville EJ, Yeager A, O'Donnell TF Jr, et al. Long-term results with the above knee popliteal expanded polytetrafluoroethylene graft. *J Vasc Surg* 1990; 11: 517-24.

24. Sottiurai VS, Jones R, Nakamura YK, Boustany C, Sue SL, Batson RC. The role of vein patch in distal anastomotic intimal hyperplasia: an histologic characterization. *Int Angiol* 1994; 13: 96-102.

25. Raptis S, Miller JH. Influence of a vein cuff on polytetrafluoroethylene grafts for primary femoropopliteal bypass. *Br J Surg* 1995; 82: 487-491.

26. Tyrrell MR, Wolfe JHN. New prosthetic venous collar anastomotic technique: combining the best of other procedures. *Br J Surg* 1991; 78: 1016-1017.

27. Suggs WD, Henriques HF, DePalma RG. Vein cuff interposition prevents juxta-anastomotic neointimal hyperplasia. *Ann Surg* 1988; 207: 717-23.

28. Da Silva AF, Carpenter T, How TV, Harris PL. Stable vortices within vein cuffs inhibit myointimal hyperplasia. *Eur J Vasc Endovasc Surg* 1997; 14: 157-163.

29. **Stonebridge PA, Prescott RJ, Ruckley CV. Randomized trial comparing infrainguinal polytetrafluoroethylene bypass grafting with and without vein interposition cuff at the distal anastomosis. *J Vasc Surg* 1997; 26: 543-50.**

30. Taylor RS, Loh A, McFarland RJ, Cox M, Chester JF. Improved technique for polytetrafluoroethylene bypass grafting: long-term results using anastomotic vein patches. *Br J Surg* 1992; 79: 348-354.

31. Ascer E, Gennaro M, Pollina RM, et al. Complementary distal arteriovenous fistula and deep vein interposition: a five-year experience with a new technique to improve infrapopliteal prosthetic bypass patency. *J Vasc Surg* 1996; 24: 134-143.

32. Dardik H, Berry SM, Dardik A, et al. Infrapopliteal prosthetic graft patency by use of the distal adjunctive arteriovenous fistula. *J Vasc Surg* 1991; 13: 685-690.

33. **Hamsho A, Nott D, Harris PL. Prospective randomized trial of distal arteriovenous fistula as an adjunct to femoro-infrapopliteal PTFE bypass. *Eur J Vasc Endovasc Surg* 1999; 17: 197-201.**

34. Brennan JA, Enzler MA, da Silva A, How TV, Harris PL. New graft design to inhibit myointimal hyperplasia in small vessel anastomoses. *Br J Surg* 1996; 83: 1383-1384.

35. Blankensteijn JD, Gertler JP, Brewster DC, et al. Intraoperative determinants of infrainguinal bypass graft patency: a prospective study. *Eur J Vasc Endovasc Surg* 1995; 9: 375-382.

36. **Miller A, Marcaccio EJ, Tannenbaum GA, et al. Comparison of angioscopy and angiography for monitoring infrainguinal bypass vein grafts: results of a prospective randomized trial. *J Vasc Surg* 1993; 17: 382-398.**

Chapter 8

37. Dalman RL, Harris EJ, Zarins CK. Is completion arteriography mandatory after reversed-vein bypass grafting? *J Vasc Surg* 1996; 23: 637-644.

38. Woelfle KD, Kugelmann U, Bruijnen H, Storm G, Loeprecht H. Intraoperative imaging techniques in infrainguinal arterial bypass grafting: completion angiography versus vascular endoscopy. *Eur J Vasc Surg* 1994; 8: 556-61.

39. Watson HR, Belcher G, Horrocks M. Adjuvant medical therapy in peripheral bypass surgery. *Br J Surg* 1999; 86: 981-991.

40. Antiplatelet Trialists' Collaboration. Collaborative overview of randomised trials of antiplatelet therapy-II: Maintenance of vascular graft or arterial patency by antiplatelet therapy. *BMJ* 1994; 308: 159-168.

41. The Iloprost Bypass International Study Group. Effects of perioperative iloprost on patency of femorodistal bypass grafts. *Eur J Vasc Endovasc Surg* 1996; 12: 363-371.

42. Arfvidsson B, Lundgren F, Drott C, Schersten T, Lundholm K. Influence of coumarin treatment on patency and limb salvage after peripheral arterial reconstructive surgery. *Am J Surg* 1990; 159: 556-60.

43. Ktretschmer GJ, Hölzenbein T, Huk I, Abela C. What is the evidence that anticoagulant treatment improves long-term patency of distal bypass? In: Greenhalgh RM, Fowkes FGR, Eds. *Trials and Tribulations of Vascular Surgery*. London: Saunders,1996: 43-52.

44. Sarac TP, Huber TS, Back MR, et al. Warfarin improves the outcome of infrainguinal vein bypass grafting at high risk of failure. *J Vasc Surg* 1998; 28: 446-57.

45. Second European Consensus Document on Chronic Critical Limb Ischaemia. *Eur J Vasc Surg* 1992; 6: Suppl A: 1-32.

Chapter 8

Improving the patency of femorodistal bypass

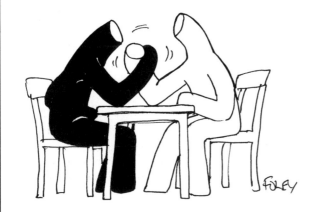

Prosthetic distal bypass for critical leg ischaemia

LD Wijesinghe
Specialist Registrar
PT McCollum
Professor of Vascular Surgery

DEPARTMENT OF VASCULAR SURGERY,
HULL ROYAL INFIRMARY, HULL

Introduction

The incidence of critical leg ischaemia in Europe is estimated to be 500-1000 per million population per year and the mortality rate in these patients is about 20% per year [1]. The most important risk factors for the development of critical ischaemia are diabetes, smoking and old age.

Jean Kunlin performed the first successful femoropopliteal vein bypass on a man with rest pain and gangrene in 1948. Since then autogenous vein has become the conduit of choice for lower limb bypass surgery. Developments in diagnostic evaluation, instrumentation, surgical technique and the economic advantages of successful bypass have encouraged the development of distal bypass for critical ischaemia. Where no suitable vein is available, surgeons have sought alternatives including autografts, allografts, xenografts, and prosthetic materials. Early enthusiasm for bovine carotid arteries, human umbilical vein (HUV) and cadaveric vessels was tempered by problems of aneurysmal dilatation, graft manufacture and preservation respectively. Dacron grafts perform well in aortoiliac reconstruction, but their disappointing results in bypasses to smaller infrainguinal vessels prompted the switch to expanded polytetrafluoroethylene (PTFE). PTFE is preferred to Dacron for several other reasons. These include less platelet activation in the early postoperative period [2], greater ease in performing thrombectomy [3], and stronger anastomotic bonding between graft and native artery [4].

Two areas of contention exist. First, some surgeons suggest that for a bypass to the above-knee popliteal artery, prosthetic grafts should be preferred over vein. Second, when no suitable vein is available, is a prosthetic graft better than a primary amputation?

Primary amputation

The estimated in-hospital cost of a successful bypass procedure is about US$ 5700, that of primary amputation US$ 13,000 and that of amputation after failed bypass US$ 25,000 [5]. Primary amputation is appropriate in certain patients with critical ischaemia such as those with a joint contracture, extensive distal necrosis, chronic paralysis of the ischaemic leg and those who are wheelchair-bound. In other patients the choice is between amputation and rehabilitation with a walking prosthesis or femorodistal bypass. The ratio of primary amputation to distal arterial reconstruction is prone to geographical variation, depending on the population, local surgical expertise and finances. Even in the absence of suitable autologous vein some surgeons advocate the use of a prosthetic graft rather than primary amputation, not only because successful bypass prolongs the amputation-free existence, but also because of the economic advantages to the community and the patient [6-9]. Although the patency of prosthetic grafts falls below that of vein, the short life expectancy of patients with severe chronic ischaemia, the economic advantage of a successful bypass and the common observation that ulcer healing,

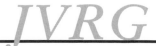

once achieved, may be permanent even if the graft occludes, are persuasive arguments for attempted reconstruction.

Experience with Dacron, PTFE and HUV

The comparison of different arterial conduits by strict scientific measures needs a randomised controlled trial. In considering femorotibial bypass for critical ischaemia, conducting such a trial poses some difficulties. First, the number of distal bypasses performed, even in major centres, is relatively low. Second, randomising between vein and prosthetic graft would present an ethical dilemma in the face of overwhelming evidence for the superiority of vein. Third, randomising only those patients who do not have suitable vein would further deplete the study population. Fourth, the limited life expectancy of the patients makes long-term follow-up difficult. At the time of writing, there are no significant randomised trials comparing any combination of PTFE, Dacron or HUV in femorotibial bypass. Therefore, information is obtained by examining randomised data of femoropopliteal grafts, and case series of femorotibial bypass operations. This process suffers from the disadvantages inherent in comparing disparate patient groups. The term critical ischaemia has been applied to a number of patients who might be described more aptly as having subcritical ischaemia [10]. This means that the patency and limb salvage rates in reported series of femorotibial bypasses could appear higher than if a strict adherence to the modern robust definition of critical ischaemia had been applied.

In the early days of prosthetic lower limb bypass, Dacron produced relatively poor results, with 5 year patencies of less than 60% to the above-knee popliteal artery and even less below the knee [11]. Kenney et al have reported a 4 year patency approaching 80% for above-knee femoropopliteal Dacron grafts which is as good as any reported series using PTFE [12]. Abbott et al, in a randomised prospective trial were unable to demonstrate a difference in patency between Dacron and PTFE for above-knee bypass at 3 years [13]. However, no randomised studies have compared PTFE and Dacron for femorotibial bypass. Despite this, PTFE is widely used as an alternative when saphenous vein is not available. The early reports of PTFE grafts were encouraging, but the long-term patency in below-knee and distal bypasses was less good [14,15]. In a randomised trial PTFE fared much worse than vein for distal bypass (49% v. 12% patency at 4 years) [16]. Several randomised trials have shown HUV grafts to have better patency than PTFE for both above- and below-knee femoropopliteal bypasses [17,18], but no randomised data are available for tibial grafts. Surgeons have been slow to adopt HUV because the grafts are subject to biodegradation, are more cumbersome to handle and are more expensive than either Dacron or PTFE.

The incidence of prosthetic graft infection is probably between 3% and 5% with a subsequent major amputation rate of 30% to 70% [19,20]. A new and particularly worrying problem is that of infection with methicillin resistant *Staphylococcus aureus*, an organism that is often endemic in nursing homes and long-stay wards where the typical patient with critical ischaemia is likely to be resident (see Chapter 28).

Adjunctive anastomotic techniques for PTFE bypass

Many explanations have been proposed for the lower patency rates of PTFE bypasses compared with vein. The mismatch in compliance between the relatively stiff prosthetic graft and the native artery, combined with iatrogenic injury caused by suturing the anastomosis, and areas of low shear stress at the heel and toe are all thought to induce myointimal hyperplasia (MIH) and therefore stenosis at the distal anastomosis. Surgical techniques have been developed in an effort to limit MIH and stem from the anastomotic vein patch described by Linton and Darling [21] and Siegman's venous cuff [22]. Miller et al described their version of the vein cuff in 1984 [23] and in 1998 this group reported a retrospective series in which PTFE femorotibial grafts achieved a 2 year primary patency of 31%. This compared with their concurrent series of vein grafts in which the 2 year primary patency was 54%. Earlier, in 1995, Raptis and Miller reported that cuffed PTFE grafts to the below-knee popliteal artery had a superior patency rate to uncuffed grafts at 36 months (57% versus 29%) [24], a finding which was later corroborated in a randomised study by the Joint Vascular Research Group (JVRG) [25]. In the JVRG study patients who had either above- or below-knee femoropopliteal bypass were randomised to have a cuffed or uncuffed distal anastomosis (Table 1). The cuff produced a significant advantage at the below-knee level, but not above the knee. When a cuffed PTFE graft occludes, the recipient artery may be spared, allowing the chance of further reconstruction [26]. However, recent evidence throws this observation into question [27]. Retrospective review of the Miller cuff in prosthetic bypasses to tibial vessels has demonstrated encouraging patency rates of 55% at 2 years [28] and 52% at 3 years [6]. Two randomised trials comparing cuffed and uncuffed PTFE distal bypasses are underway, one by the Belgian Miller Cuff Group and the other by the SCAMICOS participants in Scandinavia, but no final results will be available until late 1999.

The Taylor patch [29] and Wolfe boot [30] are modifications of the distal anastomotic vein interposition technique. Both configurations have achieved patencies comparable to those of the Miller cuff, but neither has been the subject of a randomised trial. The use of an arteriovenous fistula (AVF) at or near the distal anastomosis has been advocated in order to decrease the outflow resistance and improve blood flow through the distal anastomosis. The combination of AVF and vein interposition for femorotibial bypass has achieved a 2 year cumulative patency of 62% [31] and a 3 year primary assisted patency of 61.9% [32].

Table 1. Randomised controlled trial of Miller vein cuff in femoropopliteal bypass: 2 year results [25].

	Primary patency (%)	Secondary patency (%)	Limb salvage (%)
Above-knee popliteal			
Vein cuff (n=76)	72	76	82
No vein cuff (n=74)	70	74	91
p (Wilcoxon)	0.90	0.63	0.37
Below-knee popliteal			
Vein cuff (n=49)	52	59	84
No vein cuff (n=47)	29	35	62
p (Wilcoxon)	0.03	0.14	0.08

Table 2. Results of femorotibial bypass for critical ischaemia using PTFE.

Author	Year	n	Graft	% Primary patency (limb salvage)				
				1yr	2yrs	3yrs	4yrs	5yrs
Veith [16]	1986	98	PTFE		35 (60)		12 (61)	
		106	vein		60 (75)		49 (57)	
Tyrrell [30]	1991	55	PTFE+VC			52		
Taylor [29]	1992	83	PTFE+TP	74		58		54
Harris [31]	1993	43	PTFE+VC+AVF		62 (55)			
		179	vein		68 (69)			
Parsons [9]	1996	66	PTFE			39 (71)		28 (66)
Wijesinghe [28]	1998	51	PTFE+VC+AVF*	64 (85)	51 (80)			

VC   Miller vein cuff
AVF   distal anastomotic arteriovenous fistula
TP   Taylor patch
* AVF in 50% of patients

Conclusions

The primacy of vein as a conduit for femorodistal bypass is undisputed. The use of PTFE and other prosthetic grafts when vein is not available is based on the assumption that the patency of prosthetic grafts, although lower than that of vein, will nevertheless be high enough to tide a patient over the ischaemia. The lack of randomised trials does not allow an evidence-based choice to be made between the several non-vein bypasses currently available. However, the largest experience appears to be with PTFE. It is reasonable, on the basis of current evidence, to suggest that a PTFE femorodistal bypass should be preferred to primary amputation if vein is not available. The patency of such a graft is improved by a vein interposition technique at the distal anastomosis.

Chapter 9

Prosthetic distal bypass for critical leg ischaemia

Sound evidence

- **There is a clear advantage in successful first time femorodistal bypass over primary amputation.**

Evidence needed

- **Whether any of the various prosthetic grafts is superior.**

- **The most favourable conformation of the distal anastomosis in prosthetic bypass.**

References (randomised trials in bold)

1. Wolfe JHN. Defining the outcome of critical ischaemia. A one-year prospective study. *Br J Surg* 1986; 73: 321.
2. **Wakefield TW, Shulkin BL, Fellows EP, Petry NA, Spaulding SA, Stanley JC. Platelet reactivity in human aortic grafts: a prospective, randomized midterm study of platelet adherence and release products in Dacron and polytetrafluoroethylene conduits. *J Vasc Surg* 1989; 3: 234-243.**
3. Kram HB, Dietzek AM, Veith FJ. Optimal synthetic grafts for aortic replacement. In: Greenhalgh RM, Mannick JA (Eds). *The Cause and Management of Aneurysms.* Philadelphia: WB Saunders, 1990; pp. 340-350.
4. Quinones-Baldrich WJ, Ziomek S, Henderson T, Moore WS. Primary anastomotic bonding in polytetra-fluoroethylene graft? *J Vasc Surg* 1987; 5: 311-318.
5. Myrhe H, Fosby B, Witsoe E, Groechenig E. Cost-effectiveness of therapeutic options for critical limb ischaemia. *Critical ischaemia* 1996; 6: 37-41.
6. Wolfe JHN, Tyrrell MR. Justifying arterial reconstruction to crural vessels - even with a prosthetic graft. *Br J Surg* 1991; 78: 897-899.
7. Cheshire NJ, Noone MA, Davies L, Drummond M, Wolfe JHN. Economic options and decision making in the ischaemic lower limb. *Br J Surg* 1991; 78: A371.
8. Tyrrell MR, Grigg MJ, Wolfe JHN. Is arterial reconstruction to the ankle worthwhile in the absence of autologous vein? *Eur J Vasc Surg* 1989; 3: 429-434.
9. Parsons RE, Suggs WD, Veith FJ, et al. Polytetrafluoroethylene bypasses to infrapopliteal arteries without cuffs or patches: a better option than amputation in patients without autologous vein. *J Vasc Surg* 1996; 23: 347-356.
10. Wolfe JH, Wyatt MG. Critical and subcritical ischaemia. *Eur J Vasv Endovasc Surg* 1997; 13: 578-582.
11. Christenson JT, Eklof B. Sparks mandril, velour Dacron and autogenous saphenous vein grafts in femoropopliteal bypass. *Br J Surg* 1979; 66: 514-517.
12. Kenney DA, Sauvage LR, Wood SJ, et al. Comparison of non-crimped, externally supported (EXS) and crimped, non-supported Dacron prostheses for axillo-bifemoral and above-knee femoropopliteal bypass. *Surgery* 1982; 92: 931-946.
13. **Abbott WA, Green RM, Matsumoto T, et al. Prosthetic above-knee femoropopliteal bypass grafting: results of a multicentre randomized prospective trial. *J Vasc Surg* 1997; 25: 19-26.**
14. Charlesworth PM, Brewster DC, Darling RC, Robison JG, Hallett JW. The fate of polytetrafluoroethylene grafts in lower limb bypass surgery: a six year follow-up. *Br J Surg* 1985; 72: 896-899.
15. Whittemore AD, Kent KC, Donaldson MC, Couch MC, Mannick JA. What is the proper role of polytetrafluoroethylene grafts in infrainguinal reconstruction? *J Vasc Surg* 1989; 10: 299-305.
16. **Veith FJ, Gupta SK, Ascer E, et al. Six-year prospective multicenter randomized comparison of autologous saphenous vein and expanded polytetrafluoroethylene grafts in infrainguinal arterial reconstructions. *J Vasc Surg* 1986; 3: 104-14.**
17. **Aalders GJ, van Vroonhoven TJMV. Polytetrafluoroethylene versus human umbilical vein in above-knee femoropopliteal bypass: six-year results of a prospective randomized trial. *J Vasc Surg* 1992; 16: 816-823.**
18. **Eickhoff JH, Broome A, Ericsson BF, et al. Four years' results of a prospective randomized trial comparing polytetrafluoroethylene and modified human umbilical vein for below-knee femoropopliteal bypass. *J Vasc Surg* 1987; 6: 506-511.**
19. Durham JR, Rubin JR, Malone JM. Management of infected infrainguinal bypass grafts. In Bergan JJ, Yao JST (Eds.). *Reoperative arterial surgery.* Orlando. Grune & Stratton. 1986, pp. 359-373.
20. Yashar JJ, Weyman AK, Burnand RJ, Yashar J. Survival and limb salvage in patients with infected prostheses. *Am J Surg* 1978; 135: 499-504.
21. Linton RR, Darling RC. Autogenous saphenous vein bypass grafts in femoropopliteal obliterative arterial disease. *Surgery* 1962; 51: 62-73.
22. Siegman FA. Use of the venous cuff for graft anastomosis. *Surg Gynaecol Obstet* 1979; 148: 930.
23. Miller JH, Foreman RK, Ferguson L, Faris I. Interposition vein cuff for anastomosis of prosthesis to small artery. *Aust NZ J Surg* 1984; 54: 283-285.
24. Raptis S, Miller JH. Influence of a vein cuff on polytetrafluoroethylene grafts for primary femoropopliteal bypass. *Br J Surg* 1995; 82: 487-491.

25. Stonebridge PA, Prescott RP, Ruckley CV. Randomised trial comparing infrainguinal polytetrafluoroethylene bypass grafting with and without vein interposition cuff at the distal anastomosis. *J Vasc Surg* 1997; 26: 543-550.

26. Tyrrell MR, Wolfe JHN. Myointimal hyperplasia in vein collars for ePTFE grafts. *Eur J Vasc Endovasc Surg* 1997; 14: 33-36.

27. Renwick P, Johnson B, Wilkinson A, Galloway J, McCollum P. Limb outcome following failed femoropopliteal polytetrafluoroethylene bypass for intermittent claudication. *Br J Surg* 1999, 86: A690.

28. Wijesinghe LD, Beardsmore DM, Scott DJA. Polytetrafluoroethylene (PTFE) femorodistal grafts with a distal vein cuff for critical ischaemia. *Eur J Vasc Endovasc Surg* 1998; 15: 449-453.

29. Taylor RS, Loh H, McFarland RJ, Cos M, Chester JF. Improved technique for polytetrafluoroethylene bypass grafting: long term results using anastomotic vein patches. *Br J Surg* 1992; 79: 348-54.

30. Tyrrell MR, Wolfe JHN. New prosthetic venous collar anastomotic technique: combining the best of other procedures. *Br J Surg* 1991; 78: 1016-1017.

31. Harris PL, Bakran A, Enabi L, Nott DM. ePTFE for femorocrural bypass - improved results with combined adjuvant arteriovenous fistula? *Eur J Vasc Endovasc Surg* 1993; 7: 528-533.

32. Ascer E, Gennaro M, Pollina RM, Ivanov M, Yorkovich WR, Ivanov M, Lorensen E. Complementary distal arteriovenous fistula and deep vein interposition: A five-year experience with a new technique to improve infrapopliteal prosthetic bypass patency. *J Vasc Surg* 1996; 24: 134-43.

Chapter 9

Prosthetic distal bypass for critical
leg ischaemia

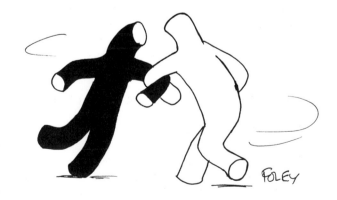

Chapter 10

Infrainguinal graft surveillance

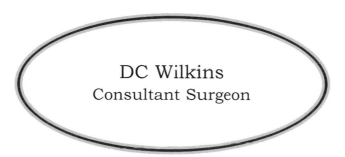

DC Wilkins
Consultant Surgeon

VASCULAR SURGICAL UNIT,
DERRIFORD HOSPITAL, PLYMOUTH

Introduction

Vascular procedures represent a considerable investment on the part of the patient, the surgeon and the Health Service. It follows that all parties have a vested interest in maximising the benefits of any vascular operation [1]. This is particularly true for infrainguinal bypass grafts where failure, leading to the loss of a leg or the onset of intractable pain, may mean a considerable degradation of a patient's quality of life. It is well established that as time passes infrainguinal grafts are susceptible to the development of stenoses. As they have become increasingly available, it is hardly surprising that ultrasound techniques for monitoring graft function and morphology now form the cornerstone of most long-term follow-up programmes. Nor is it surprising that it has become customary to treat graft-related lesions discovered in this way (Figures 1-4). However, with 5-6,000 infrainguinal by-passes being performed annually in the United Kingdom [2] this represents a substantial workload, and one that is probably still increasing.

What is the best method of graft surveillance?

Angiography, long regarded as the gold standard for detection of graft-related problems, has been superseded by ultrasonic methods of imaging [3]. These methods are also capable of measuring flow and resistance. Flow velocity used on its own is an unreliable predictor of graft function, although a flow velocity of 45cm/sec would be regarded by most surgeons as worrying. Colour duplex is often used as a screening tool to detect areas of flow disturbance requiring more detailed examination. Flow velocity measured in normal sections of the graft and compared to that in stenotic areas is then expressed as the peak systolic velocity flow ratio (PSVR). The disadvantage of relying on PSVR alone is that it does not measure the resistance to flow and may underestimate the effect of less marked stenoses [4]. This may be relevant in the sudden unheralded graft occlusion that occurs occasionally. It is possible that more use may be made of graft impedance measurement in future, but further work is needed [5].

Some surgeons still rely on clinical methods of surveillance. A variety of indicators are used. Onset or deterioration in clinical symptoms, a drop in resting ankle pressure (ABPI) or a drop in post exercise ABPI are employed in varying combinations as indicators for more detailed investigation with a view to intervention [6].

The incidence of graft stenosis

Prosthetic grafts

Since most occlusions in prosthetic grafts occur without warning, there are few proponents of regular duplex-based surveillance. Dunlop et al in a prospective

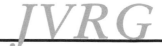

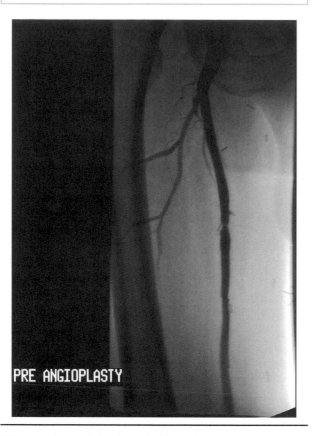

PRE ANGIOPLASTY

Figure 1. Isolated web-like stenosis in a vein graft before angioplasty.

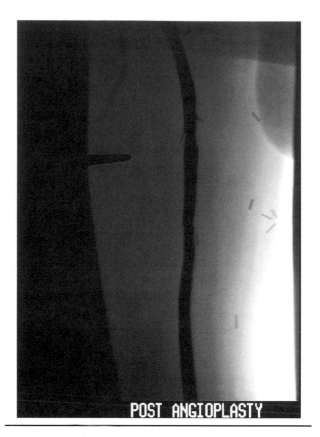

POST ANGIOPLASTY

Figure 2. Stenosis shown in Fig. 1 after balloon angioplasty.

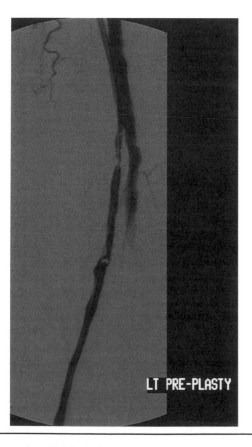

LT PRE-PLASTY

Figure 3. Multiple strictures in a vein graft before angioplasty.

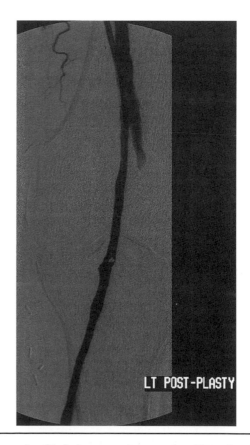

LT POST-PLASTY

Figure 4. Strictures shown in Fig. 3 after balloon angioplasty.

series found that approximately a quarter of their prosthetic infrainguinal grafts occluded unexpectedly, despite 3 monthly duplex imaging [7]. They concluded that the results did not justify the investment. Following a similar protocol, however, Aune et al [8] felt the programme was worthwhile as they calculated that up to one third of the grafts at risk of occlusion were salvaged. There are no randomised trials to settle this point.

Vein grafts

Using angiography, Szilagi et al drew attention to the problem of vein graft stenosis in 1973 [9]. There is now clear agreement from several series that the incidence of vein graft stenosis is highest during the first year after surgery and affects between 20% and 30% of all grafts [3,10,11]. The definition of what constitutes a stenosis is by no means consistent. Most vascular surgeons now regard a PSVR of >2.5, indicating a reduction of cross-sectional area of more than 70%, as significant. This is equivalent to a reduction in vessel diameter of 50%.

Are some grafts more susceptible to the development of stenoses?

Gupta et al [12] found that 23% of reversed saphenous vein grafts and 28% of composite vein grafts required revision during a 3-year interval, compared to 10% of *in situ* vein grafts. An extensive prospective study from the Netherlands [13], however, showed no such correlation but did find that small calibre vein grafts were at greater risk of developing a significant stenosis. The rate of stenosis was 60% for grafts with a minimum diameter of <3.5mm, 42% for grafts between 3.5 and 4.5mm and 25% for grafts >4.5mm. This apart, there is little evidence to suggest major differences between the different categories of autogenous vein grafts [14].

Should graft surveillance be continued for life?

There is agreement in the literature that the rate of development of graft stenoses is highest in the first 6 months, dropping considerably to a rate of approximately 3% per year thereafter. The incidence is lowest in grafts that have not developed a stenosis previously and on this basis it can be argued that surveillance of this group may safely be discontinued at this point [15]. McCarthy et al point out that there is a continuing risk of developing an associated, and equally dangerous, arterial stenosis caused by progression of either proximal or distal disease, and that this risk amounts to 10% per year [16]. On this basis it would seem sensible to continue graft surveillance indefinitely.

The indications for intervention for graft stenosis

Vein graft stenoses may be characterised by their position and morphology as well as by their severity. The following are usually, though by no means always, defined by authors: inflow, outflow, peri-anastomotic strictures and true intra-graft stenoses [2]. Most series include peri-anastomotic stenoses and stenoses in the true body of the graft under the general heading of 'vein graft stenosis'.

There is also considerable divergence of opinion on the point at which intervention is necessary. Although most series regard a PSVR >2.5 as indicative of a significant stenosis, the values used to trigger intervention are inconsistent and vary between 1.5 and 5.0. Olojugba et al [17] found that grafts with a PSVR up to 3.0 could safely be left, providing duplex imaging was carried out monthly for at least 3 months after detection. The St Mary's group defined a stenosis as having a PSVR >3:2 (equivalent to a 20% reduction in diameter), but intervened only in patients with symptoms or a reduction in ABPI of >0.2. They found that approximately 25% of the stenoses detected became 'significant requiring intervention' [3]. Although in this early series imaging took place at three month intervals, it is interesting to note that in approximately 15% of the group with a mild stenosis, considered to be non-haemodynamically significant, sudden graft occlusion still occurred [3]. Rapidly progressive stenoses are universally thought to warrant intervention and there is also general agreement in the literature that extremely tight stenoses with a PSVR >5.0 require urgent action. Despite this rather subjective, but relatively uniform approach, the effect of a stenosis on the fate of a vein graft is by no means predictable. In one study, of 22 stenoses detected while following 80 grafts by intravenous digital subtraction angiography, only five occluded, while four of the 58 with no stenoses also occluded! [18].

Which intervention?

Much work has been carried out on the nature of vein graft stenosis. The pathology includes short segment, web-like lesions associated with valve cusps, segments of vein wall thickening associated with proliferation of smooth muscle fibres (myointimal hyperplasia), fibrous strictures, and technical problems such as kinking and entrapment due to external pressure [9]. The tendency of some patients to develop multiple strictures in the same vein graft, or in bilateral grafts, raises the possibility that there may be a systemic factor, or factors, at work [19].

Authors have identified the rapidity of onset following surgery, the rate of progression and the length of a stenosis as factors that should influence the timing and type of intervention. Clinicians seeking guidance on which method of treatment to apply to the various types of stenosis will find the evidence conflicting [10]. Popular opinion suggests that long stenoses are best treated by surgical bypass and short lesions, such as those associated with valve cusps, should be treated by balloon angioplasty. Extensive series have been published, however, where enthusiastic primary treatment by either surgery or balloon angioplasty appeared to give similar results [21]. A randomised trial would be helpful in answering some of the questions regarding the optimum intervention for graft stenosis but for the present it seems that the method of treatment in individual patients should be selected on the basis of the experience, resources, commitment and expertise available locally.

The value of a graft surveillance programme

The justification for graft surveillance is that it saves legs. Since a major amputation has a severe impact on the quality of life, as well as cost implications for the community, this is a laudable aim. Until recently, however, it has been tacitly accepted that the clear improvements in secondary graft patency demonstrated in most published series equates with legs saved and so represents a health gain. While techniques of surveillance, imaging intervals and methods of treatment were still evolving, this was a reasonable assumption. Now that there is some uniformity of approach the time is ripe for a prospective, randomised trial comparing clear outcome measures such as overall amputation rates, quality of health assessment and costs between surveillance and non-surveillance groups.

The burgeoning costs of these surveillance programmes should also not be overlooked. Apart from the capital costs and vascular technologists' time, the expense associated with interventions is considerable, doubling the cost of the original procedure [22,23]. Reviewing published series between 1987 and 1995, Golledge and colleagues identified reports concerning 6257 vein grafts. Seventeen series included surveillance programmes, 26 did not. The lack of conformity between series prevented direct comparison but there was a surprising similarity in the rates of amputation between the two groups (12-13%), despite an apparent increase in patency rates in the surveillance group [2]. Further powerful evidence that graft patency does not necessarily correlate with limb salvage comes from analysis of a large series of femorodistal vein grafts [24]. Although there was a reasonable correlation between patency and amputation rate, a significant number of patients who had undergone surgery for critical ischaemia occluded their graft without losing their leg.

There have been two published prospective randomised controlled trials comparing vein graft patency using clinically based follow-up *versus* duplex-based follow-up (Table 1). Ihlberg [6] recently reported the results of a randomised prospective trial carried out in Helsinki, comprising 185 infrainguinal vein grafts. The important finding of this trial was the lack of significant difference in amputation rates between the two groups, one which had clinically based and the other duplex-based graft surveillance. The authors acknowledge various problems with protocol violations and there were also problems with the analysis. Although randomised at the time of operation, patients whose grafts occluded during the first month were excluded from the analysis of the amputation rate. There was also no quality of life examination.

Lundell et al [25] in a similar trial including 156 infrainguinal grafts, some of which were prosthetic, also reported an advantage to graft patency in the duplex surveillance group. Amputation rates were not reported. Nonetheless, despite their small size, both these trials are important indicators that the benefits to the patient of a duplex-based graft surveillance programme may not be as clear cut as expected.

The Vein Graft Surveillance Trial [26] funded by the British Heart Foundation and under way in the UK at the time of writing, should go a considerable way to addressing the uncertainties outlined above. This prospective trial will randomise patients with patent infrainguinal vein grafts at hospital discharge into either duplex or clinical surveillance groups. All patients will be followed up for 18 months. Graft patency, amputation, quality of life and cost are the main outcome measures.

Table 1. Randomised prospective trials comparing clinical with duplex-based surveillance programmes.

	Duplex follow-up	Clinical follow-up
Lundell et al [25] **n= 106 grafts** **followed to 36 months**		
Secondary patency	82%	56%
Limb salvage	not given	not given
Ihlberg et al [6] **n= 185 grafts** **followed to 12 months**		
Secondary patency	71%	84%
Limb salvage	81%	88%

Infrainguinal graft surveillance

Sound evidence

- **Autogenous vein grafts are at risk from developing a stenosis at a rate of 20-30% during the first year.**

- **Duplex surveillance of vein grafts results in an enhanced patency rate at 3 years.**

Evidence needed

- **The optimum surveillance programme.**

- **Whether an intensive duplex-based graft surveillance programme results in an overall saving of legs, improves quality of life and is value for money.**

Chapter 10

References (randomised trials in bold)

1. Harris PL. Vein graft surveillance - all part of the service. *Br J Surg* 1992; 79: 97-98.
2. Golledge J, Beattie D K, Greenhalgh R M, Davies AH. Have the results of infra inguinal bypass improved with the widespread utilisation of postoperative surveillance? *Eur J Vasc Endovasc Surg* 1996; 11: 388-92.
3. Grigg MJ, Nicolaides AN, Wolfe JHN. Femorodistal vein bypass graft stenoses. *Br J Surg* 1988; 75: 737 -740.
4. Moawad J, Brown S, Schwartz LB. The effect of 'non-critical' stenosis on vein graft longitudinal resistance and impedance. *Eur J Vasc Endovasc Surg* 1999; 17: 517-520.
5. Davies AH, Magee TR, Wyatt M, Baird R, Horrocks M. Impedance analysis versus colour duplex in femorodistal vein graft surveillance. *Eur J Vasc Endovasc Surg* 1993; 7: 14-15.
6. **Ihlberg L, Luther M, Tierala E, Lepantalo M. The utility of duplex scanning in infrainguinal vein graft surveillance: results from a randomised controlled study. *Eur J Vasc Endovasc Surg* 1998; 16: 19-27.**
7. Dunlop P, Sayers RD, Naylor AR, Bell PRF, London NJM. The effect of a surveillance program on the patency of synthetic infrainguinal bypass grafts. *Eur J Vasc Endovasc Surg* 1996; 11: 441-445.
8. Aune S, Pedersen OM, Trippestad A. Surveillance of above-knee prosthetic femoropopliteal bypass. *Eur J Vasc Endovasc Surg* 1998; 16: 509-512.
9. Szilagyi DE, Elliot JP, Hagerman JH, Smith RF, Dallomolino CA. Biologic fate of autologous vein implants as arterial substitutes. *Ann Surg* 1973; 178: 232-46.
10. Caps MT, Cantwell-Gab K, Bergelin RO, Strandness DE. Vein graft lesions: time of onset and rate of progression. *J Vasc Surg* 1995; 22: 466-475.
11. Wilson YG, Davies AH, Currie IC, et al. Vein graft stenosis: incidence and intervention. *Eur J Vasc Endovasc Surg* 1996; 11: 164-9.
12. Gupta AK, Bandyk DF, Cheanveciai D, Johnson BL. Natural history of infrainguinal vein graft stenosis relative to bypass grafting technique. *J Vasc Surg* 1997; 25: 211-225.
13. Idu MM, Buth J, Hop WCJ, Cuypers Ph, van de Pavoordt EDWM, Tordoir JMH. Factors influencing the development vein-graft related stenosis and their significance for clinical management. *Eur J Vasc Endovasc Surg* 1999; 17: 15-21.
14. Lawson JA, Tongelder MJD, Algra A, Eikelbloom B, on behalf of the Dutch BOA study group. The myth of the *in situ* graft: superiority in infrainguinal bypass surgery? *Eur J Vasc Endovasc Surg* 1998; 18: 149-157.
15. Idu MM, Buth J, Cuypers Ph, Hop WCJ, van de Pavoordt EDWM, Tordoir JMH. Economising vein-graft surveillance programs. *Eur J Vasc Endovasc Surg*; 15: 432-438.
16. McCarthy MJ, Olojugba D, Loftus IM, Naylor AR, Bell PRF, London NJM. Lower limb surveillance following autologous vein by-pass should be life long. *Br J Surg* 1998; 85:1369-1372.
17. Olojugba DH, McCarthy MJ, Naylor AR, Bell PRF, London NJM. At what peak velocity ratio should duplex-detected infrainguinal vein graft stenoses be revised? *Eur J Vasc Endovasc Surg* 1998; 15: 258-260.
18. Moody P, DeCossart LM, Douglas HM, Harris PL. Asymptomatic strictures in femoropopliteal vein grafts. *Eur J Vasc Surg* 1989; 3: 389-92.
19. McCarthy MJ, Varty K, Naylor AR, London NJM, Bell PRF. Bilateral infrainguinal vein grafts and the incidence of vein graft stenosis. *Eur J Vasc Endovasc Surg* 1998; 15: 231-234.
20. Avino AJ, Bandyk DF, Gonsalves AJ, et al. Surgical and endovascular intervention for infrainguinal vein graft stenosis. *J Vasc Surg* 1999; 29: 60-69.
21. Tennesen KH, Holstein P, Rordam L, Bulow, Helgstrand U, Dreyer. Early results of percutaneous transluminal angioplasty of failing below-knee bypass grafts. *Eur J Vasc Endovasc Surg* 1998; 15: 51-56.
22. Loftus IM, Reid A, Thompson MM, London NJM, Bell PRF, Naylor AR The increasing workload required to maintain infrainguinal bypass graft patency. *Eur J Vasc Endovasc Surg* 1998; 15: 337-341.
23. Cheshire NJW, Wolfe JHN, Noone MA, Davies L, Drummond M. The economics of femorocrural reconstruction for critical leg ischaemia with or without autogenous vein. *J Vasc Surg* 1992; 15: 167-174.
24. Watson HR, Schroeder TV, Simms MH, et al. Relationship of femorodistal bypass patency to clinical outcome. *Eur J Vasc Endovasc Surg* 1999; 17: 77-83.
25. **Lundell A, Lindblad B, Bergquist D, Hansen R. Femoro-popliteal-crural graft patency is improved by an intensive surveillance program: a prospective randomised study. *J Vasc Surg* 1995; 21: 19-27.**
26. Kirby PL, Brady AR, Thompson SG, Torgerson D, Davies AH, on behalf of the Vein Graft Surveillance Trial Participants. The vein graft surveillance trial: rationale, design and methods. *Eur J Vasc Endovasc Surg* 1999 (in press).

Infrainguinal graft surveillance

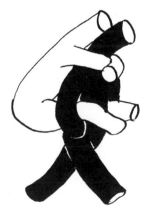

Chapter 11

Management of critical leg ischaemia: quality of life issues

J Robinson
Surgical Research Fellow
JD Beard
Consultant Vascular Surgeon

SHEFFIELD VASCULAR INSTITUTE,
NORTHERN GENERAL HOSPITAL, SHEFFIELD

Introduction

The revolution in the management of critical limb ischaemia that has taken place over recent years, with the refinement of distal bypass procedures and the development of endovascular procedures, has led many to argue that revascularisation should be attempted in all patients. Since quality of life was shown to be a useful outcome measure in vascular surgery [1] there have been many relevant studies, and most lend support to the argument that revascularisation is better than amputation. Surgeons have continued to advocate reconstructive surgery based on the poor mobility achieved by amputees in various retrospective studies [2]. However, these quality of life studies are hampered by the use of measures which impose preselected values on the patient rather than seeking to define those factors that motivate an individual, enabling them to determine their own quality of life. With the absence of a randomised controlled trial of amputation versus reconstruction there is no good scientific evidence for the superiority of either treatment.

Tools for assessing quality of life

The Quality Adjusted Life Year (QALY), which gives the concept of the value of each life year for an individual, provides a single measure of the value that a respondent attaches to their overall health status. This provided one of the earliest tools for assessing quality of life [3] and, although it has been developed to make it more applicable to clinical practice, including vascular surgery [4] (Table 1), many other tools have superseded it. The vast array of scales and profiles used by clinicians and health economists to assess quality of life range from domain specific scales, such as the Hospital Anxiety and Depression Scale and the Barthel Activities of Daily Living Index [5] (Table 2) to those which measure responses across a range of domains, such as emotional reactions and physical energy. The Nottingham Health Profile (NHP) and the Medical Outcomes Short Form 36 (SF-36) both fall into the latter category and the patient's responses are scored for each domain; 6 for the NHP and 8 for the SF-36 (Table 3) to provide a profile for each individual. The SF-36 is now widely used in many studies, and health economists are also developing a system to provide an index from this profile, thereby allowing data to be used by themselves. It has been suggested that there should be a consensus over which is the most reliable quality of life measure, resulting in the use of a single one internationally [6]. The SF-36 has been shown to be the most appropriate generic quality of life analysis tool in current use, and its use has been advocated to standardise the assessment of outcome from vascular surgery [7].

Health economists have developed the complicated (for many patients) concept of standard gamble and time trade-off [8] which provides a single utility index for cost

JVRG

Table 1. Rosser classification of quality of life, adapted for vascular patients.

Disability		
	1	None
	2	Slight social disability
	3	Severe social disability, or slight impairment at work
	4	Severe restriction at work
	5	Inability to work, elderly confined to home unless escorted
	6	Confined to chair
	7	Confined to bed
Pain	A	None
	B	Mild claudication at >200 metres
	C	Severe claudication at <200 metres or mild rest pain
	D	Severe rest pain requiring regular analgesia

Table 2. Barthel Index of Activities of Daily Living.

ACTIVITY OF DAILY LIFE	SCORE=0	SCORE=1	SCORE=2	SCORE=3
Bowels	Incontinent	Occasional accident	Continent	
Bladder	Incontinent or catheterised	Occasional accident	Continent	
Grooming	Needs help	Independent		
Toilet use	Dependent	Needs some help	Independent	
Feeding	Unable	Needs help cutting	Independent	
Transfer	Unable, no sitting balance	Major help, 1 or 2 people	Minor help	Independent
Mobility	Immobile	Wheelchair	Walks with help of 1 person	Independent, may use aid
Dressing	Dependent	Needs help	Independent	
Stairs	Unable	Needs help	Independent	
Bathing	Dependent	Independent		

benefit analyses, and they have also been instrumental in developing standardised generic instruments for describing health related quality of life from which a single index can be calculated, such as the EuroQol [9].

life, and any deterioration in this state may not be assessed by generic quality of life tools [10]. There is evidence that the SF-36 is unhelpful in assessing some of the changes in health that the elderly perceive [11] and that structured interviews reveal these differences more clearly.

Table 3. The domains of the SF-36 Questionnaire.

DOMAIN	NUMBER OF ITEMS	AREAS COVERED
Self-reported general health	5	Rating of own health and in comparison to other people
Physical functioning	10	Ability to walk, dress, kneel
Physical role limitations	4	Limits that health has on daily activities
Bodily pain	2	Severity and impact on daily activities
Mental health	5	Degree of happiness, nervousness or peacefulness
Emotional role limitations	3	Limits that 'emotional problems' has on daily activities
Social functioning	2	Impact of health or emotional problems on social activities
Energy	4	Incidence of feeling tired or energetic

N.B. An additional item (not a domain) relates to changes in health in comparison to one year ago.

The limitations of quality of life measurement in general is that it frequently measures an external value system derived from group data, so a total score may bear little relationship to the experience of an individual. Events do not necessarily retain the same meaning for individuals over time or the course of an illness, and the impact of any change is difficult to assess with a system that is confined to a few specific domains. Many of the quality of life analysis tools also have a 'floor' or 'ceiling' effect, i.e. limited ability to detect changes in poor or good health, and the SF-36 seems to have a 'floor' effect when used on patients with critical limb ischaemia. Physical role frequently scores the lowest possible, so any deterioration is undetected, and improvement must be marked to register a different score. Significant quality of life changes may thus go undetected. Using any quality of life analysis tool has particular problems in the elderly by virtue of the fact that their perception of their own health is often related to their peer group, and consequently their scores are usually higher than an objective observer might have anticipated. Individuals have different concepts of how their health state affects the quality of

More recently, tools have been developed in an attempt to assess patient-determined quality of life. These are few and have been developed by a variety of para-medical groups, including physiotherapists and psychologists. One such tool is the Schedule for the Evaluation of the Individual Quality of Life (SEIQoL), developed by psychologists at the Royal College of Surgeons in Ireland [12]. It is a system based on judgement analysis, and allows individuals to describe their lives in terms of the factors they consider important, and to measure how they rate those factors and their relative importance in their lives. The technique aims to highlight individuality whilst describing quality of life in terms which can be assessed critically. It overcomes some limitations of other quality of life tools by not imposing any external value system on the respondents, and also considers their change in priorities. Individuals are asked to nominate five areas (referred to as cues) in their life that they feel determine their quality of life, whether those cues have a positive or negative effect at that time. They are then asked to rate on a visual analogue scale how well each of those cues are at that time. Finally they are asked to rate the relative importance (referred to as weights) of each cue in their life at that time. The combination of cues, weights, and the score from the visual analogue scale are combined to give a profile for each individual.

Current evidence

A number of studies looking specifically at the quality of life in patients with critical limb ischaemia have been published over recent years.

A retrospective review of 112 patients using a questionnaire that included the Hospital Anxiety and Depression Scale compared the quality of life between revascularisation and amputation, and showed that those with attempted revascularisation had less impairment of social functioning, were less depressed and mobilised more, but there was no significant difference in their anxiety scores [13]. Another retrospective review of amputees compared to normal controls using the Nottingham Health Profile showed the former had lower scores in all modalities, but when they were adjusted for mobility the significance of the difference was lost, i.e. mobility was the only significant difference between the two groups [14].

A prospective study looked at the outcome in 150 patients admitted with critical limb ischaemia who were offered radiological intervention, surgical reconstruction or amputation [15]. The quality of life was measured at baseline, 6 and 12 months after intervention by a number of instruments including the Burford Pain Thermometer, the Hospital Anxiety and Depression Scale and the Barthel Activities of Daily Living Index. Postoperatively, patients who had a successful bypass procedure were more anxious than amputees, although they were less anxious than before surgery. Only those who underwent successful surgical reconstruction had an improvement in their depression scores. The Barthel Index was improved following both successful reconstruction and primary amputation, whilst those with failed limb salvage and bilateral amputees maintained their pre-operative, dependent status. All patients had an improvement in their pain scores, and this was statistically significant in all but those with a failed reconstruction. There was little difference in mobility prior to intervention between amputees or those who had revascularisation, but mobility increased significantly in the latter. Thus the improved quality of life of those undergoing successful revascularisation was largely the result of the improved mobility related to limb salvage. Given that on other quality of life scales amputees scored no worse than those who kept their limbs, those in whom mobility is not a priority may be best served by primary amputation.

It is clear that a successful infrainguinal reconstruction results in an improvement in quality of life, and this has been demonstrated succinctly using the SF-36 in a prospective comparative analysis of 55 patients treated for critical limb ischaemia [16]. All patients with patent grafts had an immediate and lasting improvement in physical function, physical role, pain and social functioning. Patients with an occluded graft had improved scores in pain, vitality and social functioning but no improvement in physical functioning or role. Those who required secondary amputation had similar improvements in pain, vitality, mental health and social functioning as those with a patent graft, and sometimes demonstrated higher scores for the psychological domains. Whilst this demonstrates that the time and expense incurred in infrainguinal reconstruction is justified for the improvement offered in quality of life, it also highlights the fact that amputees can also benefit from an improvement in their quality of life in all except physical domains. Some amputees do achieve good mobility and many others report an increase in their quality of life because of lack of pain or worries about their graft failing. These patients challenge the assumption that amputation reflects failure for the patient and surgeon.

When infrainguinal reconstruction is performed for limb salvage, the ideal of uncomplicated surgery, with the relief of pain, swift wound healing and a rapid return to pre-morbid function with no further surgery is rarely achieved. In one retrospective review [17], only 16 of 112 patients had the 'ideal' result, and this study quantified the proportion of patients attending clinic with delayed wound healing. Although persistence of symptoms is often related to the progression of disease in patients with a limited life expectancy, having a functioning graft may be less satisfying for the patient than it is for the surgeon.

Measuring the outcome of surgery with reference to the preservation of pre-morbid residential status is of value in the elderly whose only other option is often to move to a residential or nursing home, with major implications in terms of their loss of independence. When the outcome of lower limb revascularisation was measured in octogenarians, the primary and secondary graft patency rates were 72 and 87% at 5 years [18]. An arbitrary scoring system measuring ambulatory and residential status showed a reduction in both, although this mainly reflected the fact that more were walking assisted by a cane, crutch or walker. The percentage of non-walking patients remained the same, although the state of some individuals changed, such that a number of previous walkers became confined to bed or a wheelchair, whilst half of those patients who were previously non-walkers became ambulant. The residential status also deteriorated, with fewer living in their home, although a significant number, none of whom required nursing home care, chose to live with their family. The only predictor of improved postoperative function was the individual's baseline perception of their health. By implication, in patients with a poor preoperative level of functioning, arterial reconstruction as a means to preserving mobility and residential status may well not be justified.

In a review of the treatment options available in critical leg ischaemia, vascular reconstruction was recognised as the treatment of choice in most patients [19]. However, it was suggested that primary amputation should be considered in patients where the benefits of surgical reconstruction would be negligible, along with those in whom the chances of successful reconstruction would be small or those with progressive ischaemia. Identifying patients who might expect 'negligible benefit' can be difficult, although focusing on quality of life issues is likely to prove to be a useful method.

If the patients' perspective in determining their quality of life is considered, the results are likely to be more valid in assessing the impact of surgical intervention than the application of questionnaires that have been developed from studying various cross-sections of the population, healthy or otherwise. Patients who fail to mobilise or who are dependent on support from either family or social services will not necessarily fall into the 'poor outcome' group. Using a system that clearly highlights a patient's perspective can identify those who will not contemplate an amputation, whether it be for mobility or psychological reasons, whilst identifying those for whom preservation of the limb is not important for their quality of life.

Conclusions

In the future, the decision to perform revascularisation or primary amputation might be based on an analysis of what is best for the individual patient and not simply on technical feasibility. Such an analysis would be invaluable for identifying patients in whom the benefit of surgical arterial reconstruction would be negligible, based on their quality of life priorities and not the pre-conceived opinions of others.

Chapter 11

References

1. Humphreys W, Evans F, Williams T. Quality of Life: Is it a practical tool in patients with vascular disease? *J Cardiovasc Pharmcol* 1994; 23(Suppl. 3): S34-S36.
2. McWhinnie DL, Gordon AC, Collin J, Gray DWR, Morrison JD. Rehabilitation outcome 5 years after 100 lower-limb amputations. *Br J Surg* 1994; 81: 1596-1599.
3. Rosser RM, Watts VC. The management of hospital output. *Int J Epid* 1988; 361-68.
4. Humphreys WV, Evans F, Watkin G, Williams T. Critical limb ischaemia in patients over 80 years of age: options in a district general hospital. *Br J Surg* 1995; 82: 1361-1363.
5. Wade DT, Collin C. The Barthel ADL Index: a standard measure of physical disability? *Int Disabil Studies* 1988; 10: 64-67.
6. Beattie DK, Golledge J, Greenhalgh RM, Davies AH. Quality of Life Assessment in Vascular Disease: towards a Consensus. *Eur J Vasc Endovasc Surg* 1997; 13: 9-13.
7. Chetter IC, Spark JI, Dolan P, Scott DJA, Kester RC. Quality of life analysis in patients with lower limb ischaemia: suggestions for European standardisation. *Eur J Vasc Endovasc Surg* 1997; 13: 597-604.
8. Krabbe PFM, Essink-Bot M-L, Bonsel GJ. On the equivalence of collectively and individually collected responses: standard-gamble and time-tradeoff judgements of health states. *Med Decis Making* 1996; 16: 120-132.
9. Brazier JE, Walters SJ, Nicholl JP, Kohler B. Using the SF-36 and Euroqol on an elderly population. *Quality of Life Research* 1996; 5: 195-204.
10. Browne JP, O'Boyle CA, McGee HM, et al. Individual quality of life in the healthy elderly. *Quality of life Research* 1994; 3: 235-244.
11. Hill S, Harries U, Popay J. Is The short form 36 (SF-36) suitable for routine health outcomes assessment in health care for older people? Evidence from preliminary work in community based health services in England. *J Epidemiol Community Health* 1996; 50: 94-8.
12. Hickey A, Bury G, O'Boyle CA, Bradley F, O'Kelly FD, Shannon W. A new short form individual quality of life measure (SEIQoL-dw) application in a cohort of individuals with HIV/AIDS. *BMJ* 1996; 313: 29-33.
13. Thompson MM, Sayers RD, Reid A, Underwood MJ, Bell PRF. Quality of life following infragenicular bypass and lower limb amputation. *Eur J Vasc Endovasc Surg* 1995; 9: 310-13.
14. Pell JP, Donan PT, Fowkes FGR, Ruckley CV. Quality of life following lower limb amputation for peripheral arterial disease. *Eur J Vasc Surg* 1993; 7: 448-51.
15. Johnson BF, Singh S, Evans L, Drury R, Datta D, Beard JD. A prospective study on the effect of limb-threatening ischaemia and its surgical treatment on the quality of life. *Eur J Vasc Endovasc Surg* 1997; 13: 306-314.
16. Chetter IC, Spark JI, Scott DJA, Kent PJ, Berridge DC, Kester RC. Prospective analysis of quality of life in patients following infrainguinal reconstruction for chronic critical ischaemia. *Br J Surg* 1998; 85: 951-55.
17. Nicoloff AD, Taylor LM, McLafferty RB, Moneta GL, Porter JM. Patient recovery after infrainguinal bypass grafting for limb salvage. *J Vasc Surg* 1998; 27: 256-66.
18. Pomposelli FB, Arora S, Gibbons GW, et al. Lower extremity arterial reconstruction in the very elderly: successful outcome preserves not only the limb but also residential status and ambulatory function. *J Vasc Surg* 1998; 28: 215-25.
19. Sillesen H. Conservative treatment, amputation or revascularisation for critical limb ischaemia. *Ann Chir et Gynae* 1998; 87: 159-161.

Management of critical leg ischaemia:
quality of life issues

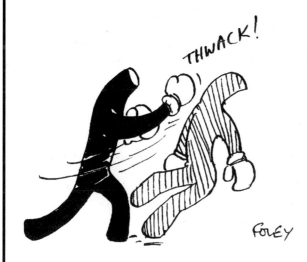

Chapter 12

Non-surgical treatment of critical ischaemia

FCT Smith
Consultant Vascular Surgeon and
Senior Lecturer

DEPARTMENT OF VASCULAR SURGERY,
BRISTOL ROYAL INFIRMARY, BRISTOL

Introduction

Critical leg ischaemia (CLI) affects approximately one in 2,500 of the population annually and carries poor long-term prognosis [1]. One year after developing CLI only 56% of patients will be alive with two legs, more than 20% will have had an amputation and 10-20% will have died from concomitant coronary or cerebrovascular disease. Surgical reconstruction with or without endovascular intervention offers the best hope of limb salvage and improved quality of life but up to 20% of patients may not be amenable to arterial reconstruction. This chapter reviews the evidence for medical and non-surgical treatments of CLI for patients in whom surgical reconstruction is not feasible.

Drug treatment

The prostanoids: the rationale

More research has been undertaken into prostanoids than any other class of drugs in the medical treatment of CLI. CLI usually occurs as a result of multi-segment arterial disease. Long-standing proximal arterial stenoses or occlusions result in vasodilation and development of collateral channels which, in CLI, progressively fail to compensate adequately for impairment of blood flow to the foot. In conjunction with disease of the larger arteries there is progressive microcirculatory impairment, largely as a result of decreased perfusion pressure. Activation of platelets and leucocytes occurs with release of growth factors, free radicals, cytokines and proteases. Vasoconstriction and endothelial cell swelling contribute to a decrease in the number of perfused capillaries. Cellular plugging of capillaries exacerbates this situation further and endothelial dysfunction is accompanied by tissue oedema. It is at this microcirculatory level that the prostanoids, which have antiplatelet, anti-leucocyte, vasodilatory and cytoprotective functions, exert their beneficial effects. Prostacyclin (PGI_2) has a short half-life of 2-3 minutes, limiting its therapeutic potential. Research has therefore concentrated on the stable prostacyclin analogue, Iloprost, which has a half-life of approximately 30 minutes. To date, Iloprost has only been available for intravascular administration, although phase three trials of an oral form have now been completed and this formulation will probably be available in the near future. PGE_1 has also been studied intensively in CLI, particularly in Germany.

Current prostanoid treatment regimens are labour intensive, involving strictly monitored intravenous infusions administered for up to 6 hours a day for several days. Gradual increases of dosage to a maximal level are titrated against vasodilatory side effects which may include facial flushing, nausea, headaches and abdominal pains. With higher doses systemic hypotension and angina may occur.

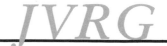

Iloprost

The effects of Iloprost in CLI have been evaluated in six large European multicentre randomised controlled studies, involving more than 700 patients with Fontaine stage III (ischaemic rest pain alone) or Fontaine stage IV (gangrene) ischaemia [2-7]. These trials have been summarised in a meta-analysis by Loosemore et al [8], and reviewed by Guilmot and Bossier [9]. Iloprost or placebo was administered intravenously at doses to a maximum of 2mg/kg/minute for 6 hours per day for the duration of each study which varied between 2 and 4 weeks. Overall, one third of patients had already undergone some previous attempt at either surgical or endovascular revascularisation. Three quarters of patients were receiving medication for heart disease and there were high prevalences of diabetes and hypertension in treatment and placebo groups in all studies. On completion of the treatment patients were judged to be responders or non-responders, according to complete pain relief in Fontaine stage III patients and healing of at least 30% of ulcer surface in patients with tissue loss (Fontaine IV). In all trials the number of responders was significantly higher in the Iloprost-treated group than in the placebo group. In each trial patients in the placebo group also improved, presumably due to the effects of adjunctive best medical treatment. Pain relief and ulcer healing have been criticised as 'soft' end-points in these trials, but in the three most recent trials the major amputation rates were also evaluated on an intention-to-treat basis [5-7]. Amputation rates were significantly lower in Iloprost-treated patients in UK and Scandinavian studies, and in all three trials analysed together by meta-analysis. In the UK and Scandinavian studies mortality or major amputation occurred in 35% of Iloprost-treated patients and in 55% of the placebo group [5,6]. The chances of a patient treated with Iloprost being alive with both legs at 6 months follow-up were significantly higher than those of a patient given placebo (P< 0.001).

Two further important studies involving Iloprost have been reported. In a European multicentre trial involving 133 patients the drug was evaluated for thromboangiitis obliterans (Buerger's Disease), against oral aspirin instead of placebo [10]. An 87% response rate occurred in the Iloprost-treated group versus a 17% response rate in the aspirin group, with benefits maintained at 6 months follow-up. Complete pain relief and ulcer healing occurred in 63% and 35% of Iloprost-treated patients, compared to 28% and 13% of the aspirin-treated group respectively. In a further trial (the Hawaii Study), involving 713 patients, in which Iloprost was used as an adjunct to healing following below knee amputation for CLI, Iloprost did not improve stump healing or re-amputation rates [11].

Prostaglandin E_1

PGE_1 suffers from a potential therapeutic disadvantage in that it is metabolised at first passage through the pulmonary circulation. Early trials therefore administered the drug by intra-arterial infusion, but this practice has largely been abandoned. In one large trial involving 267 patients that compared intravenous PGE_1 to Iloprost in patients with Fontaine IV ischaemia, there was a tendency towards increased benefit with Iloprost but this did not achieve statistical significance for survival, limb salvage, ulcer healing or relief of rest pain at 6 months [12]. Side effects occurred more frequently in the Iloprost treated group.

Other medical treatments

Conclusive evidence for benefits of other medical treatments of CLI is limited. Two drugs used extensively for treatment of claudication, naftidrofuryl (Praxilene) and pentoxifylline (Trental) have been evaluated. Microcirculatory benefits of naftidrofuryl, in terms of increased $TcpO_2$ in Fontaine III/IV patients have been reported [13,14], but in a further placebo-controlled trial in patients with rest pain, no significant clinical advantage was found in the treatment group [15]. In two multicentre (Norwegian and European) trials involving 420 patients with CLI, pentoxifylline (600 mg b.d.) or placebo was administered intravenously for up to 21 days [16,17]. Rest pain was improved by treatment in one study, but not in the other.

Other drugs used to treat CLI for which unequivocal benefits have not yet been demonstrated include antiplatelet agents, heparin, defibrinating agents (ancrod) and L-arginine, a precursor of endogenous nitric oxide (NO).

Spinal cord stimulation

Epidural Spinal Cord Stimulation (SCS) has been described as a method for the control of chronic pain and has also been employed specifically for treatment of intractable ischaemic rest pain. This technique involves conduction of low voltage electrical impulses from a pulse generator to an electrode positioned in the epidural space and thence to the spinal cord and dorsal columns. Implantation of both stimulator and electrode involves a minor surgical procedure performed under local anaesthesia and fluoroscopic control with prophylactic antibiotic cover. Stimulation produces a sensation of paraesthesia in the lower limbs, more tolerable than rest pain, and the electrode is manipulated into an optimal position for pain ablation, usually at the T10 to T12 level. The pulse generator has programmable parameters for pulse width, amplitude and frequency and these are adjusted to provide maximal pain relief using either continuous or cyclical modes. The stimulator is usually controlled by the patient using magnetic switching.

Mechanism of SCS

The proposed mechanism of pain relief is based on the pain gate theory described by Melzack and Wall in 1965. In ischaemia, both deep ischaemic and superficial pain may occur, arising from ulcers and surrounding ischaemic tissue. Nociceptive input may also be affected by neuropathy. Pain impulses are transferred by large myelinated A-type nerve fibres and C-type fibres to the cells of the substantia gelatinosa, the dorsal column fibres and to the first order communicating cells in the dorsal horn of the spinal cord. SCS induces both orthodromic and antidromic conduction of impulses. Antidromic impulses are transmitted to the dorsal horn of the spinal cord exciting the larger A-type fibres, inhibiting the first order communicating fibres and blocking nerve transmission by the smaller nociceptive C-fibres. Orthodromic impulses result in the paraesthesia perceived by the patient. Pain relief may also attenuate reflex vasoconstriction mediated through reduction in sympathetic tone, resulting in peripheral vasodilation. Roles for involvement of vasoactive neurotransmitter peptides, substance P, serotonin, vasoactive intestinal polypeptide (VIP), and other substances including prostaglandins and NO have also been proposed. However, there is a paucity of substantiative evidence supporting direct involvement of these substances as a consequence of SCS.

Uncontrolled trials of SCS

Outcome measures in uncontrolled clinical trials of SCS have concentrated principally on clinical assessments of pain reduction, healing of small ulcers and limb salvage. Ankle Doppler pressures, $TcpO_2$ readings, skin temperature recordings and capillary microscopy have been employed to detect changes in macro- and microcirculatory parameters. Ubbink and Jacobs have reviewed these trials comprehensively [18]. Claims of reduction in rest pain (60-94%), healing of ulcers less than 3cm in diameter and variable limb salvage (42-88%) over follow-up intervals ranging from less than 12 months to 4 years have been made by various authors. In most studies SCS did not increase ankle pressures. Improvements in $TcpO_2$ and skin temperature following treatment by SCS have been demonstrated in several studies, suggesting a beneficial microcirculatory effect. Further objective evidence of microcirculatory effects has been provided by Jacobs et al, who demonstrated increased capillary density and red blood cell velocity using capillary microscopy, in patients with severe ischaemia (Fontaine stage III/IV) who

responded to SCS [19]. However, the trials described above are uncontrolled. Improvements in pain scores might equally well have been achieved with analgesia or placebo treatment and quoted ranges of limb salvage in these studies are equivalent to those described in natural history studies of CLI.

Prospective randomised trials of SCS

Data from prospective randomised control trials of SCS in CLI are limited to a few principal studies. Jivegård et al randomised 26 patients with inoperable severe leg ischaemia to SCS and 25 to oral analgesic treatment in a prospective study with an 18 month follow-up [20]. No significant change in ankle brachial pressure index (ABPI), toe pressures or skin temperature occurred in either group. Using a visual analogue pain scale and semi-quantitative pain scores, significant long term pain relief occurred in the SCS group but not in the control group. At 18 months there was no significant difference in limb salvage (62% SCS versus 45% controls). However, subgroup analysis suggested significantly lower amputation rates in normotensive patients, treated by SCS. There were eight deaths in each group.

In a prospective randomised trial with one year follow-up reported by Claeys et al, patients with Fontaine stage IV ischaemia received 21 days of intravenous PGE_1 plus SCS (n = 45) or PGE_1 alone (n = 41) [21]. At 12 months total healing of foot ulcers had apparently occurred in 69% of the SCS group versus 17% of controls (P < 0.0001). Maintained increases in $TcpO_2$ were described in the SCS group, although a baseline $TcpO_2$ level of <10mmHg was found to be prognostic for poor outcome with SCS. Pain relief was reported to be significantly better in the SCS group, but there were no differences in either ABPIs or amputation rates between the two groups.

The most comprehensive data have arisen from the recent Dutch SCS Multi-centre Study Group [22]. One hundred and twenty patients with CLI (Fontaine III/IV) not suitable for vascular reconstruction were randomised to spinal cord stimulation in addition to best medical treatment or to best medical treatment alone, according to the intention-to-treat principle. Both groups were well matched, with diabetes occurring in 37% of patients. Primary outcomes were mortality and amputation, with the primary end point of limb salvage at 2 years. Median follow-up was 605 days. Some 67% of patients who had SCS were alive at the end of the study compared to 69% of controls (P = 0.96). Twenty-five major amputations were undertaken in the SCS group compared to 29 in controls (P = 0.47). The risk ratio for survival at 2 years without major amputation in the spinal cord stimulated group compared to controls was 0.96 (95% CI 0.61 - 1.51). In the SCS group, analgesic requirements were reduced, but there was no statistically significant difference in ulcer healing between the SCS group and controls. These results failed to demonstrate a significant clinical benefit for spinal cord stimulation over conservative medical treatment. Subsequent cost effectiveness studies highlighted the 26% increase in the overall cost of spinal cord stimulation over best medical treatment.

In summary, whilst spinal cord stimulation may occasionally confer benefit for an individual patient with impaired microcirculation, small ulcers or intractable rest pain, there is little unequivocal evidence to support routine use of the technique in patients with inoperable CLI.

Angiogenic revascularisation and gene therapy

Potential advantages of revascularisation of ischaemic tissue by inducing formation of new blood vessels without recourse to angioplasty or bypass are evident. Angiogenesis involves activation of quiescent vascular endothelial cells, causing sprouting of new vessels from existing ones with controlled proliferation, migration and differentiation resulting in neo-vascularisation. The feasibility of using recombinant formulations of angiogenic growth factors (including vascular endothelial growth factor [VEGF], fibroblast growth factor and platelet derived growth factor) or DNA encoding these proteins has recently been demonstrated in animal studies and early clinical trials. Isner and his colleagues first administered human plasmid DNA encoding VEGF, applied by coating an angioplasty balloon. This stimulated popliteal collateral vessel development, evident 4 weeks after gene therapy in a patient with CLI [23]. Subsequently, the same workers have employed intramuscular injections of plasmid DNA encoding phVEGF165 in an uncontrolled clinical trial involving nine patients with CLI [24]. Increases in ankle pressure indices were noted and new collateral vessel formation documented by x-ray and magnetic resonance angiography. Similar techniques have since been used to induce angiogenesis in patients with thromboangiitis obliterans (Buerger's Disease) [25]. Whilst such findings must be interpreted cautiously, recognising that therapeutic gene transfer is still in its infancy, these early clinical results herald the dawn of an exciting and novel approach to the treatment of CLI.

Conclusions

The best results of treatment of CLI are achieved by surgery alone, or in combination with endovascular intervention. Primary amputation may be a preferred option in a small subgroup of patients. The results of non-surgical treatment of CLI are largely disappointing, although administration of prostanoids or spinal cord stimulation may have a palliative role, particularly for the treatment of rest pain or small ulcers in patients with inoperable disease. Information concerning the role of oral prostanoids and the development of gene therapies are awaited.

Non-surgical treatment of critical ischaemia

Sound evidence

- Beneficial microcirculatory effects of prostanoids.

- Improvement in 'soft' clinical end points including rest pain in some patients following treatment with prostanoids or spinal cord stimulation in inoperable CLI.

Evidence needed

- Advantages of non-surgical treatment over surgical reconstruction for CLI.

- Long-term clinical improvement following non-surgical treatment of CLI.

- Improved survival following treatment with pharmacotherapy or spinal cord stimulation in CLI.

- Cost effectiveness of prostanoids or spinal cord stimulation as routine therapy in inoperable limb ischaemia.

References (randomised trials in bold)

1. Critical limb ischaemia: management and outcome. Report of a national survey. The Vascular Surgical Society of Great Britain and Ireland. *Eur J Vasc Endovasc Surg* 1995; 10: 108-13.

2. **Diehm C, Abri O, Baitsch G , et al. Iloprost a stable prostacyclin derivative, in stage 4 arterial occlusive disease. A placebo-controlled multicenter study. *Deutsch Med Wochenschr* 1989; 114: 783-788.**

3. **Brock FE, Abri O, Baitsch G, et al. Iloprost in the treatment of ischemic tissue lesions in diabetics. Results of a placebo-controlled multicenter study with a stable prostacyclin derivative. *Schweiz Med Wochenschr* 1990; 120: 1477-1482.**

4. **Balzer K, Bechara G, Bisler H, et al. Reduction of ischaemic rest pain in advanced peripheral arterial occlusive disease. A double blind placebo controlled trial with iloprost. *Int Angiol* 1991; 10: 229-232.**

5. **Norgren L, Alwmark A, Angqvist KA, et al. A stable prostacyclin analogue (iloprost) in the treatment of ischaemic ulcers of the lower limb. A Scandinavian-Polish placebo controlled, randomised multicenter study. *Eur J Vasc Surg* 1990; 4: 463-467.**

6. **U.K. Severe Limb Ischaemia Study Group. Treatment of limb threatening ischaemia with intravenous iloprost: a randomised double blind placebo controlled study. *Eur J Vasc Surg* 1991; 5: 511-516.**

7. **Guilmot JL, Diot E. Treatment of lower limb ischaemia due to atherosclerosis in diabetic and nondiabetic patients with iloprost, a stable analogue of prostacyclin. Results of a French multicenter trial. *Drug invest* 1991; 3: 351-359.**

8. Loosemore TM, Chalmers TC, Dormandy JA. A meta-analysis of randomized placebo control trials in Fontaine stages III and IV peripheral occlusive arterial disease. *Int Angiol* 1994; 13: 133-142.

9. Guilmot JL, Boissier C. Medical treatment with Prostanoids in patients with critical ischaemia. *Critical Limb Ischaemia* (Eds Branchereau A, Jacobs M). Futura Publishing Co. 1999; 9: 63-68.

10. **Fiessinger JN, Schafer M. Trial of iloprost versus aspirin treatment for critical limb ischaemia of thromboangiitis obliterans. The TAO study. *Lancet* 1990; 335: 555-557.**

11. **Dormandy J, Belcher G, Broos P, et al. Prospective study of 713 below-knee amputations for ischaemia and the effect of a prostacyclin analogue on healing. Hawaii Study Group. *Br J Surg* 1994; 81: 33-7.**

12. **Alstaedt HO, Berzewski B, Breddin HK et al. Treatment of patients with peripheral arterial occlusive disease Fontaine stage IV with intravenous iloprost and PGE$_1$: a randomized open controlled study. *Prostaglandins Leukot Essent Fatty Acids* 1993; 49: 573-578.**

13. Abendroth D, Sunder-Plassman L. Einfluss einer intra-venosen naftidrofurylbehandlung auf die Mikrozirkulation von Patienten im Stadium III und IV einer peripheren arteriellen Verschlusskrankheit. *VASA* 1988; Suppl 24: 33-37.

14. Horsch S. Uber den Einsatz von naftidrofuryl im Stadium III/IV einer peripher arteriellen Verschlusskrankheit. *VASA* 1988; Suppl 24: 38-43.

15. **Greenhalgh RM. Naftidrofuryl for ischemic rest pain: A controlled trial. *Br J Surg* 1981; 68: 265-6.**

16. **Intravenous pentoxifylline for the treatment of chronic critical limb ischaemia. The European Study Group. *Eur J Vasc Endovasc Surg* 1995; 9: 426-436.**

17. **Efficacy and clinical tolerance of parenteral pentoxifylline in the treatment of critical lower limb ischemia. A placebo controlled multicenter study. The Norwegian Pentoxifylline Multicenter Trial Group. *Int Angiol* 1996; 15: 75-80.**

18. Ubbink DT, Jacobs MJHM. Spinal cord stimulation in critical limb ischaemia. *Critical Limb Ischaemia* (Eds Branchereau A, Jacobs M). 1999; 11: 75-84.

19. Jacobs MJ, Jorning PJ, Beckers RC, et al. Foot salvage and improvement of microvascular blood flow as a result of epidural spinal cord electrical stimulation. *J Vasc Surg* 1990; 12: 354-360.

20. **Jivegard LEH, Augustinsson LE, Holm J, Risberg B, Ortenwall P. Effects of spinal cord stimulation (SCS) in patients with inoperable severe lower limb ischaemia: a prospective randomised controlled study. *Eur J Vasc Endovasc Surg* 1995; 9: 421-425.**

21. Claeys LG, Horsch S. Transcutaneous oxygen pressure as predictive parameter for ulcer healing in end-stage vascular patients treated with spinal cord stimulation. *Inter angio* 1996; 15: 344-349.

22. **Klomp HM, Spincemaille GH, Steyerberg EW, Habbema JD, van Urk H. Spinal-cord stimulation in critical limb ischaemia: a randomised trial. ESES Study Group. *Lancet* 1999 Mar 27; 353: 1040-4.**

23. Isner JM, Pieczek A, Schainfeld R, et al. Clinical evidence of angiogenesis after arterial gene transfer of phVEGF165 in patient with ischaemic limb. *Lancet* 1996 348: 370-4.

24. Baumgartner I, Pieczek A, Manor O, et al. Constitutive expression of phVEGF165 after intramuscular gene transfer promotes collateral vessel development in patients with critical limb ischemia. *Circulation* 1998 ; 97: 1114-23.

25. Isner JM, Baumgartner I, Rauh G, et al. Treatment of thromboangiitis obliterans (Buerger's disease) by intramuscular gene transfer of vascular endothelial growth factor: preliminary clinical results. *J Vasc Surg* 1998; 28: 964-73.

Non-surgical treatment of critical ischaemia

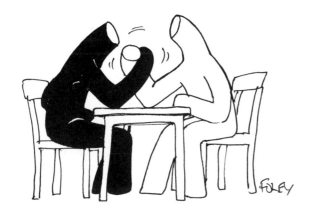

Chapter 13

Treatment of acute leg ischaemia

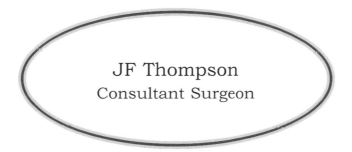

JF Thompson
Consultant Surgeon

DEPARTMENT OF SURGERY,
ROYAL DEVON AND EXETER HOSPITAL, EXETER

Introduction

Acute lower limb ischaemia is a surgical emergency, caused by embolic occlusion or in-situ thrombosis of either a native vessel, or pre-existing bypass graft. Rarely, thrombophilia, a hypercoagulable state, drugs, trauma or radiation may cause thrombosis. Thrombosis may also be a pre-morbid event, which in part explains the high mortality rate found in most series.

Emboli associated with valvular or ischaemic heart disease may lodge at the common femoral artery bifurcation or popliteal trifurcation. In the absence of collateral vessels, the ensuing ischaemia is profound, resulting in the classical presentation of a pale, paralysed, pulseless, paraesthetic and perishing cold limb. Ischaemia caused by thrombosis is more insidious.

Over the last 20 years there has been a change in the spectrum of disease. Pure emboli are rarer, due to a fall in the incidence of rheumatic heart disease and an increase in the use of anticoagulation for the treatment of atrial fibrillation. Thrombosis, on the other hand, is more common in an ageing population with peripheral vascular disease, diabetes and previous vascular reconstructions.

Historical perspective

In 1963, Thomas Fogarty introduced the balloon embolectomy catheter but, despite its use, death or amputation rates still remained at 10-20% and 20-40%

respectively [1,2]. In 1997, the Swedish national vascular registry reported 1054 acute ischaemic episodes, with 44% treated by thromboembolectomy, 31% with lysis (at least initially), 7% with distal bypass and the rest by graft revision. Thirty-day reocclusion and mortality rates were 9% and 15% for emboli and 24% and 14% for thromboses [3].

In 1978, Blaisdell proposed early heparinisation to prevent further clot propagation with delayed intervention by either bypass grafting or amputation. He suggested that this might save lives at the expense of a higher rate of limb loss [4]. Aspirin decreases the incidence of secondary vascular events in patients with arterial disease [5]; heparin and aspirin are now the accepted minimum treatment for acute ischaemia, but additional intervention is often required.

Balloon embolectomy under local anaesthetic is the gold standard for the pure embolus. Ideal candidates should have a good source for putative emboli, such as atrial fibrillation, a short history and relatively normal vessels, suggested by palpable pulses or clear biphasic Doppler signals in the normal limb. Local anaesthetic is important to avoid cardiac morbidity, particularly if a myocardial infarction was the underlying problem. Full anaesthetic monitoring is required during the operation and the whole leg should be prepared for surgery. If the result is disappointing angiography, on table lysis or angioscopy can be useful, although their true value is as yet unproven [6].

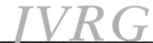

Table 1. Algorithm for the treatment of acute lower limb ischaemia [8].

Ischaemic Class	Heparin	Treatment	Angiogram	Additional intervention
I	Yes	None	Elective	None
IIa	Yes	Thrombolysis	Urgent	If causative lesion identified
IIb	Yes	Surgery	On table	If causative lesion identified
III	Yes	Delayed amputation	-	-

Unfortunately, this relatively straightforward situation, is rare. Many patients have pre-existing vascular disease and associated cardiac, renal and pulmonary dysfunction. An experienced initial assessment by a vascular specialist is vital to plan a strategy, which will often involve angiography, percutaneous thrombolysis, angioplasty or reconstructive surgery. Extra-anatomic bypass or distal grafting may be required. It is clear that the patient with acute leg ischaemia is best managed in a specialist unit [7].

The severity of ischaemia - what can wait?

In practice, very few legs need immediate intervention but it takes experience to judge which patients can wait overnight. It is important to stratify treatment according to the severity of the initial ischaemia. The Society for Vascular Surgery/International Society of Cardiovascular Surgery (SVS/ISCVS) grading system is widely accepted.

Class I ischaemia denotes a viable leg, without impairment of sensory or motor function and audible Doppler signals. Heparin is given and elective treatment, either conservative or interventional, is arranged.

Class IIa legs are marginally threatened with symptoms limited to a mild sensory loss (usually in the toes). A delay of seven to nine hours is acceptable to attempt treatment by lysis.

Class IIb legs are immediately at risk with pronounced sensory loss, mild to moderate motor loss, but audible Doppler signals. Delay is unacceptable and urgent clot extraction by aspiration or embolectomy is required. Accelerated thrombolysis may be used.

Class III legs have absent Doppler flow, paralysis, total sensory loss and irreversible tissue damage. Attempts to restore blood flow would lead to hyperkalaemia and myoglobinuria, so delayed amputation should be performed after resuscitation.

Treatment strategies based on the SVS/ISCVS grading system are summarised in Table 1.

The role of thrombolysis

The introduction of thrombolysis revolutionized the treatment of myocardial infarction. Vascular surgeons had great hopes that it would have a similar role in the management of peripheral ischaemia. After mixed success with systemic therapy, which had a high complication rate, locally directed treatment with more fibrin specific agents was introduced [9]. Thrombolysis has potential advantages over surgical methods. It is less invasive, less likely to dislodge atheromatous plaques or rupture vessels, and is capable of clearing smaller run off vessels to improve patency (Figure 1)[10].

The age of the clot is important. Whereas pure emboli can be treated using lysis as sole therapy, treatment of an in-situ thrombosis often unmasks the lesion leading to the occlusion, such as a high grade atheromatous stenosis. Such lesions may require further treatment with angioplasty or stenting if they are short, or by bypass grafting if they are longer. As a result of this many would consider lysis to be pharmacological procrastination. After early enthusiasm there has been a fall in the number of patients treated by lysis.

The Working Party on Thrombolysis have made 30 recommendations regarding the objectives, indications, type of agent, monitoring and complications of this treatment [6]. The primary end point is amputation-free survival of the patient, but several surrogate end-points

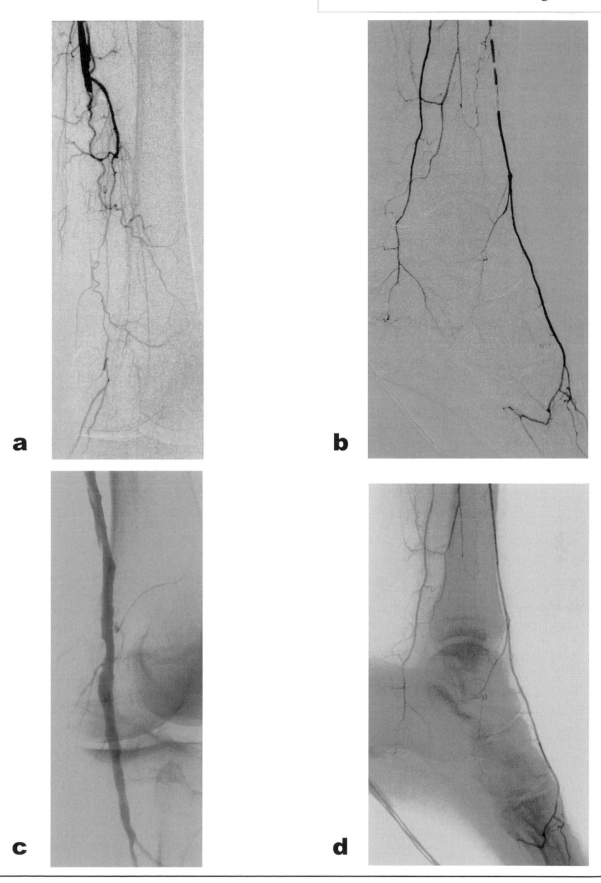

Figure 1. Intra-arterial thrombolysis. (a) Angiogram showing acute left superficial femoral artery occlusion, treated with low dose tissue plasminogen activator, 1mg/h. As the artery recanalised a mid-superficial femoral artery stenosis was revealed and treated by balloon angioplasty. (b) This caused distal embolisation into the anterior tibial artery. (c) Continued lysis for 6h resulted in patency of the femoropopliteal segment. (d) The anterior tibial artery was also cleared.

are described. There are very few data to compare dose regimens between agents. High doses are dangerous, but an initial bolus followed by an infusion is popular. Accepted dose rates are:

Tissue plasminogen activator - 1.0 mg/h
Urokinase - 240,000 IU/h for 4h then 120,000IU/h
Streptokinase - 5000 IU/h

Heparin should be given to prevent catheter-related thrombosis and aspirin improves the results of lysis. What is remarkable from the literature is the consistency of results, regardless of the agent or dose. Complication rates are also consistent, with a stroke rate of 1.2-2.1% in the STILE and TOPAS studies (see below). Clearly this is an effective but potentially dangerous treatment.

Indications for lysis

The risk of stroke or death mitigates strongly against lysis for the treatment of intermittent claudication. It is ineffective for the treatment of atheroembolus (trash) or stable ischaemia. Specific contraindications have been defined (Table 2).

Table 2. Contraindications for lysis

Absolute
- **Established cerebrovascular event within two months**
- **Active bleeding diathesis**
- **Recent gastrointestinal bleeding**
- **Neurosurgery within 3 months**
- **Intracranial trauma within 3 months**

Major
- **Cardiopulmonary resuscitation within 10 days**
- **Major surgery or trauma in the last 10 days**
- **Uncontrolled hypertension**
- **Puncture of uncontrollable vessel**
- **Intracranial tumour**
- **Recent eye surgery**

Minor
- **Hepatic failure**
- **Endocarditis**
- **Pregnancy**
- **Diabetic haemorrhagic retinopathy**

Several small studies have shown lysis to be effective in the treatment of thrombosed popliteal aneurysms, where it can be used to clear in-situ thrombosis of the run-off vessels [11]. It is also used to treat the complications of endovascular treatment such as thrombosis at an angioplasty site. The literature suggests that thrombolysis has a limited role in the resurrection of failed bypass grafts [12] unless the thrombotic occlusion is fresh (less than two weeks old). Secondary patency rates are disappointing, and revisional surgery is usually required to deal with the underlying defect. Surgical thrombectomy or replacement of the graft, if required on clinical grounds, is recommended.

Lysis may be attempted in patients with SVS/ISCVS grade IIa ischaemia, if there is time. In clinical practice the 'guide-wire' test is used. If a guide wire passes through the lesion or at least part of it, soft thrombus is present and lysis is worth trying. Complications may arise following lysis, especially if the patient is female and over 80 years of age [13]. The fresher the clot, the better the result.

Thrombolysis versus surgery

Unfortunately, randomized studies comparing surgery with lysis have been inconclusive. In a severely ischaemic group of patients there was a greater mortality in patients who had initial surgery, but no difference in limb salvage [14]. There were no differences in mortality and amputation between the lysis and surgical patients in the 392 patients included in the STILE (Surgery versus Thrombolysis for Ischaemia of the Lower Extremity) study, but this study contained large numbers of patients who presented late [15]. Post hoc analysis of surrogate end points, such as death and amputation, haemorrhage and perioperative complications, favoured surgery. Recurrent ischaemia was more common in the lysis group. When recent occlusions (<14 days) were considered separately, fewer amputations were reported in the patients who had lysis.

In the TOPAS (Thrombolysis or Peripheral Arterial Surgery) study, amputation and mortality rates were similar at discharge and at one year follow-up [16]. Although the STILE and TOPAS studies both claimed better results for graft occlusions compared to native vessel occlusions, adjuvant procedures were usually required to maintain patency.

Although it seems sensible, there are no data to support the use of long term anticoagulation after successful lysis unless atrial fibrillation was the cause.

New techniques

Clot aspiration, mechanical clot dissolving devices, and jet disrupters, alone or combined with thrombolysis have been reported [17,18]. Angioscopy has been used as an adjunct to both embolectomy and lysis, and intraoperative lysis has been used successfully to dissolve run-off thrombosis. Continuous postoperative infusion of lytic substances is associated with a high complication rate and cannot be recommended.

Conclusions

Successful management of acute leg ischaemia depends on accurate initial assessment stratification based on the severity of the ischaemia and selection of the appropriate treatment. This may be medical, surgical, or radiological and often involves a multi-disciplinary approach. The future organisation of vascular services should continue to reflect this approach.

Treatment of acute leg ischaemia

Sound evidence

- **All patients with acute limb ischaemia should receive aspirin and intravenous heparin (and probably oxygen and intravenous rehydration).**

- **The main cause of death in this group of patients is myocardial infarction. Appropriate medical and anaesthetic precautions are required.**

- **Patients should be stratified according to the severity of their ischaemia.**

- **Local anaesthetic balloon embolectomy is a safe and effective treatment for recent arterial emboli.**

- **Thrombolysis is useful to unmask the causative lesion but further intervention is frequently required.**

Evidence needed

- **A comparison of surgery or thrombolysis in the treatment of SVS/ISCVS grade IIa ischaemia of less than 14 days duration.**

- **Prospective trials of adjunctive lysis in the treatment of thrombosed popliteal aneurysm.**

- **The role of lysis in the failed bypass graft.**

Chapter 13

References (randomised trials in bold)

1. Earnshaw JJ, Hopkinson BR, Makin GS. Acute critical ischaemia of the limb: a prospective evaluation. *Eur J Vasc Surg* 1991; 4: 365-8.
2. Ericsson I, Holmberg JT Analysis of factors affecting limb salvage and mortality after arterial embolectomy. *Acta Chir Scand* 1977; 143: 237-40.
3. Jivegard L, Wingren U. Management of acute limb ischaemia over two decades: The Swedish experience. *Eur J Vasc Endovasc Surg* 1999; 18: 93-95.
4. Blaisdell FW, Steele M, Allen RF. Management of acute lower extremity ischaemia due to embolism and thrombosis. *Surgery* 1978; 84: 822-34.
5. Antiplatelet Trialists' Collaboration. Collaborative overview of randomised trials of antiplatelet treatment. Part 1: prevention of death, myocardial infarction and stroke by prolonged antiplatelet therapy in various categories of patients. *Br Med J* 1994; 308: 81-106.
6. Working party on thrombolysis in the management of lower limb ischaemia: Thrombolysis in the management of lower limb peripheral arterial occlusion - a consensus document. *Am J Cardiol* 1998; 81: 207-218.
7. Campbell WB, Ridler BMF, Szymanska TH. Current management of acute leg ischaemia: results of an audit by the Vascular Surgical Society of Great Britain and Ireland. *Br J Surg* 1998; 85: 1498-1503.
8. Rutherford RB, Flannigan DP, Gupta SK et al. Suggested standards for reports dealing with acute lower limb ischaemia. *J Vasc Surg* 1986; 4; 80-94.
9. Marder VJ. The use of thrombolytic agents: choice of patient, drug administration, laboratory monitoring. *Ann Internal Med* 1979; 90: 802-812.
10. Earnshaw JJ. Thrombolysis in acute limb ischaemia. *Ann R Coll Surg Engl* 1994; 76: 219-22.
11. Thompson JF, Beard J, Scott DJA, Baird RN, Earnshaw JJ. Intraoperative thrombolysis in the management of thrombosed popliteal aneurysms. *Br J Surg* 1993; 80: 858-9.
12. Lacroix H, Suy R, Nevelsteen A, et al. Local thrombolysis for occluded arterial grafts: is the yield worth the effort? *J Cardiovasc Surg* 1994; 35: 187-191.
13. Braithwaite BD, Davies B, Birch PA, Heather BP, Earnshaw JJ. Management of acute leg ischaemia in the elderly. *Br J Surg* 1998; 85: 217-20.
14. **Ouriel K, Shortell CK, DeWeese JA, et al. A comparison of thrombolytic therapy with operative revascularisation in the treatment of acute peripheral arterial ischaemia. *J Vasc Surg* 1994; 19: 1021-30.**
15. **The STILE investigators. Results of a prospective randomised trial; evaluating surgery versus thrombolysis for ischaemia of the lower extremity. The STILE trial. *Ann Surg* 1994; 220: 251-68.**
16. **Ouriel K, Veith F, Sasahara AA for the TOPAS investigators. A comparison of recombinant urokinase with vascular surgery as initial treatment for acute arterial occlusion of the legs. *N Eng J Med* 1998; 338: 1105-11.**
17. Fogarty T, Monofort S, Hermann C. New techniques and instrumentation for the management of adherent clot in native and synthetic vessels. *Curr Surg* 1991; 48: 123-6.
18. Overbosch E, Pattynama P, Aarts J, et al. Occluded haemodialysis shunts; Dutch multicentre experience with the hydrolysor catheter. *Radiology* 1996; 201: 485-8.

Chapter 14

The case for screening for abdominal aortic aneurysm

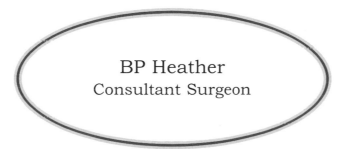

BP Heather
Consultant Surgeon

DEPARTMENT OF SURGERY,
GLOUCESTERSHIRE ROYAL HOSPITAL, GLOUCESTER

Ruptured abdominal aortic aneurysm (AAA) accounts for approximately 10,000 deaths annually in the UK [1] and there is evidence that there is an increasing incidence of the condition [2,3]. While some of the recorded deaths occur in the extremely elderly, many are seen in patients in the sixth and seventh decades of life, when such a death represents loss of considerable potential years of life. Mortality rates of between 5% and 8% are routinely reported for elective AAA repair, with a few centres claiming even better results [4,5]. In contrast, there is little evidence of any significant improvement in the outcome for surgery on ruptured aneurysms where the overall community mortality remains in excess of 80%. Improvements in surgical, anaesthetic and postoperative techniques do not appear to have produced the same benefits in outcome for ruptured aneurysms as they have for elective cases [6-9]. The reported variations in mortality after surgery for ruptured AAA probably owe more to differences in referral patterns and case selection than to treatment techniques.

The large difference in outcome between elective and emergency surgery strongly suggests that overall mortality from this condition could be reduced by an increase in the number of elective operations performed. The wider use of diagnostic ultrasound and, to a lesser extent, increased public and medical awareness of the condition, have probably produced a small increase in the incidental discovery of AAA. However, large numbers of aneurysms still remain undiagnosed and asymptomatic until they rupture: logically, the only way in which this situation can be improved is by a deliberate policy of widespread screening of the at-risk population. One randomised trial in the UK has already suggested a survival advantage in men offered screening for asymptomatic aneurysm. In 1995, Scott et al published data from the Chichester area, which showed a small but significant reduction in both the incidence of aneurysm rupture and overall aneurysm-related deaths in a group of 3205 men offered aneurysm screening, compared to a control group without screening [10]. A much larger multicentre randomised trial of aneurysm screening has now started in the south and east of England, but results from this are not expected until at least the year 2001. Nevertheless, before large scale population screening for AAA can be recommended in the context of the UK's National Health Service, fundamental questions must be answered.

Practical considerations

- Can aneurysms be detected easily and reliably?
- Does increased detection result in increased and appropriate elective operations?
- Does an increase in elective operations result in an overall reduction in aneurysm related mortality?

Financial and resource issues

- Are there sufficient funds and physical resources to carry out the screening and deal with additional workload?
- How does aneurysm screening compare with other ways in which we might use limited health care resources?

JVRG

The case for screening for abdominal aortic aneurysm

Table 1 summarises the organisation of a screening programme for asymptomatic AAA which has been running in Gloucestershire, UK since 1990 [11,12]. From a total county population of 520,000, men reaching the age of 65 years of age are invited to undergo an abdominal ultrasound scan, which is carried out by a mobile team visiting each of the county's 98 general practice premises on an annual basis. Men who were older than 65 when the programme started in 1990 were not included. This

diameters in the range 2.6 cm to 3.9 cm. These figures demonstrate that population screening by abdominal ultrasonography is capable of detecting very significant numbers of unsuspected aneurysms at reasonable cost. Perhaps even more important is the fact that 95% of men aged 65 have aortic diameters below 2.6 cm. A local study has demonstrated that these men can be almost entirely excluded from the risk of development of a significant aneurysm in the future on the basis of a single

Table 1. The organisation of Gloucestershire's aneurysm screening programme.

- **mobile team - nurse co-ordinator, radiographer, portable ultrasound scanner**
- **annual visit to each participating general practice**
- **invite each year's batch of new 65 year old men**
- **patients selected by general practice from age/sex register**
- **detailed information sheets for all patients**
- **aortic diameter <2.6cm - reassured, discharged**
- **aortic diameter 2.6 to 3.9cm - rescan in practice next year**
- **aortic diameter >3.9cm - refer to vascular surgeon**

has resulted in a steadily enlarging cohort of men offered screening. By the end of 1998, the original 65 year olds had reached the age of 73, and all men in the county between the ages of 65 and 73 had been offered the opportunity of an ultrasound scan.

Table 2. Summary of aneurysm screening in Gloucestershire 1990-98.

- **25,000 ultrasound invitations**
- **85% attendance**
- **costs approx £10 per scan**
- **99% imaging success**
- **1% of aortas >4cm diameter**

Table 2 shows an encouragingly high acceptance rate for the screening examination, probably because the programme is based in the more familiar surroundings of the general practice surgery rather than a hospital. Costs per scan are significantly below those in a hospital based ultrasound department and adequate visualisation of the abdominal aorta can be obtained in the vast majority of patients; very few require a repeat ultrasound or computed tomography for clarification. The prevalence of aortic diameter in excess of 4.0 cm is approximately 1% at the initial scan in this age group [13], and the subsequent detection rate of aneurysms above this size is at least doubled by the annual follow-up of men with aortic

scan, drastically reducing the costs of population screening by eliminating the need for further examinations [14].

The gradual introduction of aneurysm screening, by examining only new 65 year olds each year, has avoided sudden workload pressures, and the total number of aneurysm operations performed each year in the county has increased only gradually since 1990. Figure 1 demonstrates quite clearly, however, that a much greater proportion of time is now spent in performing elective surgery on aneurysms discovered in the screening programme, compared to emergency cases or those elective cases discovered incidentally.

In order to measure any beneficial effect of aneurysm screening and increased elective surgical activity, it is necessary to consider the total aneurysm-related mortality in a defined community. The figure for Gloucestershire may be calculated by including:

- all deaths outside hospital in which ruptured AAA was recorded as the cause of death, using hospital post-mortem records and the heath authority's computerised records of death certificates (available for 1994 onwards),
- all deaths in the county's hospitals caused by ruptured AAA, with or without surgery,
- all deaths following elective AAA repair.

Figure 2 shows the total aneurysm-related mortality for the county for each year from 1994 to 1998, with deaths in the 65 to 73 year old age group shown separately from

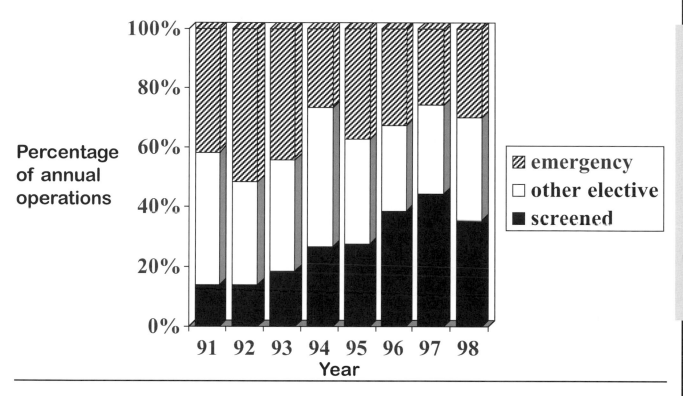

Figure 1. Proportions of aneurysm surgery categories in Gloucestershire.

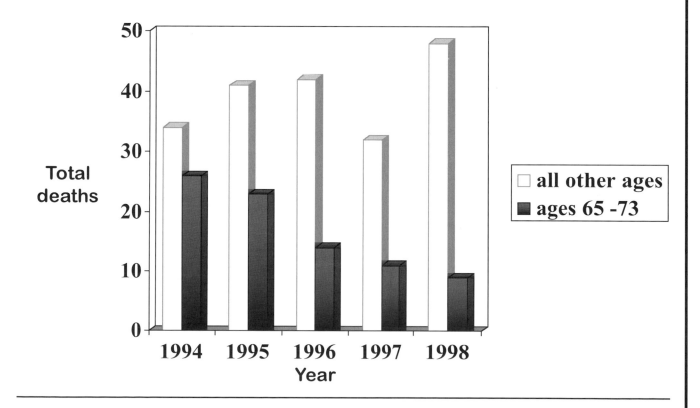

Figure 2. Total aneurysm related mortality in Gloucestershire.

The case for screening for abdominal aortic aneurysm

all other ages. The screening programme has encroached progressively on the 65 to 73 year old group during the period studied and a year by year reduction in total deaths related to AAA has been clearly noted. No such change in mortality has been observed in the age group outside the scope of the screening programme. In fact, there seems to be a trend towards a larger number of deaths in this group, possibly reflecting increased awareness of the condition amongst general practitioners. These data may be regarded as strong evidence that the screening programme has reduced overall deaths from aortic aneurysm, with the inevitable small increase in elective surgical mortality more than compensated by a larger reduction in the incidence of aneurysm rupture. The majority of aneurysm ruptures observed in the age group offered screening have occurred in the 15% of patients who did not attend their original screening invitation, emphasising the vital importance of maximising attendance rates in this or any other screening programme.

The absence, until recently, of good clinical evidence for any benefit of aneurysm screening has meant that discussions of cost/benefit have inevitably been based on theoretical calculations of possible outcomes in various groups of the population with and without screening. While such calculations are relatively easy to set up, they rely entirely on accurate data about aneurysm prevalence, growth rates, rupture risk at various sizes and operative mortality. It can be shown that relatively small changes in assumptions made in these calculations, in the absence of firm data, can have a major influence on the conclusions reached, with calculated results varying from significant benefit to clear financial and clinical disadvantage from aneurysm screening [15-18]. When calculations of cost per quality adjusted life year (QALY) gained by aneurysm screening have been made, these have ranged from £450 to £1500 [15,19], both figures are very significantly less than the cost per added QALY quoted for breast cancer screening (over £4000) [20]. It is to be hoped that accumulating data from the Gloucester and other studies will rapidly render such theoretical models redundant.

A population screening programme for AAA will inevitably result in the discovery of a number of small aneurysms and slightly enlarged aortas which are not of immediate clinical significance. Local figures on aortic size distribution at the age of 65 suggest a 5% prevalence of aorta diameter > 2.6 cm, 2.5% of > 3.0 cm and only 1% of > 4.0 cm. Clearly it would be a mistake to equate the discovery of small aneurysms with the repair of small aneurysms, particularly when the current trend seems to be towards a slightly more conservative approach regarding the size at which elective AAA repair is indicated [21,22]. Maximum benefit to the community can only be achieved by a combination of a screening programme to detect aortic abnormalities and elective repair of those aneurysms for which the risk of rupture greatly exceeds the risk of elective surgery.

Concern has been expressed that the discovery of a previously unsuspected AAA may result in unnecessary anxiety for the patient, particularly if elective repair is not performed. This has certainly not been my experience [23]. Carefully written information sheets, backed up by detailed explanation from the surgeon, can alleviate anxiety in the great majority of patients, who feel relieved that a potential problem has been discovered and is being carefully monitored. The discovery by screening of a large aneurysm in a patient who is manifestly unfit for elective repair remains a worrying problem, which might be avoided to some extent by the initial filtering of patients by their family doctor to exclude those obviously unfit for surgery. However, it should be borne in mind that the commonest cause of death in patients with large aneurysms, whose medical condition is thought to preclude elective surgery, is still rupture of the aneurysm [24-26]. Endovascular aneurysm repair may provide a suitable option for some of these medically unfit, high risk patients, and there may well be an argument for the acceptance of a higher surgical risk in such patients, even at the cost of some increase in operative mortality figures.

Overall, evidence is accumulating to support the wide adoption of aneurysm screening in men of 65 years and over. AAA is ideally suited to detection by a quick, harmless, relatively inexpensive and highly reliable test. Provided that such detection is combined with careful follow-up and thoughtful selection of appropriate cases for elective repair, a substantial reduction in premature deaths from aneurysm rupture will follow.

References (randomised trials in bold)

1. Office of Population Censuses and Surveys, *Mortality Statistics, England and Wales* London: HMSO, 1989.

2. Fowkes FGC, MacIntyre CCA, Ruckley CV. Increasing incidence of aortic aneurysms in England and Wales. *Br Med J* 1989; 298: 33-35.

3. Melton LJ, Bickerstaff LK, Hollier LH et al. Changing incidence of abdominal aortic aneurysms. A population based study. *Am J Epidemiol* 1984; 120: 379-386.

4. Veith FJ, Goldsmith J, Leather RP, Hannan EL. The need for quality assurance in vascular surgery. *J Vasc Surg* 1991; 13: 523-526.

5. Akkersdijk GJ, van de Graaf Y, Van Bockel JH, Eikelboom BC. Mortality rates associated with operative treatment of infrarenal abdominal aortic aneurysms in the Netherlands. *Br J Surg* 1994; 81: 706-709.

6. Bengtsson H, Bergqvist D. Ruptured abdominal aortic aneurysm: a population based study. *J Vasc Surg* 1993; 18: 74-80.

7. Mealy K, Salman A. The true incidence of ruptured abdominal aortic aneurysms. *Eur J Vasc Surg* 1988; 2: 405-408.

8. Johansson G, Swedenborg J. Ruptured abdominal aortic aneurysms: a study of incidence and mortality. *Br J Surg* 1986; 73: 101-103.

9. Katz DJ, Stanley JC, Zelenock GB. Operative mortality rates for intact and ruptured abdominal aortic aneurysms in Michigan: an 11 year statewide experience. *J Vasc Surg* 1994; 19: 804-815.

10. **Scott RA, Wilson NM, Ashton HA, Kay DN. Influence of screening on the incidence of ruptured abdominal aortic aneurysm: 5 year results of a randomized controlled study. *Br J Surg* 1995; 82: 1066-1070.**

11. O'Kelly TJ, Heather BP. General practice based population screening for abdominal aortic aneurysms: a pilot study. *Br J Surg* 1989; 76: 479-480.

12. Lucarotti M, Shaw E, Poskitt K, Heather B. The Gloucestershire aneurysm screening programme: the first 2 years experience. *Eur J Vasc Surg* 1993; 7: 397-401.

13. Lucarotti ME, Shaw E, Heather BP. Distribution of aortic diameter in a screened male population. *Br J Surg* 1992; 79: 641-642.

14. Emerton ME, Shaw E, Poskitt K, Heather BP. Screening for abdominal aortic aneurysm: a single scan is enough. *Br J Surg* 1994; 81: 1112-1113.

15. St Leger AS, Spencely M, McCollum CN, Moss M. Screening for abdominal aortic aneurysm: a computer assisted cost-utility analysis. *Eur J Vasc Endovasc Surg* 1996; 11: 183-190.

16. Mason JM, Wakeman AP, Drummond MF, Crump BJ. Population screening for abdominal aortic aneurysm: do the benefits outweigh the costs? *J Pub Health Med* 1993; 15: 154-160.

17. Russell JG. Is screening for abdominal aortic aneurysm worthwhile? *Clin Radiol* 1990; 41: 182-184.

18. Frame PS, Fryback DG, Patterson C. Screening for abdominal aortic aneurysm in men aged 60 to 80 years. A cost-effectiveness analysis. *Ann Intern Med* 1993; 119: 411-416.

19. Collin J. The value of screening for abdominal aortic aneurysm by ultrasound. In: Greenhalgh RM, Mannick JA Eds. *The cause and management of aneurysms.* London: Saunders, 1990.

20. Blamey RW, Hardcastle JD. The early detection of cancer. In: Russell RCG, Ed. *Recent advances in surgery* (12). Edinburgh: Churchill Livingstone, 1986.

21. **The UK Small Aneurysm Trial Participants. Mortality results for a randomised controlled trial of early elective surgery or ultrasonographic surveillance for small abdominal aortic aneurysms. *Lancet* 1998; 352: 1649-1655.**

22. Scott RA, Tisi PV, Ashton HA, Allen DR. Abdominal aortic aneurysm rupture rates: a 7 year follow-up of the entire abdominal aortic aneurysm population detected by screening. *J Vasc Surg* 1998; 28: 124-128.

23. Lucarotti ME, Heather BP, Shaw E, Poskitt KR. Psychological morbidity associated with abdominal aortic aneurysm screening. *Eur J Vasc Endovasc Surg* 1998; 14: 499-501.

24. Jones A, Cahill D, Gardham R. Outcome in patients with a large abdominal aortic aneurysm considered unfit for surgery. *Br J Surg* 1998; 85: 1382-1384.

25. Szilagyi DE, Elliott JP, Smith RF. Clinical fate of the patient with asymptomatic abdominal aortic aneurysm and unfit for surgical treatment. *Arch Surg* 1972; 104: 600-606.

26. Englund R, Perera D, Hanel KC. Outcome for patients with abdominal aortic aneurysms that are treated non-surgically. *Aus NZ J Surg* 1997; 67: 260-263.

The case for screening for abdominal aortic aneurysm

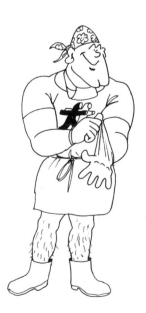

Chapter 15

The case against screening for abdominal aortic aneurysm

J Collin
Consultant Surgeon and
Reader in Surgery

THE NUFFIELD DEPARTMENT OF SURGERY,
THE JOHN RADCLIFFE HOSPITAL, OXFORD

Screening for abdominal aortic aneurysm (AAA) was first suggested in 1985 [1]. Subsequently, many local screening programmes have been established, mostly targeted at elderly men in whom the disease is common. The prevalence of AAA in men aged 65 - 74 years has been consistently confirmed and typical figures are shown in Table 1.

Underlying assumptions

The sole justification for screening for abdominal aortic aneurysm is the belief that early detection of occult aneurysms and appropriate therapy will reduce the number of life years lost from the disease. The belief is supported by no randomised controlled trials but is currently an article of faith endorsed by most vascular surgeons. The belief rests on the following unstated assumptions.

- A substantial proportion of individuals with AAA will not present in clinical practice until later than the point at which elective AAA replacement does more good than harm.

- Data exist that allow an evidence based decision to be made on the best management for each patient with an AAA.

- The number of inappropriate, non evidence based elective AAA operations performed will be too small to affect the overall benefit of screening.

- A life year lost by one man from elective operative mortality is similar in value to a life year gained by another man several years older.

- The reduced quality of life of everyone during convalescence from elective AAA surgery is more than compensated by a gain in the length of life experienced by some of them.

- It is rational for a man in his seventies to agree to an elective operation which cannot make him feel better and which will inevitably make him, temporarily, feel worse when (a) that operation carries a substantial risk of immediate death, and (b) the gain if he survives is a slightly greater chance of living into his eighties than he would have had if he had not had elective surgery.

Operative mortality

At present there is no consensus on the weighting to be given to the many factors that can influence operative mortality and subsequent life expectation. These factors are numerous and some of them are listed in Table 2. Published operative mortality rates vary widely. Higher unpublished mortality rates are anecdotally known to occur. The evidence from prospectively collected population based data indicates that the true elective AAA operative mortality is around 8% [2]. Operative

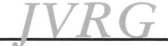

mortality for ruptured AAA is around 50% but fewer than half of those with rupture reach hospital alive [3]. Institutionally variable case selection takes place within hospitals based on age, coexistent disease, physical condition and availability of staff and resources. Overall, around 15% of patients with a ruptured AAA will survive the event.

Table 1. Prevalence of abdominal aortic aneurysm in men aged 65 - 74 years.

Max anteroposterior diameter (mm)	Prevalence (%)
2.5 - 3.9	4
4.0 - 5.4	1.5
5.5 - 14.5	0.5

Table 2. Factors affecting operative mortality and life expectancy after elective surgery for abdominal aortic aneurysm.

- Age
- Sex
- Cardiac disease
- Respiratory disease
- Other major coexistent disease
- Family history
- Cigarette smoking
- Serum cholesterol
- Serum fibrinogen

What is the risk of AAA rupture?

Many surgeons believe that rapid AAA expansion and AAA tenderness indicate an increased risk of AAA rupture, but there is no evidence to support either assumption. Other factors that might increase the risk of rupture are current cigarette smoking, obstructive airways disease or recent major surgery. Most data relate the risk of rupture to aortic aneurysm diameter. The subject is confused by the multiplicity of methods and modalities of measurement. Anteroposterior, transverse or maximum aortic diameter have been used singly, or in combination. The diameters have been obtained from abdominal palpation, radiographs, computed tomograms, magnetic resonance images and ultrasonography, all of which usually produce a different value for the same measurement.

To allow realistic comparisons of the outcome of elective surgery with the natural history of the untreated

disease one must know the annual AAA rupture and all cause mortality rates in patients with AAAs of confirmed diameter. This basic information cannot be extracted with any certainty from any of the key papers which are the cornerstone of contemporary surgical practice. Re-evaluation of these papers leads to the inescapable conclusion that the risk of rupture of a large AAA is substantially less than previously believed.

Reassessing the risk of AAA rupture

Let us assume that the death rate from all causes other than ruptured AAA in patients with AAA is 4%; that is the same as the all-cause mortality for the entire population of similar age. If one applies the assumption to the data available from the seminal papers, approximate AAA rupture rates for untreated patients with AAA may be calculated.

a. Foster et al 1969 [4]

For AAA of >6 cm diagnosed by palpation or abdominal radiography, the non-rupture deaths during follow-up were 35%, while rupture occurred in 51%. The rupture rate was therefore approximately 5.8% per annum. For AAA of <6cm the rupture rate was 1% per annum.

b. Szilagyi et al 1966 [5]

Patients with AAA of >6cm measured by various methods died during follow-up in the ratio of rupture to all other causes of 61:66. The rupture rate might therefore have been 3.7% per annum. For AAA <6cm at initial measurement the corresponding ratio was 16:29 and the probable rupture rate therefore 2.2% per annum.

c. Darling et al 1977 [6]

A review was undertaken of 24,000 autopsies with aneurysm diameters measured by unspecified methods. For AAAs of 5.1 - 7.0cm diameter, 25% were ruptured and therefore the cause of death. For aneurysms of 7.1 - 10.0cm, 46% were ruptured. The annual rupture risks were, therefore, probably 1.3% and 3.4% per annum respectively.

d. Sterpetti et al 1991 [7]

A review was made of 49,144 autopsies in Rome: 39% of AAAs of 5.1 - 6.9cm diameter and 65% of those 7.0 - 10.0cm in diameter were ruptured. The rupture rates are, therefore, likely to have been 2.6% per annum and 7.4% per annum respectively.

Comparison of surgery versus no surgery for AAA

The UK small aneurysm treatment trial [8] has confirmed that the maximum rupture risk for an AAA <5.5cm in anteroposterior diameter, measured by ultrasonography, is 1% per annum. The studies outlined above suggest that for all aneurysms >6.0 cm in diameter the risk is probably not more than 5% per annum. If we assume that (a) elective operative mortality is 8%, (b) ruptured AAA mortality is 5% per annum and (c) mortality from all other causes after successful AAA repair is 5% per annum, Table 3 may be constructed of outcome at yearly intervals for patients allocated to no treatment or early elective AAA repair (Figure 1). It can be seen that 5 years after elective AAA repair, for every 100 patients treated, there is a gain of 16 life years. Against this must be set eight immediate operative deaths and 23 life years of convalescence from the operation.

Conclusions

- It is debatable whether early elective treatment of even large aneurysms confers a clear advantage compared with no treatment.

- The great majority of patients identified by screening have small AAAs. Detection of such aneurysms exposes patients and their surgeons to the temptation of undergoing premature, unnecessary and harmful treatment.

- On current evidence, screening asymptomatic men to detect occult AAAs cannot be justified by any clear clinical benefit. In such circumstances issues of cost and affordability are irrelevant.

Table 3. Surgery versus no surgery.
Operative mortality 8%, natural mortality 10% per annum, after surgery mortality 5% per annum. 100 men in each group.

		1 year	2 years	3 years	4 years	5 years
Number of survivors	Surgery	87	83	79	75	71
	No surgery	90	81	73	66	59
	NNT (NNK)	(33)	50	17	11	8
Life years lost	Surgery	10.5	25.5	44.5	67.5	94.5
	No surgery	5	19.5	42.5	73	110.5
Net gain or (loss) of life years with surgery		(5.5)	(6.0)	(2.0)	5.5	16

NNT   number needed to treat
NNK   number needed to kill

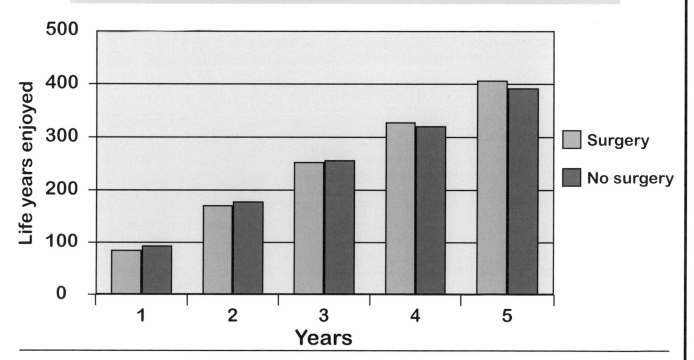

Figure 1. Surgery versus no surgery. (100 men in each group).

References (randomised trials in bold)

1. Collin J. Screening for abdominal aortic aneurysms. *Br J Surg* 1985; 72: 851-2.
2. Blankensteijn JD, Lindenburg FP, Van Der Graaf Y, Eikelboom BC. Influence of study design on reported mortality and morbidity rates after abdominal aortic aneurysm repair. *Br J Surg* 1998; 85: 1624-30.
3. Ingolby CJH, Wujanto R, Mitchell JE. Impact of vascular surgery on community mortality from ruptured aortic aneurysms. *Br J Surg* 1986; 73: 551-553.
4. Foster JH, Gobbel WG, Scott HW. Comparative study of elective resection and expectant treatment of abdominal aortic aneurysm. *Surg Gynec Obstet* 1969: 129: 1-9.
5. Szilagi DE, Smith RF, De Russo FJ, Elliott JP, Sherrin FW. Contribution of abdominal aortic aneurysmectomy to prolongation of life. *Ann* Surg 1966; 164: 678-699.
6. Darling RC, Messina CR, Brewster DC, Ottinger LW. Autopsy study of unoperated abdominal aortic aneurysms. The case for early resection. *J Cardiovasc Surg* 1976, Supp 2, Circulation 56: 161-164.
7. Sterpetti AV, Cavallaro A, Cavallari N, et al. Factors influencing the rupture of abdominal aortic aneurysms. *Surg Gynec Obstet* 1991; 173: 175-178.
8. **UK Small Aneurysm Trial Participants. Mortality results for randomised controlled trial of early elective surgery or ultrasonographic surveillance for small abdominal aortic aneurysms. *Lancet* 1998; 352: 1649-55.**

Indications for elective surgery for abdominal aortic aneurysm

AA Milne
Specialist Registrar
CV Ruckley
Professor of Vascular Surgery

DEPARTMENT OF VASCULAR SURGERY,
ROYAL INFIRMARY OF EDINBURGH, EDINBURGH

Asymptomatic abdominal aortic aneurysm

Since the respective merits of open surgery versus transluminal stent graft insertion have yet to be evaluated by clinical trial, the terms 'surgery' or 'repair', throughout this chapter, are employed to convey surgical and/or radiological intervention by whatever means are shown in due course to offer the safest and most durable prospect for the patient.

Elective repair of abdominal aortic aneurysm (AAA) is a prophylactic operation undertaken with the aim of prolonging life by preventing death from ruptured AAA. Therefore, to determine whether operation is indicated, the risk of death or major morbidity from operation must be balanced against the risk of death by rupture. Superficially this may appear to be a relatively simple equation, balancing operative risk against rupture rate, but there are many complicating factors.

Selection

Attempts to define operative risk for a population can seldom be determined from published series. Publication bias and selection bias both produce a falsely low impression of mortality rates and, consequently, the mortality rate in the surgical community as a whole is likely to be greater than it appears in the literature. Case mix is a crucial determinant of outcome and better results may be obtained by denying operation to high risk candidates. Published series seldom itemise patients who are not offered surgery. In a given series, it is generally impossible to determine how selective the surgeons have been and thus how comparable the data may be to any other surgeon's practice. When discussing surgical risks with a patient the surgeon has an obligation to advise the patient on the basis of outcomes derived from his or her own practice, not on selected series or clinical trials. Patients entered into multicentre trials do not represent the generality, since trial protocols, the surgeons' self selection or patient selection processes reduce the likelihood of unfavourable outcomes. Internal audit is the best way for an individual surgeon or surgical unit to determine operative risk, but this is only meaningful when a large enough series of patients has been analysed; this is a requirement that may take many years in smaller units, highlighting the importance of 'critical mass' in planning and auditing specialist services.

Risk

There is some evidence that may assist the estimation of individual risk of death from operation for aortic aneurysm [1]. The established risk factors are age, ischaemic heart disease, chronic obstructive pulmonary disease and renal impairment [1,8,10]. The presence of these factors is known to increase mortality rates but the precise risk of an operation for an individual patient cannot be calculated on currently available evidence.

JVRG

Estimation of the risk of rupture for an individual patient within a given time period is, at best, an informed estimate of probabilities. It is generally accepted that the major determinant for rupture is the maximum diameter of the aneurysm, but precise rupture rates for different sizes of aneurysms are not so clearly defined. Large aneurysms (>6 cm diameter) have been said to carry a high risk of rupture, of the order of 25% at one year [2]. Small aneurysms (<5 cm diameter) may rupture but do so uncommonly and several uncontrolled series have shown that, given an elective operative mortality of 5-10%, expectant management of such aneurysms represents the safer option [2-4].

Expansion rate

The mean rate of expansion of an AAA is in the order of 3 mm per year but larger aneurysms grow more quickly [5]. However, expansion rates are variable, both between different patients and within the same patient over different time periods. The risk of rupture has been shown to be related to the rate of expansion [5]. Aneurysms observed to expand rapidly, i.e. >5 mm over 6 months, are regarded as being at high risk for rupture and an indication for early surgery. This principle was incorporated within the design of both the UK Small Aneurysm Trial and the Aneurysm Detection and Management Study (ADAM) [6-7].

Compliance

The high degree of compliance of the distal aorta in normal subjects relates to the elastin content within the wall. Aneurysmal dilatation of the aorta is associated with loss of elastin fibres and an increase in collagen fibres. The wall, therefore, becomes less compliant, i.e. more stiff, as the aneurysm increases in size. There is evidence that aneurysms which do not conform to this pattern and which are more compliant than expected, or which do not become less compliant as they grow, are more likely to rupture [12].

Early surgery versus delay

The argument for early surgery runs as follows. Operation is likely to be required eventually. It is safer to intervene when the patient is younger and fitter rather than to wait until the aneurysm grows, at which point the patient may be less healthy and the operation more hazardous. The counter argument is that it is unwise to undergo a major risk of death when it could possibly be deferred for several years. For example, if the mortality rate is 5%, by deferring surgery for 2 years one patient in 20 would gain an extra 2 years of life. Furthermore, many patients with aneurysm die from other causes. Both policies have potential benefits, but it is difficult to calculate precisely the magnitude of benefit from either policy. So age considered in relation to aneurysm size

and general fitness is an equation that the surgeon must consider carefully; the options should be discussed fully with the patient.

Life expectancy must be taken into consideration. For example, a patient with disseminated malignancy and a life expectancy of 1 year would not be considered for elective surgery, even if the aneurysm were large and the patient fit for surgery, because the benefit of extended years of life would be insufficient to justify the risks of surgery. This example may be quite clear-cut, but life expectancy is usually difficult to estimate, especially when the reduction in life expectancy is due to unpredictable co-morbid conditions such as ischaemic heart disease. Even if life expectancy could be predicted accurately, the threshold beyond which surgery would become beneficial depends on many other variables.

Taking the above evidence and imponderables into account there has been a widely held view that large aneurysms over 5.5 cm in diameter should be surgically repaired, and that very small aneurysms less than 4 cm in diameter should be kept under surveillance; there was no consensus on the management of aneurysms in the range 4.0 - 5.5 cm diameter. This led to the setting up of three randomised trials. The Canadian Small Aneurysm Treatment Trial commenced in 1991 but was abandoned due to poor recruitment. The enrolled patients are still being followed and some data may become available. The Aneurysm Detection and Management (ADAM) study, being carried out in Veterans Administration hospitals in the United States, began in 1992 and was planned to run for 7 years [6]. Data should therefore be available soon. The UK Small Aneurysm Trial has recently been reported and will be discussed in some detail [7].

The UK Small Aneurysm Trial

This study randomised 1090 patients, aged 60-76 years and fit for surgery, with asymptomatic aneurysms 4.0-5.5 cm in maximum diameter on ultrasound scan to early surgery or ultrasound surveillance until the aneurysm either grew to 5.5 cm or became symptomatic, when operation was undertaken [7]. The mean follow-up was 4.6 years and the primary endpoint was death. Statistical analysis was made on an intention to treat basis and indicated no difference in mortality between the two groups (Figure 1). Cost analysis indicated that surveillance was a cheaper option than early surgery. This study was well designed and conducted and the large numbers make it statistically robust. The conclusion that aneurysms of <5.5 cm maximum diameter should be managed by ultrasound surveillance therefore appears clear-cut, but some details require further discussion.

The 30 day postoperative mortality rate for patients in the early surgery groups was 5.8% - higher than in many published series and almost three times the expected rate used in the power calculations for the study design.

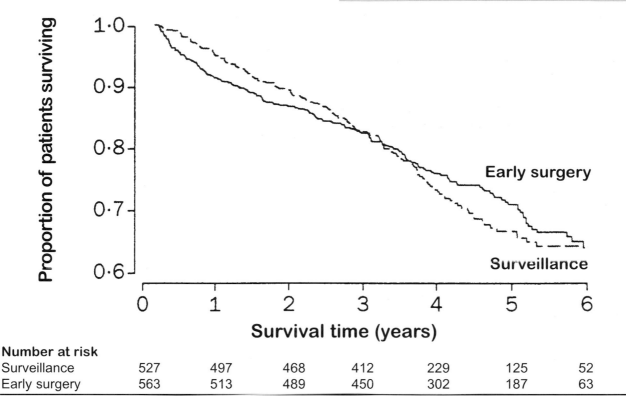

Number at risk							
Surveillance	527	497	468	412	229	125	52
Early surgery	563	513	489	450	302	187	63

Figure 1. Overall survival by treatment group from the UK Small Aneurysm Trial. No statistically significant difference between groups. (With permission from The Lancet Ltd. The UK Small Aneurysm Study Participants. Mortality results for the randomised controlled trial of early elective surgery or ultrasonographic surveillance for small abdominal aortic aneurysms. *Lancet* **1999; 352: 1649-55).**

As discussed above, publication bias favours superior results which are unrepresentative of the outcomes in the wider surgical community. The trial mortality rate is similar to other unselected multicentre studies [8]. However, surgeons who are consistently able to achieve mortality rates significantly lower than that in the trial may argue that early surgery in their hands is likely to confer a long-term benefit.

The trial was not stratified for age and aneurysm size, but some subgroup analysis was carried out. This indicated that younger patients (aged 60-66 years) and patients with larger aneurysms (4.9-5.5 cm) may have some benefit from early surgery, although the benefit did not reach statistical significance. This may lead some surgeons to recommend surgery when aneurysms reach 5.0 cm, especially in younger patients judged to be at relatively low operative risk; this may be a reasonable approach if it concurs with the patient's preference. The ADAM trial is stratified for age, sex and aneurysm size and subgroup analysis is planned. Therefore more evidence on this particular subject may be available soon.

Finally, as with any randomised trial, the results cannot be extrapolated to patients who fall outwith the trial's inclusion criteria and the trial protocol must be rigorously followed if the similar results are to be achieved in normal practice. For example, the results cannot be applied to patients aged <60 years in whom there remains uncertainty about whether early repair is the better option. The adherence to the ultrasound surveillance programme was excellent in the trial and similar standards must be attained in normal practice if surveillance is to be as safe as indicated in the trial.

Although the clinician can present the evidence and offer advice, the final decision lies with the patient. Some patients find that living with a 'time-bomb' in the abdomen is a considerable burden of anxiety. Such patients may prefer to get the surgery over with, even when it involves considerable risk, so that they can get on and enjoy their lives. There is evidence to support this from the UK Small Aneurysm Study; quality of life analysis showed that those undergoing early surgery had an improvement in health perception compared with those undergoing surveillance [9].

Future studies

The large randomised trials of conservative versus surgical management provide high quality evidence to underpin broad management policies for patients with asymptomatic aneurysm, but more evidence is still required to allow better estimation of risk of rupture and risk of surgery when weighing therapeutic options in the balance with individual patients. As noted above, the growth rate of aneurysms is highly variable, but there is no way to estimate the rate of growth in any individual. One candidate marker for aneurysm growth is aortic wall compliance which can be measured noninvasively using specialised ultrasound scanning equipment [12]. There are ongoing studies investigating the relationship between aortic wall compliance and aneurysm growth and rupture rate. A number of publications have identified risk factors for adverse outcome after elective aneurysm repair [1]. There have also been attempts to devise scoring systems, but none has been widely adopted [10]. The development of a scoring system validated on large prospective series of patients would be a valuable aid in clinical decision making for patients with AAA.

Symptomatic aneurysm

AAA may cause symptoms of pain or produce distal embolisation. Pain is usually felt in the abdominal or lower lumbar region and is constant in nature. It may be referred to groin, genitalia or thigh. Painful or tender aneurysms should be repaired in patients fit for surgery, not only for pain relief but also because of the possibility of contained rupture or the threat of impending rupture.

The two difficulties in a patient with pain and an aneurysm are, first, to determine whether the aneurysm is the cause of the pain rather than some other intra-abdominal pathology or musculoskeletal disorder and, second, whether the aneurysm has already leaked. There is some evidence to suggest that outcome is worse with emergent operation within 4 hours of admission and that surgery is safer when delayed for up to 7 days [11]. This does not necessarily mean, however, that surgery for the symptomatic aneurysm should be delayed. Difference in outcome may not only reflect the less favourable circumstances under which the urgent surgery may be undertaken but also the more serious pathology in urgently operated cases; failure to operate timeously may be a death sentence. The decision whether it is safe to defer operation can be a difficult one and computed tomography (CT) has not proved to be entirely reliable as a guide [13]. A careful history and abdominal palpation is required; if in doubt, clinical judgment should over-ride CT imaging.

Distal embolism usually presents with multiple small infarcted patches on the lower legs and feet, commonly described as trash foot. Operation is indicated to prevent tissue loss. Very rarely intact aneurysms can cause disseminated intravascular coagulation which can present as a bleeding disorder. Such patients may be stabilised on low dose heparin prior to operation if fit.

Coincidental occlusive and aneurysmal disease

In patients undergoing aorto-iliac or renovascular reconstruction for occlusive disease it is usually prudent to undertake repair of a coincidental aortic aneurysm, even when it is below the size that would normally be considered for repair on its own merits.

Conclusions

Patients with asymptomatic aneurysms of <5 cm maximum diameter should be followed by ultrasound surveillance at intervals of 6 months and should be operated on if growth exceeds 5 mm in any 6 month period and the patient is fit. Asymptomatic aneurysms of >5.5 cm maximum diameter should be repaired unless there are strong contraindications. There remains a grey area between 5.0 and 5.5 cm where it can be argued that operation should be advised for patients who are relatively young and otherwise healthy, and where patients' wishes should weigh importantly. Symptomatic aneurysms should be operated on urgently if the pain is acute and assessment suggests the possibility of localised leak. If, on the other hand, the symptoms have been present for a number of days and the patient is stable, surgery should be undertaken on the next available elective list rather than as an 'out of hours' emergency.

Indications for elective surgery for abdominal aortic aneurysm

Sound evidence

- **Patients with AAA >5.5cm and fit for surgery should be offered early surgery.**

- **Patients with AAA <5.0cm aged >60 years should undergo ultrasound surveillance.**

Evidence needed

- **Should young patients (aged <60 years) with aneurysm >4.0cm undergo early surgery or surveillance?**

- **Should fit patients with aneurysm 5.0 - 5.5cm undergo early surgery (in a unit with excellent audited results) or surveillance?**

References (randomised trials in bold)

1. Johnston KW, Scobie TK. Multicenter prospective study of nonruptured abdominal aortic aneurysms. *J Vasc Surg* 1988; 7: 69-81.
2. Johansson G, Nydahl S, Olofsson P, Swedenborg J. Survival in patients with abdominal aortic aneurysms. Comparison between operative and non-operative management. *Eur J Vasc Surg* 1990; 4: 497-502.
3. Scott RA, Wilson NM, Ashton HA, Kay DN. Is surgery necessary for abdominal aortic aneurysm less than 6 cm in diameter. *Lancet* 1993; 342: 1395-6.
4. Brown PM, Pattenden R, Vernooy C, Zelt DR, Gutellius JR. Selective management of abdominal aortic aneurysms in a prospective measurement program. *J Vasc Surg* 1996; 23: 213-22.
5. Bengtsson H, Bergqvist D, Ekberg O, Ranstam J. Expansion pattern and risk of rupture of abdominal aortic aneurysms that were not operated on. *Eur J Surg* 1993; 159: 461-7.
6. Lederle F, Wilson SE, Johnston GR, et al. Design of the abdominal aortic Aneurysm Detection and Management Study. *J Vasc Surg* 1994; 20: 296-302.
7. **The UK Small Aneurysm Study Participants. Mortality results for the randomised controlled trial of early elective surgery or ultrasonographic surveillance for small abdominal aortic aneurysms. *Lancet* 1999; 352: 1649-55.**
8. Katz DJ, Stanley JC, Zelenock GB. Operative mortality rates for intact and ruptured aortic aneurysms in Michigan: an eleven-year statewide experience. *J Vasc Surg* 1994; 19: 804-15.
9. **The UK Small Aneurysm Study Participants. Health service costs and quality of life for early elective surgery or ultrasonic surveillance for small abdominal aortic aneurysms. *Lancet* 1998; 352: 1656-60.**
10. Steyerberg EW, Kievit J, de Mol Van Otterloo JC, van Bockel JH, Eijkemans MJ, Habbema JD. Perioperative mortality of elective aortic aneurysm surgery. A clinical prediction rule based on literature and individual patient data. *Arch Int Med* 1995; 155: 1998-2004.
11. Cambria RA, Gloviczki P, Stanson AW, Cherry KJ, Bower TC, Pairolero PC. Symptomatic, non-ruptured abdominal aortic aneurysms: are emergent operations necessary? *Ann Vasc Surg* 1994; 8: 121-6.
12. Wilson K, Bradbury AW, Whyman MR, et al. Relationship between abdominal aortic aneurysm wall compliance and clinical outcome: a preliminary analysis. *Eur J Vasc Endovasc Surg* 1998; 15: 472-7
13. Adam DJ, Bradbury AW, Stuart WP, et al. The value of computed tomography in the assessment of suspected ruptured abdominal aortic aneurysm. *J Vasc Surg* 1998; 27: 431-7.

Chapter 16

Indications for elective surgery for
abdominal aortic aneurysm

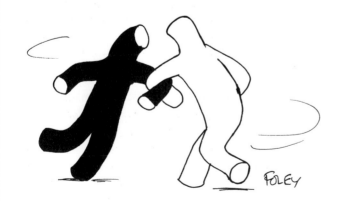

Chapter 17

Endovascular aneurysm repair: state of the art 2000

MG Wyatt
Consultant Surgeon
J Rose
Consultant Radiologist

NORTHERN VASCULAR CENTRE,
FREEMAN HOSPITAL, NEWCASTLE UPON TYNE

Introduction

Parodi et al performed the first endovascular abdominal aortic aneurysm repair (EVAR) in 1990 [1]. He showed, when balloon expandable stents were sutured to the partially overlapping ends of a tubular knitted Dacron graft, that friction seals were created which fixed the ends of the graft to the vessel wall. This resulted in exclusion of the aneurysm from the circulation, allowing normal flow through the graft lumen. He described this treatment in five patients and concluded that further developments and more clinical trials were needed before this technique could become of wide use.

Since this initial report, aortic stent grafts have developed rapidly, from homemade to commercially produced devices, and from tube grafts to aorto-uni-iliac and bifurcated devices. Stent grafts may be modular (more than one piece), or non-modular (one-piece) designs. The metallic stent may be placed on the outside or inside of the graft material. The graft may be fully stented or incorporate stents just at its extremities. In addition, the top of the device may be constructed with graft material and/or metal stent up to the renal arteries or with bare metal designed to cover the renal arteries, allowing for improved proximal fixation.

In the nine years since Parodi's early report, approximately 230 articles have appeared describing the use of endovascular aortic stent graft combinations for the treatment of abdominal aortic aneurysm (AAA). Unfortunately, to date no randomised controlled trial of endovascular versus conventional repair of AAA has been reported. Although EVAR has been shown to be feasible in the short term, longer-term failures are significant and evidence for the efficacy of EVAR remains weak.

The evolution of EVAR

Tube grafts

Initial stent grafts were homemade tube devices consisting of an 'extra-large' Palmaz stent and a thin polyester graft attached at the mid-portion of the stent. These produced good results in animals [2], but it was soon appreciated that a second stent was required to seal the distal end of the graft. These modified tube grafts were used by Parodi in 38 patients but, as most aortic aneurysms did not have a distal neck or cuff, a high leak rate ensued.

Between 1992 and 1996, May's group from Sidney, Australia were also experimenting with EVAR [3] and reported the results of 136 implantations. Initially tube devices were implanted into 50 patients and analysis using Kaplan-Meier curves demonstrated a success probability at 40 months of only 50%, compared to 80% for non-tube devices. Following similar reports from

101

JVRG

several centres, and with the realisation that only 5% of AAAs were suitable for treatment with tube grafts, the use of these devices has largely withered.

Aorto-uni-iliac grafts

Several centres were involved with the development of aorto-uni-iliac (AUI) devices [4,5]. Hopkinson from Nottingham, described the use of a Dacron graft secured at both ends with a self-expanding Gianturco stent [6]. This method was successful in excluding 25 of 30 (83%) aortic aneurysms with a 30-day mortality rate of 6.6%.

In Leicester, Bell et al were describing similar work using a tapered AUI graft prepared from an 8mm thin-walled expanded polytetrafluorethylene tube graft predilated proximally to 35mm and tapered distally to 15mm [7]. The proximal graft was sutured to a pre-dilated Palmaz stent, mounted on a balloon and backloaded into a packaging sheath. Early results showed success in 52 of 60 patients treated (87%), with aneurysm exclusion in 49 (82%) and a peri-operative mortality rate of 3% [8]. AUI devices are now commercially available and are marketed by several companies.

Bifurcated grafts

One of the disadvantages of the AUI device is that it uses only one side of the iliac bifurcation, and so requires occlusion of the contralateral iliac system and insertion of an extra-anatomic femoro-femoral bypass graft. Although this procedure may be carried out with minimal additional morbidity, it does involve potential inherent problems such as anastomotic stricture, graft occlusion and a small risk of cross-over graft infection [9]. The gold standard of open aneurysm repair is able to maintain anatomical normality and does not involve destruction of the contra-lateral iliac system. For this reason many centres, including our own, have preferred to use bifurcated stent grafts in preference to AUI devices.

Non-modular designs

Chuter et al described the first clinical experience with bifurcated aortic stent grafts in 1994 [10]. The graft was a traditional Dacron bifurcated graft with modified self-expanding Gianturco stents sutured proximally and to both iliac limbs distally. Early results using this graft were promising, with technical success in 39 of 42 patients (92%), but by 3 years 26% of grafts had failed [11]. The primary reasons for failure were graft thrombosis due to kinking and proximal stent migration. The first commercial bifurcated device was developed by Endovascular Technologies. Based on a graft designed and patented by Lazarus [12], this was the only device to gain Food and Drug Administration approval in the United States of America. The graft had two identical limbs with self-expanding stents sewn on to the distal ends [13]. One of

the limitations of this device was that each limb was identical in length and diameter. Although still available, it may, in my opinion, be suitable for the repair of only about 10% of AAAs.

Modular designs

With the obvious limitations of one-piece design, several companies began to design modular bifurcated devices, which could be custom built to fit an individual patient's anatomy. The first of these was the MinTec Stentor device. The graft consisted of two components, a main body with a uni-lateral limb and a contralateral limb. The main body was inserted via one iliac system to lie within the body of the aneurysm sac. The contralateral limb was introduced from the opposite groin to form the bifurcated graft. The two components were held together by radial force. The Stentor graft introduced a second new design feature in that it was supported along its entire frame by a self-expanding Nitinol stent, as opposed to just at the proximal and distal ends. The device was subsequently modified to produce the Vanguard device, but recently it was temporarily withdrawn following reports of ligature breakage, stent kinking and distortion, and limb dislocation [14]. Following extensive testing and analysis of follow-up data, the graft has now been re-marketed.

Several other companies have developed or acquired modular bifurcated devices and, although the early outcome is acceptable, medium and long-term results are still awaited (Figure 1) [15-18]. The problems associated with the Vanguard device are likely to affect most modular systems, but continued development in graft design should eventually minimise these drawbacks.

The Newcastle EVAR experience

Our own experience of EVAR includes 100 aortic stent grafts implanted between December 1995 and July 1999. Bifurcated grafts have been used when possible; only 9% of patients received an AUI device (Table 1). Patient, aneurysm and operative details are summarised in Table 2.

Initial results

EVAR was successful in 99 of the 100 attempted deployments. One patient required an open conversion following immediate migration of the top stent of a Leicester AUI device (Figure 2). No commercially available devices have been associated with conversion to open repair. Two patients have undergone laparotomy for banding of significant proximal leaks, with a mortality of 50% (Figure 3). Three distal leaks sealed spontaneously and, of two patients with lumbar vessel refilling, one sealed and one required embolisation. Complications of EVAR have included transient renal failure (2), microemboli to toes (1), minor methicillin-resistant *Staphylococcus aureus* wound infection (1),

Table 1. Types of endovascular aortic aneurysm repair device implanted in Newcastle.

Aorto-uni-iliac		**Talent**	5
		Zenith	2
		Palmaz (Leicester)	2
Bifurcated			
	Non modular	**EVT**	4
		Endologix	1
	Modular	**Stentor/Vanguard**	54
		Zenith	17
		Talent	6
		Excluder	4
		AneuRx	4
		Stenford	1

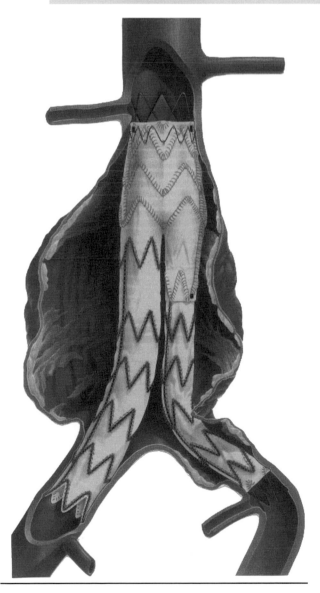

Figure 1. Diagram showing a modular bifurcated device used to exclude an abdominal aortic aneurysm (Talent, World Medical).

transient femoral nerve palsy (1), transient ischaemic attack (1), false femoral aneurysm (2) and distal embolism requiring embolectomy (1). Seven patients died within 30 days of their operation (one after proximal banding, one from cerebral haemorrhage and five from cardiac events). Four of these patients were American Society of Anesthesiologists fitness category IV (ASA). There has been one late stent-related death due to rupture following proximal migration.

Follow-up

All patients have been followed-up for between 1 and 43 months according to Eurostar criteria (Chapter 18). Two late migrations (one Stentor device at 33 months and one Talent device at 6 months), neither of which were

Table 2. **Patient demography, aortic anatomy and operative details for 91 men and nine women having EVAR in Newcastle.**
(Values are medians with ranges in parentheses unless otherwise stated).

Age	**72 years**	**(45-89 years)**
ASA	**I-III (95%)**	**IV (5%)**
Aneurysm diameter	**5.9 cm**	**(4.2-9.2 cm)**
Diameter of proximal necks	**2.2 cm**	**(1-10 cm)**
Operative time	**120 min**	**(60-380 min)**
Blood loss	**200 ml**	**(30-2500 ml)**
Postoperative stay	**3 days**	**(2-27 days)**

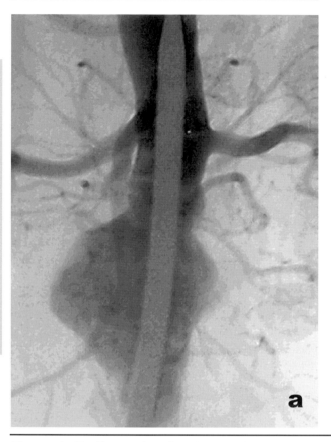
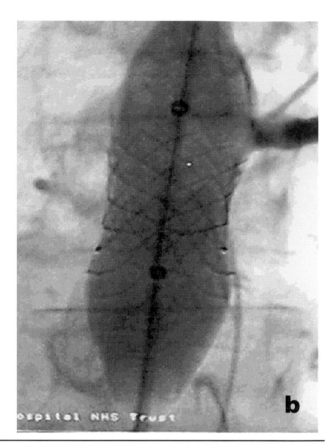

Figure 2. Radiographs showing deployment of a Leicester aorto-uni-iliac device into an aneurysm with a long neck. (a) Despite adequate balloon dilation (b) the top stent migrated requiring conversion to open operation.

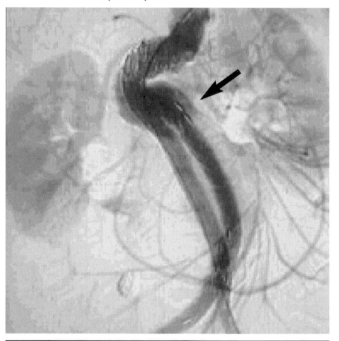

Figure 3. Radiograph showing a Vanguard bifurcated stent graft deployed within a tortuous aortic neck. There is a large endoleak (arrow), which was successfully banded at open operation. The patient had severe ischaemic heart disease and died from a myocardial infarction three days later. This degree of neck tortuosity should be treated very cautiously by endovascular repair.

associated with endoleak, were treated with proximal cuffs. Four distal endoleaks have occurred between 18 and 24 months and all had further endovascular repair with limb extensions or embolisation. A total of ten have suffered graft limb occlusion (Table 3).

EVAR today

On the basis of experience and on review of the available literature, it is apparent, with careful patient selection and co-operation between surgeons and interventional radiologists, that satisfactory early and medium term results can be obtained from EVAR. The morbidity and mortality associated with the procedure are acceptably low (3% peri-operative mortality in ASA I-III patients), and most patients can return to the open ward after operation, to be discharged 2 or 3 days later. There are few data on the results of EVAR for ASA IV patients (severe cardiorespiratory impairment or contained rupture), but it is this group in which the peri-operative mortality remains high [19,20,21]. Local and regional anaesthetic techniques may reduce mortality, but this remains to be verified [22,23]. Only a randomised controlled trial will determine whether these sick patients should undergo EVAR, but it is our impression that this group generally does badly.

Table 3. Graft limb occlusions.

Cause	Number		Treatment
Operative (iatrogenic)	2		Cross-over graft
Recurrent thoracic emboli	1		Embolectomy
Iliac disease	4	2 early	Cross-over graft
		2 late	Endovascular repair
Graft distortion/dislocation	3	(12-18 months)	Cross-over graft (2)
			No treatment (1)

Endoleak remains a major problem of EVAR (Figure 4). It implies failure to exclude the aneurysm and an associated increased risk of aneurysm growth and eventual rupture [24]. In addition to endoleaks that are present from the time of operation (primary endoleaks), all series of endo-grafts are showing evidence of the continued development of perigraft flow with time (secondary endoleaks). Endoleaks may be classified as follows [25]: Type I - related to the graft device itself; Type II - retrograde flow from collateral branches; Type III - due to fabric tears, graft disconnection or disintegration, and Type IV - flow through graft wall associated with graft wall porosity.

The reported incidence of primary endoleak varies between 5 and 44%. Approximately half of these heal spontaneously, but their occurrence may be dependent on the type of device used and the experience of the operating team. Nevertheless, the frequency and completeness of follow-up may influence the observed incidence [26]. A recent meta-analysis of 23 publications revealed that of 1118 patients with successfully implanted endovascular aortic grafts, 270 experienced endoleaks (24%), of which 17% were primary and 7% secondary [27]. The majority arose from the distal attachment site (36%) and were persistent with time (37%). The incidence of endoleak for tube, bifurcated and AUI devices was 35%, 20% and 18% respectively. These figures are alarming because the presence of an endoleak implies that the aneurysm is not excluded from the systemic circulation and remains a danger. In the presence of endoleak, 86% of aneurysms continue to increase in diameter and these patients remain at risk of rupture. Of note, side branch endoleaks rarely seem to lead to progressive aneurysm dilation [28], but aneurysm growth with lumbar endoleaks has occasionally been reported [27].

The endovascular treatment of AAA is an evolving field, but another worrying outcome identified by the above meta-analysis was that when older devices were excluded from analysis, the endoleak rate remained the same at 25%. In addition, it remains difficult to predict at the time of identification of an endoleak whether the aneurysm sac will continue to expand, remain the same or reduce in size. Furthermore, reports of diameter increase and rupture in the absence of obvious endoleak are of concern [29,30].

EVAR in the future

The 1990s have shown that the repair of AAA using an endovascular technique is feasible. It is associated with a reduced physiological disturbance than open repair [31,32] and the early and intermediate results remain acceptable [24,33]. In addition, endovascular repair is associated with less peri-operative discomfort and the postoperative stay can be as little as 2 days. The mortality rate (3-8%) and complication rate (10-20%) are similar to those of the open procedure with the exception of continued perfusion of the aneurysm sac (endoleak).

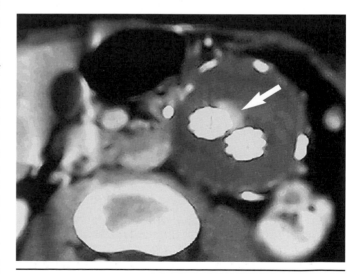

Figure 4. Contrast enhanced computed tomogram showing a junctional endoleak (arrow).

New devices

At least ten types of device have been made commercially available in the UK up to the present time. Three of these have been superseded or withdrawn from the market and a further three or four devices are in the process of development. This situation highlights the fact that no single stent-graft has yet proven to be ideal and that graft design remains an evolving and controversial area. For instance, it appears appropriate to attempt to preserve aortic anatomy, but less than 40% of AAAs are suitable for treatment using bifurcated aortic stent grafts. A greater number, perhaps two thirds, of aneurysms may be treated using AUI devices, but these should probably be reserved for patients with anatomy unsuitable for bifurcated devices.

Recent data have suggested that aneurysm sacs distort and shorten with time and that this results in kinking and possible limb dislocation of modular devices (Figure 5) [14]. This is true for all modular devices; care should be taken during deployment to allow for adequate overlap of the contralateral limb and placement of the limbs well down into the iliac orifices, as close as possible to the iliac bifurcations. It would seem appropriate to use a non-modular device if possible, as the join associated with modularity is a weakness in stent design.

It is not known whether aortic stent grafts should be fully stented or incorporate metallic stents just at the extremities. The disadvantage of non-supported limbs is that they kink with sac distortion. Types of fully stented grafts that employ suture material to link adjacent strands of metal may disintegrate with movement, although the significance of such 'suture breakage' is as yet unclear. Stent design that depends on a more direct link between metal segments, by interweaving the wires, seems more prudent in the longer term.

A major problem encountered with all available devices is distal migration of the top of the graft; this is associated with continued expansion of the aortic neck. In an attempt to improve proximal fixation and to minimise subsequent migration, devices with suprarenal attachments are being developed, designed to fit larger, shorter aneurysmal necks. An uncovered Gianturco stent forms the proximal anchor of the Perth bifurcated system and has been deployed across the renal arteries with no deleterious effects in 85% of the cases recently described by Lawrence-Brown et al [34]. Several other studies have confirmed that it is possible to cover the renal arteries with bare metal stent in the short term without adverse effect on renal function [35,36]; the long-term effects of this practice are unknown (Figure 6).

Further work is continuing into the design of more sophisticated systems for suprarenal fixation. These

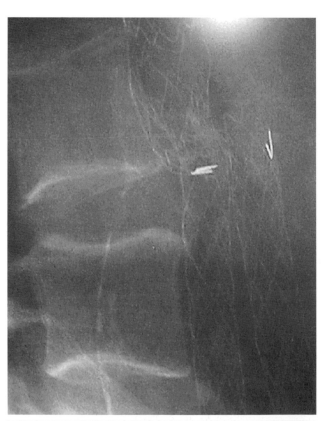

Figure 5. Plain radiograph showing dislocation of the contralateral limb of a Vanguard device. This resulted in an endoleak at 18 months which was treated using a further covered stent to bridge the gap.

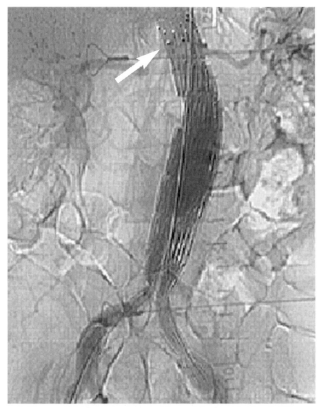

Figure 6. Radiograph showing deployment of a Zenith modular bifurcated device. Note the presence of the uncovered stent above the renal arteries (arrow).

might improve long-term endoleak-free survival by successfully utilising the often (relatively) normal 'island' of aortic wall in the region of the visceral arterial origins. It is likely that aortic stent-grafts will eventually be available with side-branches [37]. Such devices could then extend the range of endovascular repair into the treatment of juxta-renal and thoraco-abdominal aneurysms.

Trials

At present, hard data concerning the long-term suitability of EVAR are simply not available. Major registries, such as the European Collaborators Group for Stent-graft Techniques for Abdominal Aortic Aneurysm Repair (Eurostar) and the UK Registry for Endovascular Treatment of Aneurysms (RETA) collate prospective data from most centres undertaking EVAR. It will, however, require a randomised controlled trial to determine whether or not endovascular techniques can improve on the gold standard of open repair for the treatment AAA.

Two randomised controlled trials of EVAR are scheduled to commence shortly. They will be multicentre and are to be funded by the National Health Service Health and Technology Assessment. EVAR 1 will randomise patients over 60 years old (ASA I-III) with non-ruptured infrarenal AAAs of over 5.5 cm diameter either to open repair or to EVAR, provided the anatomy of the AAA is suitable for either treatment. EVAR 2 will consider patients who are unfit for surgical repair (ASA IV). These patients will be randomised either to EVAR plus best medical treatment or to best medical treatment alone.

All centres with experience of over 20 EVAR procedures will be eligible for inclusion in the trial and results will be monitored by RETA (Chapter 18). Each trial will compare EVAR against the current best alternative in terms of mortality, durability, safety and cost, as well as generic and patient-specific health related quality of life. Eleven hundred patients will be entered over 4 years, 800 in EVAR 1 and 300 in EVAR 2. The trials will indicate the degree of safety, efficacy and durability of new EVAR systems as they are introduced. The hope is that it may be possible to reduce the cost of treatment of all AAAs and provide potential to reduce bed occupancy and increase patient satisfaction. Until these trials are reported, one must rely on the Eurostar and RETA registries to provide continued short, medium and long-term follow-up data. At present, aortic stent graft insertion is a technological advance in the treatment of AAA whose clinical benefit remains unproven.

Chapter 17

Endovascular aneurysm repair

Sound evidence

- **Endovascular repair of abdominal aortic aneurysm is feasible and gives acceptable early results (with limited physiological disturbance and short hospital stay).**

- **In the intermediate term there is a significant failure rate (25%).**

- **Only 5% of abdominal aortic aneurysms are suitable for repair with a tube graft; the majority require a bifurcated design (or aorto-uni-iliac repair).**

- **Endoleaks remain a major problem, even with modern devices.**

Evidence needed

- **The late results of repair of abdominal aortic aneurysm by endovascular means are unknown.**

- **No randomised controlled trial of endovascular repair has yet been completed (but at least two will commence before the year 2000).**

Chapter 17

References

1. Parodi JC, Palmaz JC, Barone HD. Transfemoral intraluminal graft implantation for abdominal aortic aneurysms. *Ann Vasc Surg* 1991; 5: 491-9.

2. Laborde JC, Parodi JC, Clem MFC et al. Intraluminal bypass of abdominal aortic aneurysm: Feasibility study. *Radiology* 1992; 184: 185-90.

3. May J, White GH, Yu W, et al. Importance of graft configuration in outcome of endoluminal aortic aneurysm repair: a 5-year analysis by the life table method. *Eur J Vasc Endovasc Surg* 1998; 15: 406-411.

4. Ivancev K, Chuter TAM, Risberg B. The Ivancev-Malmo system of endovascular aneurysm exclusion. In Hopkinson B, Yusef SW, Whitaker SC, Veith F (Eds). *Endovascular Surgery for Aortic Aneurysms*. London: WB Saunders 1997: 150-163.

5. Parodi JC, Criado FJ Barone HD et al. Endoluminal aortic aneurysm repair using a balloon expandable stent-graft device: a progress report. *Ann Vasc Surg* 1994; 8: 523-529.

6. Yusef SW, Whitaker SC, Chuter TA et al. Early results of endovascular aortic aneurysm surgery with aortouniiliac graft, contralateral iliac occlusion, and femorofemoral bypass. *J Vasc Surg* 1997; 25: 165-72.

7. Thompson MM, Sayers RD, Nasim A, Boyle JR, Fishwick G, Bell PRF. Aortomonoiliac endovascular grafting: difficult solutions to difficult aneurysms. *J Endovasc Surg* 1997; 4: 174-81.

8. Thompson MM, Boyle JR, Fishwick G, Bell PRF. Aorto-uni-iliac endovascular repair utilizing ePTFE and balloon-expandable stents - The Leicester experience. In: *Indications in Vascular and Endovascular Surgery*. Greenhalgh RM (Ed.). WB Saunders. London. 1998: 229-240.

9. Brown AS, Rose JDG, Wyatt MG. What is the case for the bifurcate modular stent-graft for abdominal aneurysms. In: *Indications in Vascular and Endovascular Surgery*. Greenhalgh RM (Ed.). London 1998: 251-259.

10. Chuter TA, Donayre C, Wendt G. Bifurcated stent-grafts for endovascular repair of abdominal aortic aneurysm. Preliminary case reports. *Surg Endosc* 1994; 8: 800-802.

11. Chuter TA, Wendt G, Hopkinson BR et al. European experience with a system for bifurcated stent-graft insertion. *J Endovasc Surg* 1997; 4: 13-22.

12. Lazarus HM. Endovascular grafting for the treatment of abdominal aortic aneurysms. *Surg Clin North Am* 1992; 72: 959-968.

13. Broeders IAMJ. The Endovascular Technologies system. In Hopkinson BR, Yusef SW, Whitaker SC, Veith F (Eds.). *Endovascular surgery for aortic aneurysms*. London 1997; 104-121.

14. Harris P, Brennan J, Martin J et al. Longitudinal aneurysm shrinkage following endovascular repair: a source of intermediate and late complications. *J Endovasc Surg* 1999: 11-16.

15. Zarins CK, White RA, Schwarten D et al. AneuRx stent graft versus open repair of abdominal aortic aneurysms: multicentre prospective clinical trial. *J Vasc Surg* 1999; 29: 306-308.

16. Biasi GM, Iglionica MR, Mereglaglia D et al. European multicentre experience with modular device (Medtronic AneuRx) for the endoluminal repair of infrarenal abdominal aortic aneurysms. *J Mal Vasc* 1998; 23: 374-380.

17. Ulfacker R, Robison JG, Brothers TE, Pereira AH, Sanvitto PC. Abdominal aortic aneurysm treatment: preliminary results with the Talent stent-graft system. *J Vasc Interv Radiol* 1998; 9: 51-60.

18. Allen BT, Hovsepian DM, Reilly RM et al. Endovascular stent grafts for aneurysmal and occlusive vascular disease. *Am J Surg* 1998; 176: 574-580.

19. Chandrasekar R, Nott DM, Enabi L, Harris PI, Bakran A. Successful repair of a ruptured abdominal aortic aneurysm in a cardiac transplant patient. *Eur J Vasc Surg* 1994; 8: 750-751.

20. Yusef SW, Whitaker SC, Chuter TA, Wenham PW, Hopkinson BR. Emergency endovascular repair of leaking aortic aneurysm. *Lancet* 1994; 344: 1645.

21. Chuter TA, Gordon RL, Reilly LM et al. Abdominal aortic aneurysm in high-risk patients: short to intermediate term results of endovascular repair. *Radiology* 1999; 210: 361-365.

22. Aadahl P, Lundbom J, Hatlinghus S, Myhre HO. Regional anaesthesia for endovascular treatment of abdominal aortic aneurysms. *J Endovasc Surg* 1997; 4: 56-61.

23. Henretta JP, Hodgson KJ, Mattos MA et al. Feasibility of endovascular repair of abdominal aortic aneurysms with local anaesthesia with intravenous sedation. *J Vasc Surg* 1999; 29: 793-798.

24. Brewster DC, Geller SC, Kaufman JA et al. Initial experience with endovascular aneurysm repair: comparison of early results with outcome of conventional open repair. *J Vasc Surg* 1998; 27: 992-1003.

25. White GH, May J, Waugh RC, Chaufour X, Yu W. Type III and type IV endoleak: toward a complete definition of blood flow in the sac after endoluminal repair. *J Endovasc Surg* 1998; 5: 305-309.

26. Harris P, Dimitri S. Predicting failure of endovascular aneurysm repair. *Eur J Vasc Surg* 1999; 17: 1-2.

27. Schurink GWH, Aarts NJM, van Bockel JH. Endoleak after stent-graft treatment of abdominal aortic aneurysm: a met-analysis of clinical studies. *Br J Surg* 1999; 86: 581-587.

28. Resch T, Ivancef K, Lindh M et al. Persistent collateral perfusion of the abdominal aneurysm does not lead to progressive change in aneurysm diameter. *J Vasc Surg* 1998; 28: 242-249.

29. Torselli GB, Klenk E, Kasprzak B, Umscheid T. Rupture of abdominal aortic aneurysm previously treated by endovascular repair. *J Vasc Surg* 1998; 28: 184-187.

30. Alimi YS, Chakfe N, Rivoal E et al. Rupture of an abdominal aortic aneurysm after endovascular graft placement and aneurysm size reduction. *J Vasc Surg* 1998; 28: 178-183.

31. Boyle JR, Thompson JP, Thompson MM et al. Improved respiratory function and analgesia control after endovascular aneurysm repair. *J Endovasc Surg* 1997; 4: 62-65.

32. Thompson MM, Nasim A, Sayers RD et al. Oxygen free radical and cytokine generation during endovascular and conventional aneurysm repair. *Eur J Vasc Endovasc Surg* 1996; 12: 70-75.

33. Lawrence-Brown M, Sieunarine K, Hartley D, van Schie G, Goodman MA, Prendergast FJ. The Perth HLB bifurcated endoluminal graft: a review of the experience and intermediate results. *Cardiovasc Surg* 1998; 6: 220-225.

34. Lawrence-Brown MM, Hartley D, MacSweeney ST et al. The Perth Endoluminal bifurcated graft system - development and early experience. *Cardiovasc Surg* 1996; 4: 706-712.

35. Maclerewicz J, Walker SR, Vincent R et al. Perioperative renal function following endovascular repair of abdominal aortic aneurysm with suprarenal and infrarenal stents. *Br J Surg* 1999; 86: 696.

36. Malina M, Brunkwall J, Ivancev K, Lindblad B, Risberg B. Renal arteries covered by aortic stents: clinical experience from endovascular grafting of aortic aneurysms. *Eur J Vasc Surg* 1997; 14: 109-113.

37. Iwase T, Hosokawa H, Suzuki T, Inoue K. Endovascular replacement of branched stent-grafts with sidearms extending into renal, superior mesenteric and coeliac arteries for treatment of aortic aneurysms. *J Vasc Int Radiol* 1999; 2:280.

Chapter 18

The evidence for endovascular aneurysm repair

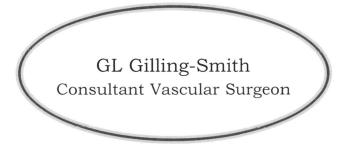

GL Gilling-Smith
Consultant Vascular Surgeon

REGIONAL VASCULAR UNIT,
ROYAL LIVERPOOL UNIVERSITY HOSPITAL, LIVERPOOL

Introduction

Abdominal aortic aneurysm remains a significant cause of premature death. Rupture of the aneurysm is associated with an in-hospital mortality of around 50% but many patients die before reaching hospital so that the overall community mortality is estimated to exceed 90%. There is, therefore, a compelling argument for prophylactic surgical intervention in patients who are considered at risk of aneurysm rupture.

Since the early 1950s, such patients have been offered surgical replacement of the aneurysmal segment of their aorta with a prosthetic graft. Conventional open repair has proved very effective, with survivors enjoying near normal life expectancy. It remains, however, a highly invasive and physiologically stressful procedure which, unsurprisingly, is associated with significant operative morbidity and mortality. In addition, patients commonly require several months of convalescence and rehabilitation before they feel as well as, and are as active as they were before surgery.

In recent years it has become possible to offer selected patients a minimally invasive endovascular alternative to conventional open repair. Rather than replacement of the aneurysmal segment, endovascular repair relies on isolation of the aneurysm from the circulation by intraluminal deployment of a covered stent-graft introduced via the femoral arteries. Laparotomy and aortic cross-clamping are thus avoided and the duration of lower limb ischaemia minimised. Such a reduction in physiological stress might be expected to result in a significant reduction in operative morbidity and mortality, and a more rapid return to pre-operative activity and well-being than after conventional operation. But there remain many important questions to be answered before this new technology can be recommended for widespread use: is it technically feasible, is it widely applicable, is it safe and does it work? Indeed, what evidence is there that endovascular repair is an acceptable alternative to conventional open operation?

The evidence

Much has been said and written about endovascular aneurysm repair since the technique was first described in 1991. Unfortunately, little of this can be cited as objective or reliable scientific evidence. Numerous reports of single centre experiences containing relatively small numbers of patients testify to surgeons' and radiologists' enthusiasm for this new technique, but such reports should be viewed with caution as they focus on preliminary learning-curve experience when there is, of course, an inevitable bias towards optimistic reporting of encouraging results. There are only a few reports of larger or multicentre experience and absolutely no prospective randomised comparisons between endovascular and conventional open repair. Currently the best available sources of data are national and international registries, such as the UK Registry for

JVRG

The evidence for endovascular
aneurysm repair

Endovascular Treatment of Aneurysms (RETA) and the Eurostar databases.

RETA is managed by the Joint Working Party of the Vascular Surgical Society of Great Britain and Ireland and the British Society of Interventional Radiologists. Submission of data to the Registry is voluntary, but it is the stated aim of both societies to collect data on all endovascular procedures performed within the UK. Stent-graft manufacturers have recently been asked to submit details of all endografts supplied to UK clinicians and this may, in time, permit the Joint Working Party to estimate the number of endovascular procedures that are not reported. Data have been collected since January 1996 and these include information on all patients (whether fit or unfit), all devices (whether commercially available or home-made) and all types of intervention (whether elective, urgent or emergency). The most recent report from the Registry provides details of 557 patients treated in 29 centres during a 3 year period (1996 - 1998). Centre experience ranges from 1 - 112 cases, with a median of 10 cases.

The European Registry of Stent-graft Techniques for Abdominal Aortic Aneurysm Repair (Eurostar) was established at a meeting of European collaborators in Liverpool in February 1996. Major vascular centres throughout Europe have been invited to submit information on all endovascular procedures performed. Data on patients treated before 1st July 1996 have been collected retrospectively but data on patients treated thereafter have been collected prospectively on an intention-to-treat basis. Since 1st July 1996 patients considered unfit for conventional repair have been excluded from the Registry, as have those treated with home-made devices that do not possess a CE mark. At the time of the last data analysis, the Eurostar Registry included details of 1,557 patients treated over 5 years (1994-1998) in 38 Centres in 11 countries. Fourteen of these centres had treated between 16 and 50 patients, 21 had treated fewer than 15 and three had treated over 50.

Both registries require the completion of standardised case record forms. These include details of patients and aneurysms treated (or scheduled for treatment), details of all interventions performed including any adjuvant procedures, and a record of operative and postoperative complications. Participating centres are also required to submit the results of regular clinical and radiological follow-up examinations.

Is endovascular repair technically feasible?

That it is possible to compress a covered stent-graft into a relatively narrow delivery system, to pass such a delivery system into the aorta via the femoral and iliac arteries, and then to deploy the stent-graft within the aorta is beyond doubt. What is less certain is the proportion of

patients and aneurysms that may be treated by this technique (applicability), and the incidence of technical failure in patients in whom endovascular repair is considered feasible.

Successful endovascular repair relies on the isolation of the aneurysm from both pressure and flow. This, in turn, mandates anastomotic zones wherein the stent-graft forms a secure seal against relatively normal aortic or iliac artery wall. Endovascular repair cannot, therefore, be performed if the neck of an infrarenal aneurysm is too short, too wide or heavily diseased and calcified. Similarly, aneurysmal disease of both common iliac arteries precludes endovascular repair unless the surgeon is prepared to extend the limbs of the stent-graft into both external iliac arteries and so sacrifice flow into both internal iliac arteries. It should also be remembered that endovascular repair will only be successful if the stent-graft can be delivered and deployed in the correct position. Narrow, tortuous and/or heavily calcified iliac arteries may prevent endovascular access to the aorta, while marked angulation of the proximal aorta may prevent accurate deployment of the stent-graft.

There have been relatively few studies of applicability. During the early experience in Liverpool, a small in-house study was conducted into patient suitability; of 117 patients with abdominal aortic aneurysm who presented over a 12 month period, only 27 (23%) were anatomically suitable for treatment with a commercially available modular bifurcated stent-graft (Vanguard, Boston Scientific Limited). Applicability has increased both with increasing experience and with the availability of other endovascular devices and delivery systems, but over 50% of patients remain unsuitable for endovascular repair.

Applicability can be increased by adopting an extra-anatomic approach to endovascular repair. One or other common iliac artery is first occluded by coil embolisation, deployment of an endovascular occluder or extra-peritoneal ligation of the artery. The aneurysm is then isolated by deployment of a tapered aorto uni-iliac graft into the contralateral iliac artery. The procedure is completed by conventional femoro-femoral crossover bypass. Such an extra anatomic approach is not, however, universally condoned.

Finally, applicability is claimed by some to be increased if the surgeon is prepared to deploy an uncovered stent across the renal artery origins. This is said to permit fixation of the proximal portion of the stent-graft even if the infrarenal neck is short. Unfortunately, proponents of this approach seem to overlook the fact that a very short contact zone between infrarenal aorta and stent-graft is unlikely to result in a secure and durable seal. It is quite likely that applicability is being increased at the expense of efficacy.

If a patient is considered to be anatomically suitable for endovascular repair, it is usually possible to deploy the stent-graft in the desired position. Although technical problems with the device or delivery system are reported in up to 13% of procedures, they can usually be overcome by additional endovascular intervention. The reported rate of immediate or early conversion to open repair is less than 5%. Interestingly, the rate of conversion is higher with aorto uni-iliac devices (8.3%) than with commercially available tube or bifurcated devices (3.3%). The rate of conversion has also decreased significantly with increasing experience, from 7.6% in 1996 to 1.7% in 1998 (unpublished RETA data).

Is endovascular repair safe?

Morbidity and mortality after endovascular repair are both reported to be low. The overall 30-day mortality among patients entered in the Eurostar database is 3.2% and is, unsurprisingly, lower in patients considered fit for conventional repair (2.3%) than in those who are not (12.5%). The RETA database confirms this finding. Mortality is also lower in patients treated with commercially available tube or bifurcated devices (3.3%) than in those treated with home-made aorto uni-iliac devices (12%). This difference is statistically significant even if a simple logistic regression model is employed to adjust for differences in age, anaesthetic risk, indications for repair and aneurysm diameter (RETA). Both databases also underline the dangers of conversion to open-repair. Death was reported in nine of 28 (32%) patients converted in the UK (RETA) and in 20% of patients converted throughout Europe (Eurostar).

The introduction of a delivery system into the common femoral artery has the potential to cause significant injury to the femoral and/or iliac arteries. There is also the possibility that the passage of the delivery system through the aneurysm sac may dislodge aneurysm thrombus thereby precipitating distal embolisation and lower limb ischaemia, but the incidence of such complications has been lower than expected. Although bruising in the groins is common, particularly if a percutaneous approach is employed for the contralateral limb, significant arterial trauma or iliac dissection has been reported in less than 2% of interventions. The incidence of distal embolisation is uncertain, but the reported incidence of critical lower limb ischaemia following endovascular repair is less than 1% and the incidence of amputation 0.1%.

The expectation of low systemic morbidity seems to have been realised. The RETA database records an overall incidence of medical complications of 18.3%. Unfortunately, this includes relatively minor complications, such as pyrexia of unknown origin (which is common after endovascular repair but usually mild and self-limiting), as well as prolonged ileus and respiratory tract infection. The incidence of renal failure is reported at 4% and this, perhaps, reflects the potential for mal-deployment of an endograft to interfere with renal artery blood flow. The incidences of major cardiac, pulmonary and cerebrovascular complications are not reported separately. The Eurostar database records a similar overall incidence of systemic complications (13%), with the incidences of cardiac, pulmonary and cerebrovascular complications reported as 4, 3 and 1% respectively.

Is endovascular repair effective?

As with conventional open repair, the primary aim of endovascular aneurysm repair is quite simply to prolong life by preventing death from aneurysm rupture. It may be argued, therefore, that endovascular repair can only be deemed to have failed if the patient dies as a consequence of aneurysm rupture. However, observation until death from presumed rupture is neither an ethical nor a particularly reliable follow-up strategy, since patients with aneurysms are, in general, elderly and so prone to sudden death from a variety of causes. In order to determine whether or not endovascular repair is effective, it must be determined whether or not the aneurysm remains at risk of rupture. Unfortunately, this is not simple.

Many published reports have focused on the problem of endoleak which has been defined as 'persistent or recurrent blood flow within the aneurysm sac but outside the stent-graft'. Endoleaks may be primary or secondary and are classified according to site. Type I contains graft related endoleaks which may occur at the proximal or distal junctions between the endograft and native artery wall, or at the junction between the components of a modular graft. Type II endoleaks are due to persistent or recurrent reperfusion of the aneurysm sac from patent lumbar or inferior mesenteric arteries.

Endoleaks are relatively common. Primary endoleaks are reported in 6% of patients in the RETA database and 18% of patients in the Eurostar database; the RETA database classifies only those endoleaks that persist at the time of discharge whereas the Eurostar database includes all endoleaks observed prior to discharge. Up to 40% of primary endoleaks seal spontaneously; the remainder are either treated by secondary intervention or persist at the time of last follow-up. A further 12% of patients develop secondary endoleaks during follow-up and it is important to note that the incidence of such endoleaks does not decrease significantly with duration of follow-up.

An endoleak is clear evidence of persistent or recurrent communication between the circulation and the aneurysm sac and for this reason is often considered to be evidence of treatment failure. Perhaps more worryingly, freedom from endoleak is by implication considered to represent successful treatment. This assumes, of course, that all patients with endoleak remain at risk of rupture while those without demonstrable endoleak are free of any form of communication between the aneurysm sac and the circulation.

There is general agreement that Type I anastomotic endoleaks maintain intrasac pressure and should, therefore, be treated by secondary intervention. The significance of Type II (side branch) endoleaks is, however, less certain. Many of these occur in association with a shrinking aneurysm and so must be assumed to be at less than systemic arterial pressure. It is difficult to believe that such endoleaks are clinically significant. The situation is complicated further by the observation that intrasac pressure can be maintained by low flow endoleaks that cannot be visualised on conventional postoperative or follow-up computed tomography or angiography. It is also known that thrombus can transmit pressure and there is growing concern that a sealed endoleak may, in fact, continue to maintain intrasac pressure.

What is becoming clear is that the presence or absence of endoleak is not a hard end-point. In particular, absence of endoleak cannot be equated with treatment success. Attention is now being focused on the problem of endotension which is defined as 'persistent or recurrent pressurisation of the aneurysm sac'. This is certainly a more realistic measure of treatment success or failure, but the problem is that at present there is no way of measuring intrasac pressure directly during follow-up. For the time being we must rely on observation of the aneurysm sac itself. Continued expansion of the aneurysm almost certainly indicates maintenance of significant intrasac pressure, while shrinkage almost certainly indicates abolition or reduction of intrasac pressure. Failure of an aneurysm either to shrink or expand may indicate depressurisation, but then again it may very well not. We simply do not know.

The Eurostar registry requires participants to monitor aneurysm diameter during follow-up but compliance has been very poor and data on aneurysm size are currently available for fewer than 10% of the patients entered into the database. Analysis of the available data reveals a shrinking aneurysm in 65%, an expanding aneurysm in 22% and no significant change in 13%. Increase in aneurysm diameter is more common in patients with a history of endoleak than in those without, but the relationship between evolution of the aneurysm sac and endoleak is inconsistent, as aneurysm expansion may be observed in patients without endoleak and aneurysm shrinkage in patients with endoleak.

It is probably fair to conclude that endovascular repair is effective for at least a while in a majority of patients. Whether it will continue to be effective in the longer term remains unknown, as does the true incidence of treatment failure.

Conclusions

There is good evidence that endovascular repair is technically feasible in selected patients and is associated with relatively low morbidity and mortality. However, there is little or no evidence to support the contention that endovascular repair is as effective as conventional open operation. A prospective randomised trial of endovascular versus conventional repair in fit patients (EVAR 1) and endovascular versus no repair in unfit patients (EVAR 2) was started during 1999 but it is not scheduled to report for at least 5 years. There are no published analyses of the two databases (RETA and Eurostar) on which much of this chapter rests, but the reader may find reports by Blum et al [1], Cuypers et al [2] and Schurink et al [3] of interest.

The evidence for endovascular aneurysm repair

Sound evidence

- Endovascular repair is technically feasible in selected patients and is associated with relatively low morbidity and mortality.

- Rates of conversion to open repair have fallen with increasing experience (to less than 5%).

- Conversion to open repair is associated with high mortality (20 - 32%).

- Endoleaks are common.

Evidence needed

- Whether endovascular repair is as effective as conventional open operation.

- The significance of Type II (side branch) endoleaks is largely unknown.

- The significance of failure of an aneurysm sac to shrink after endoluminal repair is unknown.

Acknowledgements

I thank Dr. Steven Thomas, Endovascular Fellow at the Northern General Hospital in Sheffield, for making available the 3 year report from the RETA database, and Dr. Phillippe Cuypers of the Eurostar Data Registry Centre in Eindhoven, the Netherlands, for making available data from the January 1999 analysis of the Eurostar database.

References

1. Blum U, Voshage G, Lammer J et al. Endoluminal stentgrafts for infrarenal abdominal aortic aneurysms. *New Engl J Med* 1997; 336: 13 - 20.

2. Cuypers P, Buth J, Harris P et al. Realistic expectations for patients with stentgraft treatment of abdominal aortic aneurysms: results of a European multicentre registry. *Eur J Vasc Endovasc Surg* 1999; 17: 507 - 516.

3. Schurink G, Aarts N, van Bockel J. Endoleak after stent-graft treatment of abdominal aortic aneurysm: a meta-analysis of clinical studies. *Br J Surg* 1999; 86: 581 - 587.

Chapter 18

The evidence for endovascular
aneurysm repair

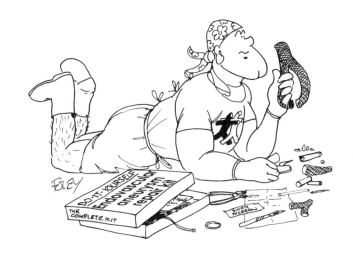

Chapter 19

Safer thoraco-abdominal aneurysm repair

MJ Brooks
Research Fellow
JHN Wolfe
Consultant Vascular Surgeon

REGIONAL VASCULAR UNIT,
ST. MARY'S HOSPITAL, LONDON

Introduction

Thoraco-abdominal aortic aneurysms are often considered uncommon, as the number presenting for elective repair is less than 5% that of infrarenal aneurysms. The true incidence, while difficult to estimate with certainty, may be higher, as a study of aneurysm deaths in Swansea showed one in four ruptured aortic aneurysms had a supra-renal component [1]. The number of patients in whom thoraco-abdominal aneurysms are detected may also increase as computed tomography (CT) and ultrasonography become routine investigations. Conservative management of such aneurysms is associated with a poor prognosis; actuarial survival of patients with a 5cm diameter thoraco-abdominal aortic aneurysm may be as low as 40% at 1 year and 13% at 5 years [2]. In comparison the outcome of surgery can be good, with an 80% 5 year actuarial survival reported by the best centres [3].

Thoraco-abdominal aneurysm repair is a major undertaking, often in patients who are elderly with limited organ reserve and concurrent disease. In addition to the surgical trauma of an extensive dissection are added the physiological insults of a proximal aortic cross-clamp, massive blood loss, hypothermia and visceral ischaemia/reperfusion. The repair of ruptured thoraco-abdominal aneurysms has been reported to carry an in-hospital mortality of 75% even in experienced centres [4]. The results of elective repair are better, despite a significant incidence of respiratory failure, renal impairment, paraplegia, myocardial infarction and multiple organ dysfunction in the peri-operative period (Table 1).

Pre-operative assessment

Since the repair of thoraco-abdominal aneurysms carries considerable morbidity and mortality, the judgement on whom to operate, and the guidance given to patients, constitutes an important component of their surgical management. As data increase it becomes easier to recognise patients with an unacceptable risk from elective surgery. Pre-operative assessment must also identify patients in whom the peri-operative risk can be reduced. The St. Mary's Hospital experience by 1993 (130 patients) was that aneurysm rupture, aneurysm extent, chronic aortic dissection, pre-operative renal impairment, chronic obstructive airways disease and abnormal spirometry were pre-operative risk factors associated with increased mortality [5]. In Crawford's larger experience (1509 patients), aneurysm symptoms, peptic ulcer disease and cerebrovascular disease were additional predictors of poor outcome [3].

Aneurysm imaging

Imaging is used to predict the risk of aneurysm rupture if left untreated and to allow pre-operative planning of the repair. Contrast-enhanced spiral CT gives most

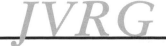

Table 1. Recent published series reporting outcome after open repair of aneurysms of the descending and thoraco-abdominal aorta.

Technique Author, year	Number n	Renal Impairment % (n)	Paraplegia % (n)	30 day Mortality % (n)
Simple cross-clamp	**2620**	**15.3 (401)**	**10.9 (286)**	**11.2 (293)**
Cambria et al 1997 [35]	160	10 (16)	6.9 (11)	9.4 (15)
Grabitz et al 1996 [37]	122	12.7 (15)	7.4 (9)	14.7 (18)
Mauney et al 1996	91	11(10)	9.9 (9)	13.2 (12)
Galloway et al 1996	24	7.7 (6)	3.7 (1)	10.3 (8)
Coselli 1994 [25]	309	7.1 (22)	7.4 (23)	5 (20)
Gilling-Smith et al 1994	130	15.4 (20)	6.1 (8)	27.7 (36)
Acher et al 1994 [42]	110	11(12)	2.7 (3)	7.3 (8)
Scheinin et al 1994	71	5.6 (4)	8.5 (6)	11.3 (8)
Svensson et al 1993 [3]	1251	18.8 (235)	14.2 (178)	8 (100)
von Sesenger 1993 [18]	42	6.6 (6)	9 (3)	8.8 (8)
Cox et al 1992 [4]	129	27 (33)	21 (25)	34.9 (45)
Cooley and Baldwin 1992	31	25.8 (8)	12.9 (4)	12.9 (4)
Hollier et al 1988	150	9.8 (14)	4 (6)	7.3 (11)
Open distal anastamosis	**95**	**4.2 (4)**	**7.4 (7)**	**12.6 (12)**
Scheinin et al 1994	71	5.6 (4)	8.5 (6)	11.3 (8)
Cooley and Baldwin 1992	24	0 (0)	4.2 (1)	16.6 (4)
Gott shunt	**366**	**2.4 (9)**	**0 (0)**	**12 (44)**
Verdant et al 1995 [27]	366	2.4 (9)	0 (0)	12 (44)
Left heart bypass	**698**	**10.8 (76)**	**12.0 (84)**	**11.6 (81)**
Schepens et al 1996	172	10.4 (18)	8.2 (14)	10.5 (18)
Grabitz et al 1996 [37]	102	6.8 (7)	6.8 (7)	6.8(7)
Galloway et al 1996	54	7.7 (6)	4.2 (2)	10.3 (8)
Coselli 1994 [25]	63	11.1(7)	1.6 (1)	5 (20)
Svensson et al 1993 [3]	258	13.2 (34)	21.7 (56)	8.9 (23)
von Sesenger 1993 [18]	49	4.4 (4)	9 (4)	9.8 (5)
Cardiopulmonary bypass	**51**	**2.2 (1)**	**6.5 (3)**	**9.8 (5)**
Kouchoukos et al 1995 [15]	51	2.2 (1)	6.5 (3)	9.8 (5)
	3830	**12.8 (491)**	**9.9 (380)**	**11.4 (435)**

information about aneurysm size, extent, dissection and wall thickness. Identification of an aortic dissection is particularly important, as surgery may be technically difficult and the risk of paraplegia is increased. Selective intercostal angiography has been proposed to locate the important arterial supply to the spinal cord, but this investigation has a morbidity (anterior spinal artery emboli) and is not widely practised [6]. No other useful techniques are available for pre-operative intercostal localisation.

It is the authors' practice to obtain an aortic angiogram to assess accurately the aneurysm neck and identify visceral, particularly renal, origin stenoses. As the appropriate software becomes available, magnetic resonance angiography may provide this information without exposing the patient to ionising radiation and contrast medium.

Cardiovascular investigation

Occlusive coronary artery disease and left ventricular hypertrophy are common in these patients. Detection of occult disease may be particularly important as supra-coeliac aortic cross-clamping induces significant myocardial ischaemia and left ventricular strain. In a retrospective study of routine coronary angiography prior to thoraco-abdominal aneurysm repair, 60% of patients with no cardiac history had a greater than 30% coronary artery stenosis [4].

A history of angina or myocardial infarction and the resting electrocardiogram are insensitive predictors of cardiac complications [5]. Exercise testing is rarely helpful in detecting occult ischaemia, as exercise tolerance is often limited by peripheral vascular disease and poor respiratory reserve. Radionucleotide myocardial perfusion imaging and echocardiography with pharmacological stress are non-invasive means of excluding ischaemic heart disease. Dobutamine stress echocardiography has been shown to be sensitive and specific in vascular patients [7]. The introduction of pharmacological stress echocardiography in all patients, with pre-operative intervention for significant coronary disease, has been associated with a reduction in peri-operative mortality of 20% in our recent experience [5]. A small retrospective study of coronary revascularisation prior to thoraco-abdominal aneurysm repair has shown that coronary artery bypass grafting can be performed safely in these patients, with peri-operative mortality as low as that of patients with normal coronary anatomy [4]. Coronary angiography can be technically difficult in these patients and is associated with the risks of aortic dissection, contrast induced nephropathy and cholesterol embolisation. This last problem is under-appreciated in patients with aneurysm disease.

Pulmonary investigation

Pulmonary complications are common after thoraco abdominal aneurysm repair. Respiratory function is impaired postoperatively by the surgical incision, division of the diaphragm, collapse of the left lung, pulmonary haemorrhage and ischaemia/reperfusion associated adult respiratory distress syndrome (ARDS). One fifth of patients will require prolonged postoperative ventilation, and one third of these will die [3,5]. Smoking, chronic obstructive airways disease and impaired spirometry are independent predictors of postoperative mortality. Pre-operative FEF_{25} (forced expiratory flow rate at 25% of total expired volume) has been shown to be an independent and specific predictor of postoperative respiratory failure [3,8]. The correlation between FEF_{25} and the risk of respiratory failure mortality is linear; no threshold exists below which operation can be considered unsafe. A large thoracic aneurysm may itself be the cause of compromised respiratory reserve.

Local practice is to perform spirometry on all patients, to identify those at increased respiratory risk who will benefit from pre-operative physiotherapy and bronchodilator therapy. Cessation of smoking is encouraged 3 months prior to operation. To reduce sedation requirements in the early postoperative period an elective tracheostomy is made at the time of aneurysm repair in patients with poor respiratory function, or on the first postoperative day if the patient remains ventilator-dependent. An attempt should also be made to confine the incision to the chest or abdomen alone [9]. It is disappointing that we have been unable to show a significant benefit from the introduction of a subcostal (transabdominal) incision for Type IV thoraco-abdominal aneurysm repair [10]. Epidural anaesthesia is used routinely which, despite the lack of evidence of its benefit, again reduces sedation and aids chest physiotherapy. The use of fresh blood may reduce the risk of ARDS and a short radial incision in the diaphragm is used rather than total diaphragmatic transection to maintain function.

Renal investigation

There is a trend towards higher mortality in patients with impaired pre-operative renal function [5]. Serum creatinine, radionucleotide excretion renogram and aortic angiogram are used to screen for renal disease. Renal artery stenoses may be present in up to one third of patients. Prior to operation nephrotoxic drugs are discontinued and patients are well hydrated. It is preferable to correct any renal artery stenosis at the time of aortic reconstruction, since such stenosis is frequently due to thrombus at the orifice within the aortic wall [11]. Angioplasty of a lesion of this type may be dangerous and ineffective.

Operative technique

Prior to aortic reconstruction the proximal aorta must be cross-clamped. Cross-clamp placement results in proximal hypertension and distal ischaemia. Proximal hypertension is controlled by pharmacological agents or the shunting of blood. The drugs commonly used are the vasodilators isoflurane, sodium nitroprusside and glyceryl trinitrate. These agents further reduce visceral and spinal cord perfusion, which may be important, as visceral ischaemia and subsequent reperfusion are thought to be important causes of postoperative complications, including renal failure, paraplegia, the systemic inflammatory response syndrome, ARDS and multiple organ dysfunction [12,13,14]. Once the aorta is clamped, reconstruction is almost universally performed using the inlay technique first described by Crawford (Figure 1). Aneurysmal dilatation and rupture of the native aortic patches is a theoretical complication of this technique; every effort must be made to suture close to the visceral origins while leaving them widely patent. A number of techniques have been developed to reduce left ventricular strain and protect the viscera and spinal cord during aortic cross-clamping.

Distal perfusion

Techniques to reduce cardiac afterload and maintain distal organ perfusion have been used since thoraco-abdominal aneurysm repair was first performed in the 1950s. More recently, the development of heparin-

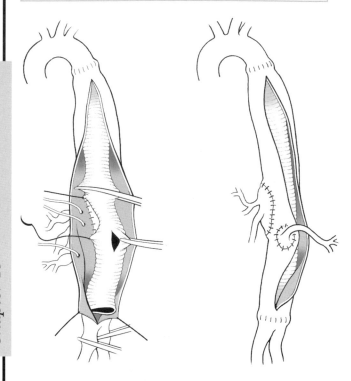

Figure 1. Aortic reconstruction using Crawford's inlay technique.

bonded extracorporeal circuits has reduced the need for systemic heparinisation; this is an important advance since bypass was previously associated with coagulopathy and significantly increased blood loss [15,16]. The authors use a heparin-bonded left heart bypass circuit with a centrifugal pump from the left atrium to the left femoral artery for repair of an extensive aneurysm. Other distal perfusion techniques include femoral vein to femoral artery bypass with a centrifugal pump and membrane oxygenator, axillofemoral bypass, a side graft from the proximal aortic graft with perfusion catheters to the superior mesenteric artery and coeliac axis, atrial-distal perfusion with selective visceral catheterisation and full cardiopulmonary bypass. Bypass circuits containing membrane oxygenators still require full systemic heparinisation. The benefits of distal perfusion techniques are summarised in Table 2.

As the benefit of distal perfusion has never been established in a randomised controlled trial, conclusions must be drawn from retrospective data. In a retrospective series by Svensson et al containing 832 operations (247 left heart and 28 cardiopulmonary bypass) mortality was 4% after left heart bypass, 9% after simple clamp and sew and 11% after cardiopulmonary bypass [17]. Von Segesser et al report similar mortality in a retrospective series of 5.3%, 19% and 10% respectively [18]. In most retrospective studies full cardiopulmonary bypass, compared to left heart bypass, is associated with significantly increased rates of pulmonary haemorrhage and mortality despite a trend towards protection from paraplegia and renal failure [15,16,19,20].

The protective effect of left heart bypass on the kidneys is unclear. While a reduction in postoperative renal failure has been noted in most retrospective studies of left heart bypass [3,18], one study showed an increased rate of renal impairment [21]. It has been proposed that the protective effect is lost if adequate flow rates are not maintained [22]. In Svensson et al's initial experience, bypass did not reduce paraplegia rates, but a reduction in paraplegia has been reported more recently in retrospective studies of bypass and cerebrospinal fluid (CSF) drainage in extensive aneurysm repairs [23-26]. Passive shunts have been shown to prevent proximal hypertension, maintain distal perfusion and reduce paraplegia, but they lack some of the benefits of bypass, most importantly flow rate control and incorporation of a heat exchanger for re-warming [27].

In a non-randomised prospective study of selective visceral perfusion containing 72 patients, in which retrograde aortic flow was maintained by left heart bypass and visceral flow by selective catheterisation of the visceral vessels, renal impairment was reduced and no patient developed organ dysfunction [28]. However, in a recent smaller prospective non-randomised study of the same technique, blood loss increased and renal failure was not reduced [29]. Achieving adequate flow rates through small distal catheters appears to have been a problem in the latter study; significant haemolysis and turbulence were observed.

Hypothermia

Hypothermia reduces tissue oxygen demands and thereby protects organs, including the spinal cord, during ischaemia, but complications, including arrhythmias and coagulopathy develop [30]. Profound hypothermia (<30°C) with cardiac standstill is widely used for repair of the ascending aorta and arch. Moderate hypothermia (33-35°C), achieved by ambient cooling or extracorporeal heat exchanger, is preferred for most thoraco-abdominal aneurysm repairs. Cooling appears to be effective in protecting the kidneys and spinal cord [15,31].

The systemic complications of hypothermia have lead to interest in local and regional cooling. The kidney has been cooled by infusion of cold heparinised saline (a medullary temperature of 15°C can be achieved) but without benefit in a retrospective study [21]. This technique has never been evaluated in a controlled trial and, because of the risk of renal artery dissection during passage of the infusion cannula, it is not a method to be recommended. Epidural spinal cooling has been shown to be effective in the baboon and feasible in man, but numbers are too small to determine its clinical value [32,33]. The authors have had difficulty producing effective spinal cooling using this technique. Local current practice is to use ambient cooling to achieve a core temperature of 32-33°C during ischaemia.

Table 2. Distal perfusion.

Advantages	Disadvantages
Reduced proximal hypertension	Increased operative time
Reduced left heart strain	Coagulopathy (platelet activation/ heparin administration)
Reduced visceral and lower limb ischaemia	Arrhythmias
Reduced de-clamp hypotension and acidosis	Traumatic cannulation
Reduced pharmacological intervention	Air embolus/embolic stroke
Prevents a rise in CSF pressure	Interference with the operative field
Allows unhurried anastomosis with intercostal and lumbar re-implantation	Shunt dislodgement
Aids cooling/re-warming	Bleeding from cannulation sites
Access for rapid volume infusion	Back-bleeding from lumbar arteries

Intercostal and lumbar artery re-implantation

The blood supply to the spinal cord is segmental from a single anterior and two posterior spinal arteries. These arteries are supplied sequentially by the vertebral, deep cervical, costovertebral, intercostal and lumbar arteries. In the middle third the anterior spinal arteries are small and a single dominant artery (artery of Adamcowitz) is believed to supply this segment from an origin between T9 and T12. In an early retrospective study intercostal re-implantation was associated with a significant reduction in the incidence of paraplegia after high risk type II thoraco-abdominal aneurysm repair [34]. However, the benefit of intercostal re-implantation has since been questioned as postoperative angiography has revealed that three quarters of the implanted intercostals in that study had occluded. Furthermore, comparable paraplegia rates have been reported without intercostal re-implantation [35]. The authors believe that an attempt should be made to incorporate large lumbar and intercostal arteries in either the proximal anastomosis or visceral patch; in extensive repairs a 6mm side graft should be anastomosed to the artery of Adamkiewicz or to a similar large intercostal artery. Simple inspection of large diameter vessels without back bleeding does not identify all important arteries. Hydrogen stimulation (injection of aortic segments with hydrogen-saturated saline and measurement from a spinal electrode), spinal somatosensory evoked potentials (SSEPs) and myogenic motor evoked potentials are being used in some centres to identify important intercostal arteries. The loss of SSEPs for over 30 minutes in a prospective study was highly predictive of the development of paraplegia [36]. In a large retrospective study of 167 patients the loss of SSEPs within 15 minutes of aortic cross-clamp placement was associated with a significant increase in paraplegia, especially in those in whom intercostal re-implantation did not result in the return of SSEPs [37]. However, as temperature, anaesthetic agents and CO_2 retention all alter SSEPs potentials, false positives are common [36,38]. The loss of transcranial motor evoked potentials has also been shown to predict paraplegia in a prospective study [39]. Interestingly, in a retrospective study oversewing, as opposed to re-implantation, of back bleeding lumbar arteries resulted in the return of SSEPs (presumably by reducing spinal artery hypotension) [40].

Spinal drainage

Local experience is that paraplegia occurs in 21% of Crawford Type II repairs, with rates as high as 41% reported by other centres [5,41]. Archer et al showed a reasonable correlation between actual and expected rates of paraplegia, regardless of operative technique [42]. Spinal cord perfusion is a balance between local arterial, venous and CSF pressure. In three randomised trials in animals, continuous dural drainage to maintain CSF pressure below 10 cm H_2O has been shown to reduce the incidence of paraplegia when a high aortic cross-clamp is applied [43-45]. In a large randomised trial of CSF drainage in man, the paraplegia rate was not reduced by the withdrawal of a median 52ml of CSF prior to aortic cross-clamp placement [41]. This study has been criticised as the volume of CSF drained was small and postoperative CSF pressure was not controlled. Three subsequent studies using historical controls, two with pharmacological intervention in addition to continuous CSF drainage, have shown a reduction in paraplegia rates in the intervention groups [42,44,46].

In one fifth of patients paraplegia develops in the early postoperative period, usually during a period of hypotension [3]. Meticulous haemodynamic monitoring at this time is essential. CSF drainage carries the theoretical risks of extradural haematoma and cerebral herniation but there are no case reports of such problems in practice.

Management of coagulopathy

Thoraco-abdominal aortic aneurysm repair is frequently complicated by coagulopathy, an important cause of intra-operative mortality. Coagulopathy develops as a result of multiple factors including blood loss, haemodilution, disruption of vascular endothelium, anticoagulant administration, transfusion of stored blood products, hypothermia, extracorporeal bypass, and ischaemia reperfusion, and associated complement and platelet activation. Clotting factors and fibrinogen are depleted (hepatic ischaemia is believed to interfere with prothrombin metabolism) and platelet function is compromised. Extracorporeal bypass causes platelet activation, coagulation factor consumption and thrombocytopaenia [47]. The early administration of clotting products (including fibrinogen and prothrombin) and platelets is essential. Surgical technique must minimise blood loss by meticulous haemostasis, the use of coated grafts and rapid over-sewing or balloon occlusion of calcified, non-contractile, lumbar and sac vessels.

The authors use a cell washing device for all repairs to reduce transfusion requirements for stored blood products. Ideally this device is used in conjunction with a rapid infusion pump to cope with the wide haemodynamic changes which occur during the operation. In our own and Crawford's experience the rate of distal thrombosis is far outweighed by the 30% of patients who suffer haemorrhagic complications [3,5]; if heparin is given (usually at a dose of 1 mg/kg) the activated clotting time must be monitored carefully. Aprotinin is currently given to correct heparin overdose and a number of other agents, including aminocaproic acid and desmopressin acetate are currently under investigation for the correction of coagulopathy.

Current challenges

Prevention of paraplegia

Paraplegia remains a significant and devastating complication of thoraco-abdominal aneurysm repair. Distal perfusion in conjunction with spinal drainage and moderate hypothermia appear to have reduced the incidence of paraplegia after Type I and II thoraco-abdominal aneurysm repair when comparison is made with historical controls [24,25]. The effect of these interventions on the incidence of paraplegia is illustrated in two large studies (Figure 2) [48,49].

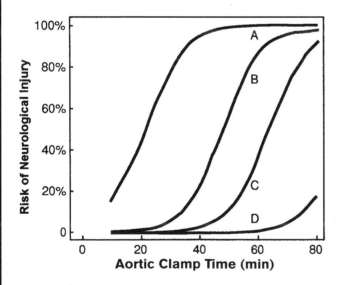

Logistic regression curves for A: No adjunct, B: Spinal drain and intrathecal papaverine, C: Hypothermia, D: Spinal fluid drainage, hypothermia and intrathecal papaverine.

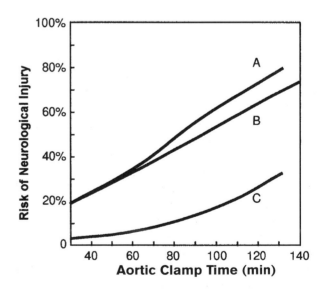

Relationship between A: No adjunct, B: Single cross clamp, C: Distal perfusion and hypothermia and outcome (Type II aneurysms only).

Figure 2. Strategies to prevent paraplegia after repair of a high risk thoraco-abdominal aortic aneurysm. Logistic regression curves show the relationship of aortic cross-clamp time and risk of neurological injury.

The benefit of monitoring SSEPs and intercostal re-implantation has not been proven in a prospective randomised trial. Such monitoring has been criticised, as spinal ischaemia first affects the anterior motor horns, not the dorsal columns. Early evidence from animal experiments suggested that motor evoked potentials may actually be a less sensitive and specific predictor of paraplegia than SSEPs [50]. The difficulty of interpretation of evoked potentials and the high rate of false positives mean that they are unlikely to gain widespread acceptance. An easily reproducible and sensitive technique is required. A number of pharmacological agents appear to protect the cord from ischaemia reperfusion injury in animal models but their clinical role has yet to be defined (Table 3).

Renal protection

The main determinants of postoperative renal function are successful renal revascularisation and intra-operative renal ischaemia time. Renal failure is uncommon if the aortic cross-clamp time is less than 30 minutes. Hypothermia and distal perfusion, with adequate flow, are probably effective for renal protection. The administration of prostaglandin E1, angiotensin converting enzyme inhibitors and free radical scavengers have not been shown to protect the kidneys in animal studies.

Pharmacological intervention

Visceral ischaemia reperfusion injury is believed to be a cause of multiple organ dysfunction after thoraco-abdominal aneurysm repair. Aortic cross-clamp time has been shown to predict the risk of paraplegia, renal failure and organ dysfunction [3]. Visceral ischaemia is associated with cellular dysfunction, leading to the build up of toxic products and the generation of pro-inflammatory cytokines, arachadonic acid breakdown products and oxygen derived free radicals. Gut mucosal integrity is compromised and bacterial products (endotoxin and proteoglycans) enter the circulation. A correlation exists between peak plasma endotoxin and the development of organ dysfunction [51]. Visceral reperfusion may wash toxic products and cytokines from the splanchnic bed and stimulate a systemic inflammatory response mediated by the neutrophil. In animals, leukocyte sequestration in the lung is characteristic of reperfusion. Significantly greater up-regulation of the neutrophil adhesion receptor CD11b, which mediates neutrophil adhesion to lung endothelium, is seen intra-operatively in patients who subsequently develop organ dysfunction [51,52]. It is too early to predict if these pathways can be used for therapeutic intervention, but the role of endotoxin, neutrophil activation and endothelial adhesion warrant further study. A number of pharmacological agents capable of protecting organs during ischaemia reperfusion are currently under investigation.

Endovascular repair

The exclusion of aneurysms by a transluminal covered endoluminal stent was first proposed by Dottener in 1969. The authors' experience with endoluminal stents in the thoracic aorta is limited; we have used them successfully for the exclusion of two aneurysms, but a third patient died from early rupture of a false aneurysm at the distal fixation point. The largest published series of endoluminal stents for descending thoracic aneurysms is 44 patients from Stanford, USA [53] In only one third of patients presenting with a thoraco-abdominal aortic aneurysm was the aneurysm anatomy suitable for endovascular repair. The stent used was a self expanding wire stent with a mean (expanded) diameter of 3.6 cm. Stent placement was achieved by a femoral or infrarenal aortic approach with a second catheter passed by a radial approach. Stent placement was often technically difficult, with a significant incidence of left subclavian occlusion, requiring carotid subclavian bypass and inadequate distal fixation needing a second distal stent. In 90% of patients the aneurysm sac was successfully thrombosed. Peri-operative mortality in patients often unfit for open repair was 7%. Two patients developed paraplegia. With follow-up at a median of only 12 months and with one patient having already died from late aneurysm rupture it is too early to predict the durability of this procedure. Until the long-term outcome is known the authors believe that endoluminal repair should be reserved for patients with suitable aneurysm anatomy who are unfit for open aneurysm repair.

Table 3. Pharmacological agents of potential benefit in attenuating spinal cord injury during thoraco-abdominal aortic aneurysm repair.

Intrathecal	
Vasodilators	**Papaverine**
Opiate antagonists	**Naloxone**
Systemic	
Anti-inflammatory	**Methylprednisolone**
Free radical scavenger	**Mannitol**
	Superoxide dismutase
	Desferrioxamine
N-methyl-D-aspartate Antagonists	**Allopurinol**
	Thiopental
	Fluarizine

Conclusions

Patients presenting with thoraco-abdominal aortic aneurysms constitute a high risk population with an already reduced life expectancy from cardiovascular, pulmonary and renal disease. Aneurysm repair involves an extensive surgical dissection and proximal aortic clamping. The patient is subjected to the physiological insults of left ventricular strain, visceral ischaemia and reperfusion, massive blood loss, coagulopathy and hypothermia. Even with meticulous surgical technique, respiratory and renal function is compromised in the early postoperative period. It is no surprise, despite improvements in anaesthetic and surgical technique, that thoraco-abdominal aneurysm repair continues to be associated with significant mortality and morbidity.

Improvements in outcome have resulted from retrospective review of the work from those relatively few centres with a large experience. In recent years, the role of cerebrospinal fluid drainage and left heart bypass has become established in this way. Currently, attention is focused on endovascular repair, pharmacological intervention, management of coagulopathy and the detection of spinal ischaemia as means to improve outcome further.

Safer thoraco-abdominal aneurysm repair

Sound evidence

- Renal impairment and impaired pulmonary function preoperatively are associated with increased postoperative mortality.

- Coronary revascularisation can be performed safely prior to thoraco-abdominal aneurysm repair and may reduce mortality.

- Spinal drainage can be performed safely, and in conjunction with pharmacological agents is of benefit in reducing paraplegia in Type I and Type II repairs.

- Paraplegia, renal failure and mortality all increase if a simple cross-clamp is applied without distal perfusion for greater than 40 minutes.

- Moderate hypothermia protects the spinal cord and kidneys during ischaemia.

- Profound hypothermia with cardiopulmonary bypass is associated with increased mortality.

Evidence needed

- Optimum method of screening for occult cardiac disease, and indications for intervention.

- Need to re-implant intercostal arteries.

- The optimum technique for spinal cord monitoring.

- Benefit of local renal and spinal cooling.

- Benefit of selective visceral cannulation and perfusion.

- Long-term outcome of endovascular techniques.

References (randomised trials in bold)

1. Ingoldby CJ, Wujanto R, Mitchell JE. Impact of vascular surgery on community mortality form ruptured aortic aneurysms. *Br J Surg* 1986; 73: 551-3.

2. Bickerstaff LK, Pairolero PC, Hollier LH, et al. Thoracic aortic aneurysms: a population-based study. *Surgery* 1982; 92: 1103-8.

3. Svensson LG, Crawford ES, Hess KR, Coselli JS, Safi HJ. Experience with 1509 patients undergoing thoraco-abdominal aortic operations. *J Vasc Surg* 1993; 17: 357-70.

4. Cox GS, O'Hara PJ, Hertzer NR, Piedmonte MR, Krajewski LP, Beven EG. Thoraco-abdominal aneurysm repair: a representative experience. *J Vasc Surg* 1992; 15: 780-8.

5. Gilling-Smith GL, Worswick L, Knight PF, Wolfe JHN, Mansfield AO. Surgical repair of thoraco-abdominal aortic aneurysms: 10 year's experience. *Br J Surg* 1995; 82: 624-9.

6. Williams GM, Perler BA, Burbick JF, et al. Angiographic localisation of spinal cord blood supply and its relationship to postoperative paraplegia. *J Vasc Surg* 1991; 13: 23-33.

7. McEnroe CS, O'Donnell TF, Yeager A, Konstam M, Mackey WC. Comparison of ejection fraction and Goldman risk factor analysis to dipyridamole-thallium 201 studies in the evaluation of cardiac morbidity after aortic aneurysm surgery. *J Vasc Surg* 1990; 11: 497-504.

8. Gracey DR, Divertie MB, Didier EP. Preoperative pulmonary preparation of patients with chronic obstructive pulmonary disease. A prospective study. *Chest* 1979; 76: 123-9.

9. Gilling-Smith GHL, Wolfe JHN. Transabdominal repair of type IV thoraco-abdominal aortic aneurysms. *Eur J Vasc Endovasc Surg* 1995; 9: 112-13.

10. Brooks MJ, Bradbury AW, Wolfe JHN. Elective repair of Type IV thoraco-abdominal aortic aneurysms by a subcostal (trans-abdominal) approach. *Eur J Vasc Endovasc Surg* (In Press).

11. Chan Y-C, Al-Kutoubi MA, Wolfe JHN. Do not be fooled by angiography in renovascular disease. *Eur J Vasc Endovasc Surg* 1998; 16: 78-9.

12. Harward TR, Welborn MB, Martin TD, et al. Visceral ischaemia and organ dysfunction after thoraco-abdominal aortic aneurysm repair. A clinical and cost analysis. *Ann Surg* 1996; 223: 729-36.

13. Pastores SM, Katz DP, Kvetan V. Splanchnic ischaemia and gut mocosal injury in sepsis and the multiple organ dysfunction syndrome. *Am J Gastroenterol* 1996; 91: 1697-1710.

14. Grace PA. Ischaemia-reperfusion injury. *Br J Surg* 1994; 81: 637-47.

15. Kouchoukos NT, Daily BB, Rokkas CK, Murphy SF, Bauer S, Abboud N. Hypothermic bypass and circulatory arrest for operations on the descending thoracic and thoraco-abdominal aorta. *Ann Thorac Surg* 1995; 60: 67-77.

16. Kieffer E, Koskas F, Walden R, et al. Hypothermic circulatory arrest for thoracic aneurysmectomy through left sided thoracotomy. *J Vasc Surg* 1994; 19: 457-63.

17. Svensson LG, Crawford ES, Hess KR, Coselli JS, Safi HJ. Variables predictive of outcome in 832 patients undergoing repairs of the descending thoracic aorta. *Chest* 1993; 104: 1248-53.

18. Von Segesser LK, Killer I, Jenni R, Lutz U, Turina MI. Improved distal circulatory support for repair of descending thoracic aortic aneurysms. *Ann Thoracic Surg* 1993; 56: 1373-80.

19. Crawford ES, Coselli JS, Safi HJ. Partial cardiopulmonary bypass, hypothermic circulatory arrest, and posterolateral exposure for thoracic aortic aneurysm operation. *J Thorac and Cardiovasc Surg* 1987; 94: 824-7.

20. Safi HJ, Miller CC, Subramaniam MH, et al. Thoracic and thoraco-abdominal aneurysm repair using cardiopulmonary bypass, profound hypothermia, and circulatory arrest via left side of the chest incision. *J Vasc Surg* 1998; 28: 591-8.

21. Svensson LG, Coselli JS, Safi HJ, Hess KR, Crawford ES. Appraisal of adjuncts to prevent acute renal failure after surgery on the thoracic or thoraco-abdominal aorta. *J Vasc Surg* 1989; 10: 230-9.

22. Ataka K, Okada M, Yoshimura N, et al. Clinical study of optimal bypass flow for temporary bypass with centrifugal pump in surgical treatment of aneurysm of the descending thoracic aorta. [Japanese] *Nippon Kyobu Geka Gakkai Zasshi* 1994; 42: 879-85.

23. Svensson LG, Grum DF, Bednarski M, Cosgrove DM, Loop FD. Appraisal of cerebrospinal fluid alterations during aortic surgery with intrathecal papaverine administration and cerebrospinal fluid drainage. *J Vasc Surg* 1990; 11: 423-9.

24. Safi H, Hess KR, Randall M, et al. Cerebrospinal fluid drainage and distal aortic perfusion: reducing neurological complications in repair of thoraco-abdominal aortic aneurysm types I and II. *J Vasc Surg* 1996; 23: 223-8.

25. Coselli JS. Thoraco-abdominal aortic aneurysms: experience with 372 patients. *J Cardiovasc Surg* 1994; 9: 638-47.

26. Lawrie GM, Earle N, DeBakey ME. Evolution of surgical techniques for aneurysms of the descending thoracic aorta: twenty-nine years experience with 659 patients. *J Cardiovasc Surg* 1994; 9: 648-61.

27. Verdant A, Page A, Cossette R, Dontigny L, Page P, Balliot R. Surgery of the descending thoracic aorta: spinal cord protection with the Gott shunt. *Ann Thorac Surg* 1988; 46: 147-54.

28. Najafi H. Descending aortic aneurysectomy without adjuncts to avoid ischaemia. 1993 update. *Ann Thorac Surg* 1993; 55: 1042-5.

29. Leijdekkers VJ, Wirds JW, Vahl AC, et al. The visceral perfusion system and distal bypass during thoraco-abdominal aneurysm surgery: an alternative for physiological blood flow? *Cardiovasc Surg* 1999; 7: 219-24.

30. Bush HL, Hydo LJ, Fisher E, Fantini GA, Silane MF, Barie PS. Hypothermia during elective abdominal aortic aneurysm repair: the high price of avoidable mortality. *J Vasc Surg* 1995; 21: 392-402.

31. Svensson LG, Hess KR, Coselli JS, Safi HJ. Influence of segmental arteries extent, and atriofemoral bypass on postoperative paraplegia after thoraco-abdominal aortic operations. *J Vasc Surg* 1994; 20: 255-62.

32. Rokkas CK, Sundaresan S, Shuman TA, et al. Profound systemic hypothermia protects the spinal cord in a primate model of spinal cord ischaemia. *J Thorac Cardiovasc Surg* 1993; 106: 1024-35.

33. Davison JK, Cambria RP, Vierra DJ, Columbia MA, Koustas G. Epidural cooling for regional spinal cord hypothermia during thoraco-abdominal aneurysm repair. *J Vasc Surg* 1994; 20: 304-10.

34. Svensson LG, Patel V, Robinson MF, Ueda T, Roehm JO, Crawford ES. Influence of preservation or perfusion of intraoperatively identified spinal cord blood supply on spinal motor evoked potentials and paraplegia after aortic surgery. *J Vasc Surg* 1991; 13: 355-65.

35. Cambria RP, Davison JK, Zanetti S, L'Italien GL, Atamian S. Thoraco-abdominal aneurysm repair: perspectives over a decade with the clamp-and-sew technique. *Ann Surg* 1997; 226: 294-305.

36. Laschinger JC, Cunningham NJ, Catinella FP, Nathan IM, Spencer FC. Detection and prevention of intra-operative spinal cord ischaemia after cross-clamping of the thoracic aorta: use of somatosensory evoked potentials. *Surgery* 1982; 92: 1109-17.

37. Grabitz K, Sandmann W, Stuhmeier K, et al. The risk of ischaemic spinal cord injury in patients undergoing graft replacement for thoraco-abdominal aortic aneurysms. *J Vasc Surg* 1996; 23: 230-240.

38. Crawford ES, Mizari EM, Hess KR, Coselli JS, Safi HJ, Patel VM. The impact of distal aortic perfusion and spinal somatosensory evoked potential monitoring on prevention of paraplegia after aortic aneurysm operation. *J Thorac Cardiovasc Surg* 1988; 95: 357-367.

39. Jacobs MJ, Meylaerts SA, de Hann P, de Mol BA, Kalman CJ. Strategies to prevent neurologic deficit based on motor-evoked potentials in type I and II thoraco-abdominal aortic aneurysm repair. *J Vasc Surg* 1999; 29: 48-57.

40. Shiiya N, Yasuda K, Matsui Y, Sakuma M, Sasaki S. Spinal cord protection during thoraco-abdominal aortic aneurysm repair: results of selective reconstruction of the critical segmental arteries guided by evoked spinal cord potential monitioring. *J Vasc Surg* 1995; 21: 970-5.

41. Crawford ES, Svensson LG, Hess KR, et al. A prospective randomised study of cerebrospinal fluid drainage to prevent paraplegia after high risk surgery on the thoraco-abdominal aorta. *J Vasc Surg* 1991; 13: 36-46.

42. Acher CW, Wynn MM, Hoch JR, Popic PM, Turnipseed WD. Combined use of spinal fluid drainage and naloxone reduces risk of paraplegia in thoraco-abdominal aneurysm repair. *J Vasc Surg* 1994; 19: 236-48.

43. Svensson LG, Von Ritter CM, Groeneveld HT, et al. Cross-clamping of the thoracic aorta. Influence of aortic shunts, laminectomy, papaverine, calcium channel blocker, allopurinol, and superoxide dismutase on spinal cord blood flow and paraplegia in baboons. *Ann Surg* 1986; 204: 38-47.

44. McCullough JL, Hollier LH, Nugent M. Paraplegia after thoracic aortic occlusion: influence of cerebrospinal fluid drainage. Experimental and early clinical results. *J Vasc Surg* 1988; 7: 153-60.

45. Elmore JR, Gloviczki P, Murray MJ, et al. Spinal cord injury in experimental thoracic aortic occlusion: investigation of combined methods of protection. *J Vasc Surg* 1992; 15: 789-98.

46. Safi HJ, Bartoli S, Hess KR, et al. Neurologic deficit in patients at high risk with thoraco-abdominal aortic aneurysms: the role of cerebrospinal fluid drainage and distal perfusion. *J Vasc Surg* 1994; 20: 434-44.

47. Harrow JC. Management of coagulopathy associated with cardiopulmonary bypass. In: *Cardiopulmonary Bypass Principles and Practice*, Ed. Gravlee GP, Davis RF, Utley JR. Williams and Wilkins, Baltimore, 1993, 436-66.

48. Svensson LG, Hess KR, D'Agostino RS, et al. Reduction of neurological injury after high-risk thoraco-abdominal aortic operation. *Ann Thorac Surg* 1998; 66: 132-8.

49. Safi HJ, Winnerkvist A, Miller CC, et al. Effect of extended cross-clamp time during thoraco-abdominal aortic aneurysm repair. *Ann Thorac Surg* 1998; 66: 1204-9.

50. Elmore JR, Gloviczki P, Harper CM, et al. Failure of motor-evoked potentials to predict neurological outcome in experimental thoracic aortic occlusions. *J Vasc Surg* 1991; 14: 131-9.

51. Foulds S, Cheshire NJ, Schachter M, Wolfe JH, Mansfield AO. Endotoxin related early neutrophil activation is associated with outcome after thoraco-abdominal aortic aneurysm repair. *Br J Surg* 1997; 84: 172-7.

52. Hill GE, Mihalakakos PJ, Spurzen JR, Baxter TB. Suprarenal, but not infra-renal, aortic cross clamping upregulates neutrophil integrin CD11b. *J Cardiothorac Vasc Anaes* 1995; 9: 515-8.

53. Mitchell RS, Dake MD, Semba CP, et al. Endovascular stent-graft repair of thoracic aortic aneurysms. *J Thorac and Cardiovasc Surg* 1996; 111: 1054-60.

Chapter 19

Chapter 20

Duplex imaging for varicose veins

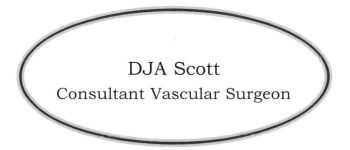

DJA Scott
Consultant Vascular Surgeon

DEPARTMENT OF VASCULAR SURGERY,
ST. JAMES'S UNIVERSITY HOSPITAL, LEEDS

Introduction

Varicose veins affect 10-15% of men and 20-25% of women in the Western World [1]. The pathogenesis of varicose veins is multifactorial but is in part due to valve failure at one of three main sites: the saphenofemoral junction (SFJ), the saphenopopliteal junction (SPJ) and/or perforating veins.

This chapter reviews the evidence on duplex imaging for varicose veins. The indications for duplex imaging remain controversial. The argument for duplex imaging is based upon the 'gold standard' label and the assumption that such a diagnostic test will optimise operations for varicose veins and reduce the incidence of recurrence. There is, however, little hard evidence to support either of these claims. The major factors affecting recurrence rates are the skill of the surgeon, the type of surgery undertaken and the alterations in venous haemodynamics following superficial venous surgery.

Tests for varicose veins before duplex imaging

In the past, the diagnosis of valve failure and subsequent superficial venous reflux was based upon a variety of clinical tests including the cough, tap impulse, tourniquet, Perthe's and the Brodie-Trendelenburg tests [2-4]. Several studies have investigated the value of these tests. McIrvine et al compared Doppler ultrasound with standard clinical tests in assessing primary saphenofemoral incompetence [3]. They reported that the usual clinical tests (cough, tap and thrill) were inaccurate. The combination of hand-held Doppler (HHD) and tourniquet testing provided the most simple and rapid means of detecting SFJ incompetence. In another study, Kim et al compared clinical tests against duplex imaging in 44 patients with primary varicose veins and noted similar findings [4].

Table 1. Sensitivity and specificity of clinical tests versus hand-held Doppler (HHD) assessment of varicose veins (from Kim et al [4]).

	Sensitivity	Specificity
Clinical tests		
Cough	0.59	0.67
Tap test	0.18	0.92
Trendelenburg test	0.91	0.15
Perthe's test	0.97	0.20
HHD tests		
SFJ incompetence	0.97	0.73
LSV incompetence	0.82	0.92
SPJ incompetence	0.80	0.90

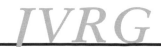

Effects of modern investigations on referral patterns and waiting lists

All of the above clinical tests have been superseded by the use of the HHD. When Doppler findings are equivocal, duplex imaging is necessary. As a consequence, there has been an increase in the number of patients referred for duplex imaging and a reduction in the number of patients directly placed on the waiting list for surgery (Table 2).

an interest in vascular surgery. By the beginning of 1994 there were four full time vascular surgeons providing a dedicated service for both arterial and venous disease (Figure 1). At the beginning of 1994 duplex imaging was provided by a single radiologist with an interest in ultrasound. As the practice increased there were increasing demands within the hospital to appoint a vascular technologist. This was fuelled by a dramatic increase in the number of requests for venous scans and an increasing waiting list for duplex imaging and subsequent surgery. Despite this, the overall number of varicose vein operations has slowly increased, in keeping with the Health Authority

Table 2. Changing management of patients referred with varicose veins with the advent of duplex imaging (from Pleass et at [5]).

	1992	1993	1994
Total referred	194	193	222
Secondary investigation (duplex/venography)	33 (16%)	77 (40%)	91 (41%)
Waiting list (no tests)	105 (47%)	56 (29%)	64 (29%)
Long saphenous surgery	104 (84%)	111 (83%)	92 (76%)
Short saphenous surgery	7 (6%)	14 (10%)	25 (21%)

At St James's University Hospital there has been a progressive increase in the number of operations for varicose veins. Of particular note is the increasing number of saphenopopliteal and revisional saphenofemoral ligations. In 1992-3 there were two general surgeons with

contract. We have investigated the effect on quality of life in patients with varicose veins waiting for duplex imaging. No difference was noted in quality of life whilst on the waiting list between the initial consultation and follow-up, as measured by Short Form 36 and/or Euroqol.

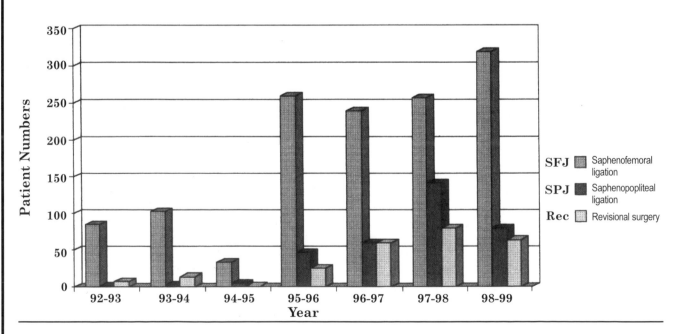

Figure 1. Varicose vein surgery performed at St James's University Hospital, Leeds.

Comparison of hand-held Doppler and duplex imaging

Numerous studies have evaluated the role of HHD in the examination of varicose veins. All these studies have used duplex imaging as the 'gold standard'. The technique of HHD venous assessment can be taught and interpreted with some degree of confidence [6]. After tuition, Bladin, a resident medical officer, studied three consecutive groups of ten patients with varicose veins. At the SFJ there was a high false positive rate (20%) in the second set of patients but this fell to 5% in the third set. This was attributed to misinterpretation of short (physiological) duration reflux. The findings at the SPJ were consistent with the known difficulties of assessing reflux in the popliteal fossa. We have recently compared HHD examination by a consultant vascular surgeon with examination by a basic surgical trainee in a series of 125 patients (190 legs). There were 99 women and 26 men. Consultants examined 115 legs and trainees 75. A comparison between clinical findings and duplex results is shown in Table 3. There was good agreement (kappa) between HHD and duplex at the SFJ, long saphenous vein (LSV) and short saphenous vein (SSV) of 0.62, 0.62 and 0.61 respectively. In the case of the SPJ the kappa value was 0.47. The conclusion was that there was no significant difference between the consultants and trainees in their assessment of varicose veins.

Table 3. HHD vs duplex imaging of varicose veins: overall results for consultants and trainees.

	Sensitivity	Specificity	Chi square	p value
SFJ	86%	82%	0.45	0.5
LSV	93%	72%	0.28	0.6
SPJ	60%	89%	0.04	0.8
SSV	77%	96%	0.53	0.46

Duplex imaging of primary varicose veins

Wills et al reported a series of 188 patients referred to a single vascular specialist in Australia [7]. Recurrent disease accounted for 39% of cases, 31% had an ulcer and the remainder had primary varicose veins. All patients underwent HHD and duplex imaging. A total of 315 legs were assessed. Some 63% had SFJ incompetence, 19% SPJ reflux, 30% perforator incompetence and 8% deep venous incompetence. If patients thought to have had SFJ reflux alone on HHD had undergone saphenofemoral ligation, stripping of the LSV and multiple stab avulsions, 29% of sites with reflux detected on duplex imaging would have been left untreated.

Darke et al, in study of 100 consecutive legs with primary uncomplicated varicose veins compared duplex imaging with HHD [8]. Of the 87 legs with long saphenous reflux on duplex, all but four were correctly assessed by HHD, giving a sensitivity and specificity of 95% and 100% respectively. There were 21 legs with SPJ incompetence on duplex; by contrast HHD had a sensitivity and specificity of 90% and 93%. On the basis of these results Darke recommended that it is prudent that all patients with reflux detected in the popliteal fossa should undergo duplex imaging because of the multiplicity and complexity of patterns of reflux there.

Similarly, Kent and Weston confirmed that HHD has a low positive predictive value in the popliteal fossa [9]. Selective use of duplex imaging was recommended in legs with suspected SPJ reflux. If no reflux was detected in the popliteal fossa or posterior thigh, surgery based on HHD results was appropriate in 94% of legs, excessive in 5% and inadequate in 1%.

Campbell et al reported a similar, but more pragmatic approach, based upon HHD findings in 1997 [10]. In 122 legs with primary varicose veins, HHD correctly identified 89 of the 98 legs with SFJ reflux. In the remaining nine legs, six had a competent SFJ and five had low level reflux. In the case of the popliteal fossa, HHD correctly identified incompetence in 28 of the 39 legs. However, reflux within the SSV was more likely to be detected than popliteal vein reflux. Campbell concluded that HHD is a satisfactory screening test, particularly for SFJ incompetence.

In our own study from a specialist vascular teaching hospital service, HHD compared with duplex imaging at the SFJ, SPJ and thigh perforator region had accuracies of 73%, 77% and 51% respectively [11]. These HHD studies were done principally by a consultant vascular surgeon and the duplex imaging by either a vascular technologist or a radiologist. Despite this, in primary varicose veins, surgery based upon the HHD alone would have left residual sites of reflux in 24% of patients.

The results and subsequent conclusions in these reports are very variable and may reflect an author's bias towards the provision of a venous service within their hospital. Ideally, a patient with varicose veins should be assessed prior to their outpatient visit by duplex imaging. In practice, HHD is an accurate method of screening patients with primary varicose veins, and identifying patients suitable for SFJ ligation, LSV stripping and multiple stab avulsions. It is strongly argued that patients with reflux in the popliteal fossa should undergo duplex imaging to rule out deep venous insufficiency and anatomical abnormalities prior to short saphenous surgery.

Duplex imaging for recurrent varicose veins

It is estimated that up to 20% of patients who undergo saphenofemoral ligation will develop recurrent varicose veins. Glass reported that with careful surgical technique this recurrence rate could be as low as 1% at 5 years[12]. Reoperative varicose vein surgery is technically more demanding and is associated with a greater morbidity [13]. Patients with recurrent varicose veins have multiple different patterns of reflux.

Englund reported a series of 202 patients with recurrent varicose veins studied over six years [14]. The majority of patients were women, with a mean age of 52 years. The distribution of reflux detected on duplex imaging is shown in Table 4. In addition, calf perforator incompetence was common (69%), as was incompetence within the gastrocnemius veins (9%), though these sites were rarely affected in isolation.

Labropoulos et al reported investigation of 123 unselected patients who had previously undergone varicose vein surgery [15]. They found that reflux was confined to the SFJ and/or LSV in 29% of legs. After SPJ ligation, reflux was present in 75% of legs compared to 64% of legs where the SSV had been stripped.

In 1993 Bradbury et al reported a study of 118 patients with recurrent varicose veins [16]. It was noted that, of the 71 patients undergoing a repeat groin dissection, only 28% had a properly ligated SFJ, 44% had an intact mid thigh perforator and 73% an intact LSV. In addition, only four of the 45 patients with SPJ reflux had undergone previous SPJ ligation.

Bradbury and colleagues also investigated 36 consecutive patients who had previously undergone SFJ ligation for primary uncomplicated varicose veins [17]. All patients had clinical assessment, HHD, duplex and varicography. Two main types of recurrence were noted at the time of surgery; an intact SFJ, suggesting inadequate previous surgery, or varices arising from a thigh perforator or abdominal and/or perineal vein, (cross-groin collaterals). On the basis of the results Bradbury recommended that clinical examination and HHD should be the principal methods of assessment for recurrent varicose veins. Duplex imaging was useful for evaluation of perforator disease but in this study was often inadequate due to scarring and distortion from previous surgery. Varicography could be reserved for complicated cases.

Duplex imaging of recurrent short saphenous veins

Tong and Royle studied 70 legs with recurrent varicose veins following SSV surgery [18]. Incompetence in the SSV was the major cause (61%) of reflux within the popliteal fossa. Four types of recurrence were identified at the level of the popliteal fossa: (i) intact SPJ and SSV, (ii) varicosities in the popliteal fossa communicating with the SSV stump, (iii) residual SSV communicating with the popliteal vein via a tortuous recurrent vein and (iv) residual SSV with no communication with the popliteal vein.

In addition to reflux at the level of the SPJ and in the SSV, there were two other major sites of reflux: incompetence of a gastrocnemius vein (34%) and popliteal vein incompetence (21%)

In summary, recurrent varicose veins have several causes including inaccurate initial diagnosis, progression of disease, inadequate initial surgery, altered venous haemodynamics and neovascularisation. The majority of vascular surgeons now recommend duplex imaging prior to any surgical decision.

Table 4. Causes of recurrent veins by duplex imaging in 202 legs (from Englund [14]).

SFJ and LSV intact and incompetent	**45%**
Thigh perforator and LSV incompetent (No SFJ)	**16.5%**
LSV intact and incompetent (No SFJ)	**10%**
SPJ intact and incompetent	**10%**
Isolated thigh perforator incompetence	**4%**

Other uses of duplex imaging

The variable anatomy of veins in the popliteal fossa and the multiple potential sites for reflux highlight the need for accurate marking of the site of venous reflux prior to surgery. Engel et al in 1991 showed that preoperative marking of the saphenopopliteal junction was highly effective; only one out of 66 legs had a negative surgical exploration [19]. Preoperative duplex may also be used to mark an incompetent thigh perforator prior to surgical intervention. The recent interest in subfascial endoscopic calf perforator ligation has also rekindled the concept of identifying calf perforators preoperatively by duplex imaging (see Chapter 23).

Despite increasing use of duplex imaging there is little evidence of a reduction in varicose vein recurrence rates. There are several possible explanations. Inadequate surgery has in the past been blamed on the inexperience of a junior surgeon. This may reflect a failure of preoperative diagnosis or inadequate surgery. Fortunately the majority of trainees now record training in surgery for both primary and recurrent varicose veins [20]. Turton et al reported that appropriate surgery undertaken by a trained junior surgeon could successfully abolish all preoperative sites of reflux [21].

One confounding factor became apparent from an 18 month prospective observational study of 46 patients with primary SFJ reflux. All were studied by duplex imaging prior to, and at 6 weeks and 1 year after varicose vein surgery [22]. New sites of reflux were present at six weeks in nine legs (20%), despite adequate surgery. This resolved in five patients at 1 year. In the 37 patients with no reflux at 6 weeks, follow-up imaging at 1 year identified three patients with recurrent reflux: one with neovascularisation at the groin, one with SPJ reflux and one with an incompetent medial thigh vein. On the basis of work by Bjordal it was felt that the sudden haemodynamic alteration to venous return in the superficial and deep veins resulting from varicose vein surgery might 'overload' those remaining veins with an inherent weakness in either the wall or valve [23]. This was further supported by Darke et al who reported that no patient presented with a varicosity arising from a perforating vein independently of either saphenous system after venous surgery [8].

Conclusions

The role of duplex imaging for varicose veins is still under evaluation. In many ways it is the ideal method, being non-invasive, simple and reproducible. It has come to be regarded as the 'gold standard'. Yet very little high quality work exists to evaluate its clinical role with respect to other tests. The fact that increasing use of duplex imaging has not led to a measurable reduction in varicose vein recurrence rates is not surprising as so many other factors are involved. Consensus is emerging from authors of open studies. It is agreed that duplex is of value in the assessment of recurrent varicose veins being considered for surgery. For primary uncomplicated varicose veins, the use of duplex imaging for all patients would place a huge burden on overstretched vascular laboratories. Initial screening with a hand held Doppler is accurate in patients with saphenofemoral incompetence alone. Many vascular surgeons believe that patients with any reflux signal on HHD in the popliteal fossa should undergo duplex imaging to enable an accurate diagnosis and to rule out deep venous insufficiency. Patients with complicated varicose veins, such as those with a previous deep venous thrombosis may also benefit. Duplex imaging is valuable in preoperative marking, particularly in the popliteal fossa where the anatomy of the saphenopopliteal junction is variable.

Duplex imaging for varicose veins

Sound evidence

- **Hand-held Doppler evaluation is reliable for detecting saphenofemoral incompetence.**

- **Hand-held Doppler evaluation is not very reliable in assessing the cause of saphenopopliteal incompetence.**

Evidence needed

- **Whether the use of duplex imaging reduces the rate of varicose vein recurrence.**

Chapter 20

References

1. Callum M. Epidemiology of varicose veins. *Br J Surg* 1994; 81: 167-73.

2. The Veins. Laufman H. Clion Chirurgica. Silvergirl, inc, *Texas* 1986 : 32-33.

3. McIrvine AJ, Corbett CRR, Aston NO, Sherriff EA, Wiseman PA, Jamieson CW. The demonstration of saphenofemoral incompetence; Doppler ultrasound compared with standard clinical tests. *Br J Surg* 1984; 71: 509-10.

4. Kim J, Richards S, Kent PJK. Clinical examination of varicose veins - a validation study. *Ann R Coll Surg Engl* (in press).

5. Pleass HCC, Holdsworth JD. Audit of introduction of hand held Doppler and duplex ultrasound in the management of varicose veins. *Ann R Coll Surg Engl* 1996; 78: 494-496.

6. Bladin C, Royle JP. Acquisition of skills for use of Doppler ultrasound and the assessment of varicose veins. *Aust N Z J Surg* 1987; 57: 225-226.

7. Wills V, Moylan D, Chambers J. The use of routine duplex scanning in the assessment of varicose veins. *Aust N Z J Surg* 1998; 68: 41-4.

8. Darke SG, Vetrivel S, Foy DMA, Smith S, Baker S. A comparison of duplex scanning and continuous wave Doppler in the assessment of primary and uncomplicated varicose veins. *Eur J Vasc Endovasc Surg* 1997; 14: 457-61.

9. Kent PJ, Weston MJ. Duplex scanning may be used selectively in patients with primary varicose veins. *Ann R Coll Surg Engl* 1998; 80: 388-9.

10. Campbell WB, Niblett PG, Ridler BMF, Peters AS, Thompson JF. Hand-held Doppler as a screening test in primary varicose veins. *Br J Surg* 1997; 84: 1541-1543.

11. Mercer KG, Scott DJA, Berridge DC. Preoperative duplex imaging is required before all operations for primary varicose veins. *Br J Surg* 1998; 85: 1495-7.

12. Glass GM. Prevention of recurrent saphenofemoral incompetence after surgery for varicose veins. *Br J Surg* 1989; 76: 1210.

13. Critchely G, Handa A, Harvey A, Harvey MR, Corbett CRR. Complications of varicose vein surgery. *Phlebologie* 1994; 9: 125.

14. Englund R. Duplex scanning for recurrent varicose veins. *Aust N Z J Surg* 1996; 66: 618-20.

15. Labropoulos N, Touloupakis E, Giannoukas AD, Leon M, Katsamouris A, Nicolaides AN. Recurrent varicose veins: investigation of the pattern and extent of reflux with colour flow duplex scanning. *Surgery* 1996; 119: 406-9.

16. Bradbury AW, Stonebridge PA, Ruckley CV, Beggs I. Recurrent varicose veins: correlation between preoperative clinical and hand held Doppler ultrasonographic examination, and anatomical findings at surgery. *Br J Surg* 1993; 80: 849-851.

17. Bradbury AW, Stonebridge PA, Callam MJ, et al. Recurrent varicose veins: assessment of the saphenofemoral junction. *Br J Surg* 1994; 81: 373-5.

18. Tong Y, Royle J. Recurrent varicose veins after short saphenous vein surgery: a duplex ultrasound study. *Cardiovasc Surg* 1996; 4: 364-7.

19. Engel AF, Davies G, Keeman JN. Preoperative localisation of the saphenopopliteal junction with duplex scanning. *Eur J Vasc Surg* 1991; 5: 507-9.

20. Turton EPL, Whiteley MS, Berridge DC, Scott DJA. Calman, venous surgery and the vascular trainee. *J R Coll Surg Edinb* 1999; 44: 172-6.

21. Turton EPL, McKenzie S, Weston MJ, Berridge DC, Scott DJA. Optimising a varicose vein service to reduce recurrence. *Ann R Coll Surg Engl* 1997; 79: 451-4.

22. Turton EPL, Scott DJA, Richards SP, et al. Duplex-derived evidence of reflux after varicose vein surgery: neoreflux or neovascularisation? *Eur J Vasc Endovasc Surg* 1999; 17: 230-233.

23. Bjordal RI. Circulation patterns in incompetent perforating veins in the calf and in the saphenous system in primary varicose veins. *Acta Chir Scand* 1972; 138: 251-261.

Chapter 21

Improving the results of varicose vein surgery

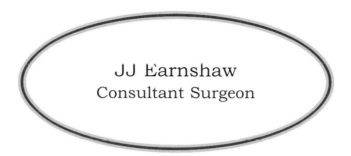

JJ Earnshaw
Consultant Surgeon

DEPARTMENT OF SURGERY,
GLOUCESTERSHIRE ROYAL HOSPITAL, GLOUCESTER

Introduction

There is a general belief that the results of varicose vein surgery are poor. This is reflected in the pessimism (or realism) among general practitioners who refer patients for a specialist opinion. While no other elective surgical operation bears such a high perceived risk of disease recurrence, there is very little objective information about actual recurrence rates following varicose vein surgery. The main problem is that it is extremely difficult to agree a general classification for recurrent veins. Each patient has a different outlook on their individual pattern of venous abnormality and no two could agree on the resulting disability. Improving the results of varicose vein surgery is an important challenge; at present approximately 20% of all varicose vein surgery is for recurrent veins. In the author's practice 16% of operations are for recurrent veins (Figure 1). Not only is recurrence a disappointment and a nuisance for patients, reoperation is harder for the surgeon and fraught with more potential complications.

Two things have happened in the past decade that have had a major influence on varicose vein surgery. First, surgical specialisation has led to trained vascular surgeons performing an increasing amount of the venous surgery in the United Kingdom. Second, the science of varicose vein surgery has advanced rapidly with the advent of duplex imaging, resulting in accurate, non-invasive diagnosis of both anatomical and haemodynamic venous abnormalities.

The cause of recurrent varicose veins

Several studies have examined the causes of recurrence after varicose vein surgery [1-3]. Many early studies blamed inadequate groin dissection by poorly trained or inexperienced surgeons. There is little doubt that the increase in venous surgery undertaken by specialist vascular surgeons who have the confidence to operate at the saphenofemoral junction (SFJ) should affect recurrence rates in future, although there has been no demonstrable effect as yet.

Most patients with recurrent veins have incompetence in the long saphenous vein (LSV) due either to a mid thigh perforating vein or recurrent incompetence at the SFJ. In Gloucester, on follow-up duplex imaging it was found that neovascularisation was the cause of recurrent saphenofemoral incompetence in approximately two thirds of patients [4]. Neovascularisation is the growth of incompetent, thin walled veins from the ligated SFJ (it may also occur from the upper end of the ligated LSV) to reconnect to any residual thigh vein, such as the LSV or the anterior thigh vein if the LSV has been stripped. Although it is not disputed that a leash of veins connecting the SFJ and the LSV is frequently found when the groin is explored for recurrent veins, it has been argued that these are not 'new' veins but rather existing small collateral veins that have expanded in response to

JVRG

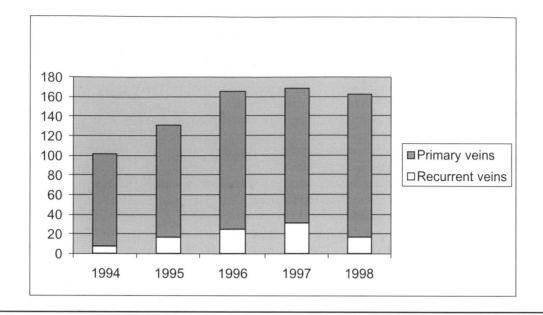

Figure 1. Author's varicose vein operations 1994-98.

saphenofemoral ligation. It has, however, been shown in a histological study that the veins found at the groin during reoperative surgery are immature and thin walled, and so are likely to be due to neovascularisation [5]. When veins recur after repeat operation, the cause of recurrence is still likely to be neovascularisation [6]. Indeed this seems to occur more frequently after reoperation than after primary varicose vein surgery. Little is known about recurrence rates after short saphenous varicose vein surgery but it is suspected that they are even higher than after LSV operations. Neovascularisation is seen too in the popliteal fossa.

One recently uncovered cause of recurrent veins after successful ligation in the superficial venous system is changing venous haemodynamics. In a study from Leeds, routine duplex imaging 6 weeks after varicose vein surgery showed that there were new sites of superficial incompetence in 20% of legs [7]. It was assumed that operation had altered venous haemodynamics and rendered weak valves incompetent.

Strategies to reduce the recurrence rate after varicose vein surgery

The two main methods that a surgeon should use to minimise disease recurrence after varicose vein surgery are, first, to obtain an accurate preoperative diagnosis and, second, to perform appropriate and technically successful surgery. There does not seem to be any variation in recurrence rates relating to the indication for surgery, although recurrence does seem to be more frequent after reoperative surgery.

Clearly, recurrence is more likely if an incorrect operation is performed. Improving the accuracy of preoperative diagnosis should be beneficial, although there are no trials of objective testing that confirm this. The level of venous reflux is usually diagnosed by a combination of clinical examination and tourniquet testing. The addition of hand-held Doppler ultrasonography has improved diagnosis and is now used routinely by vascular surgeons in the outpatient clinic. The advent of colour duplex imaging has brought new controversy. Venous disorders may now be diagnosed anatomically and haemodynamically, and mapped before operation. While the burden of this work on vascular laboratories would be immense if duplex scanning became routine for all patients with varicose veins, omitting it would be indefensible if such imaging could be shown to improve results. Until randomised evidence is available, a sensible compromise is to screen patients with a hand-held Doppler ultrasound probe and to use duplex imaging for recurrent veins, complicated cases or patients with a reflux signal in the popliteal fossa.

Surgery for long saphenous vein disease

In some branches of surgery it has been possible to show convincingly that having an operation done by an expert/specialist improves the outcome. No evidence is yet available for venous surgery, partly because of the difficulty in defining and measuring recurrence. It is believed that careful saphenofemoral ligation is the most important part of LSV surgery. Certainly this is the area with the highest potential for localised recurrence and it is the most technically challenging part of the operation for an inexperienced surgeon. If it is accepted that neovascularisation is a significant problem after saphenofemoral ligation, then it is important to remove any residual veins near the SFJ so there is nothing for neovascular veins to rejoin. Tributaries should not simply be tied adjacent to the SFJ but should be dissected back to their first branch before ligation. A technique used by the author is diathermy avulsion of tributaries back to and beyond the first branch, which has the advantage of speed and simplicity. The medial deep perforating branch remains a conundrum. Some surgeons deny that this has any role in recurrent veins, others believe it should always be divided.

The single component of the varicose vein operation clearly shown to affect outcome is routine stripping of the LSV to knee level. In several randomised trials, stripping reduced the risk of recurrent veins and improved venous haemodynamics [8-15]. In the Gloucester study of 100 patients undergoing LSV surgery, patients randomised to routine stripping had a 6% reoperation rate after 6 years, compared to 20% for those who had saphenofemoral ligation alone. Stripping has several potentially beneficial effects. It abolishes any connection with mid-thigh perforating veins that might subsequently become incompetent. In addition, if neovascularisation does occur in the groin, it has nowhere to join to cause recurrence. For the latter reason it is also important to remove any other residual thigh veins. The LSV may be bifid and, if so, both vessels should be removed. The anterior thigh vein is commonly identified during groin exploration for long saphenous varicose veins; it may be stripped but it is often possible to remove 10-15cm by careful avulsion through the groin wound.

The morbidity associated with routine stripping has discouraged some surgeons, but this may be minimised by perforate invagination (PIN) or inversion stripping [16], or sequential avulsion [17]. Some argue that the LSV should be preserved for future use in arterial bypass surgery, however, a varicose vein is seldom useful. Selective retention of a non-varicose, non-incompetent LSV (on duplex imaging) might be advantageous in this respect but runs the risk of increasing the recurrence rate [18].

The creation of a barrier at the SFJ has been suggested as a way of reducing recurrence due to neovascularisation. Glass was one of the first to describe the use of a Mersilene mesh in the groin to try to prevent recurrent varicosities [19]. His work was reported before the introduction of duplex imaging, but use of a mesh sutured over the ligated SFJ reduced the rate of clinical recurrence from 25% to 1% after 4 years. Thomson preferred to avoid the use of prosthetic material in the groin and suggested using a patch of cribriform fascia

turned back and over the SFJ [20]. Both he and Glass have reported recurrence rates under 5% using this method [19,20]. Locally in Gloucester, we have used a 2cm polytetrafluoroethylene (PTFE) patch in the manner of Glass (Figure 2). While no randomised data exist, neovascularisation appears to be minimised using this technique, although not abolished altogether [6].

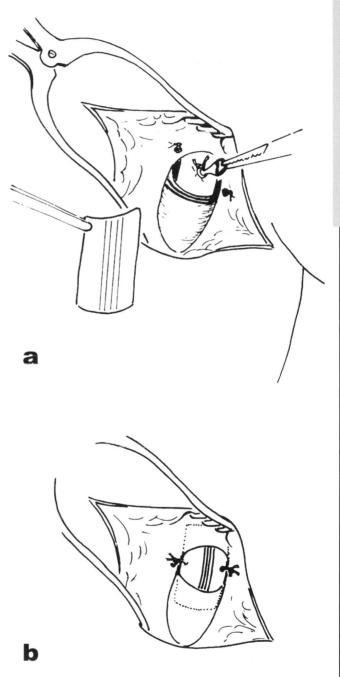

Figure 2. PTFE patch saphenoplasty. (a) Flush saphenofemoral ligation with the PTFE patch ready for insertion. (b) PTFE patch sutured to tissue either side of the common femoral vein; the upper and lower ends are then tucked underneath the cribriform fascia. (Reproduced with permission from Phlebology 1998; 13: 10-13).

Surgery for short saphenous vein disease

Short saphenous vein (SSV) surgery is technically more challenging. The aim is to ligate the SSV at the saphenopopliteal junction (SPJ) by careful dissection at its origin, while avoiding damage to neurovascular structures in the popliteal fossa. All patients should be warned explicitly about this potential complication before operation. The anatomy of the SPJ is very variable and it may lie several centimetres above the skin crease. It is helpful to have the junction marked preoperatively using duplex scanning, but this may be confusing because in a supine patient it may be lower than when marked with the patient erect. Patients with recurrent SSV disease often have a leash of veins emanating from the popliteal fossa to join the SSV, analogous to neovascularisation in the groin. Similarly, stripping the SSV might be a logical way to reduce recurrence, but the risk of damage to the sural nerve is high in historical series. It is the author's practice to avulse the top 10cm of the vein by inserting a finger behind it through the main wound and dissecting its upper part for accurate avulsion through a separate stab incision 10cm distally. One common problem in the popliteal fossa is the presence of gastrocnemius veins. These may be confused with the SPJ unless dissection is thorough. Gastrocnemius veins are thin-walled and fragile, and do not avulse well. They should be ligated and divided as they are a significant cause of recurrent varicosities. Little is known about the incidence of recurrent SSV disease. It is suspected that it is high and this may be a fruitful area for future investigation.

Operations for recurrent veins

Recurrence rates after reoperation may be higher than after surgery for primary varicosities. Morbidity is also higher, principally due to wound complications such as infection or seroma. Accurate preoperative diagnosis with duplex imaging is essential.

For recurrent saphenofemoral incompetence, the aim should be to clear 2-3cm of the common femoral vein at the SFJ. A variety of surgical methods exist based on dissection through virgin tissue. The lateral approach from the direction of the common femoral artery is the most popular. Flush religation is important as is stripping of any residual LSV. The LSV may need preoperative marking if it is not visible.

Barrier methods have also been investigated for treatment of recurrent varicosities. In the Gloucester series, neovascularisation remained the commonest cause of further recurrence after reoperation for recurrent LSV disease [6]. Prosthetic material has been employed (Dacron or PTFE). Living tissue has also been used but, in a randomised trial of the effect of routine use of a pectineus flap versus control, there was no difference in subsequent recurrence [21]. The Gloucester PTFE patch has been used in 43 patients (70 legs) with a 2 year recurrence rate of 11% (unpublished data). It has yet to be tested in a randomised trial.

Minimising complications

Optimising results also entails minimising complications. The principal complications are haematoma, bruising and infection. The most feared is deep vein thrombosis. No study has ever shown that routine antibiotic prophylaxis is worthwhile for varicose vein surgery. Infection is commoner when a venous ulcer is present and it is the author's practice to give a single dose of intravenous co-amoxiclav (Augmentin) to these patients. The commonest site for haematoma is in the thigh strip track. Reducing the size of the stripper head or using PIN stripping reduces the size of the stripper exit site but does not decrease the size of any haematoma [16]. Performing varicose vein surgery under tourniquet reduces blood loss and the duration of surgery, and also decreases the size of any postoperative haematoma [22]. There are many different regimens for postoperative bandaging but there does not seem to be any advantage in prolonging this beyond one week after surgery [23].

The possibility of deep vein thrombosis after varicose vein surgery arouses much anxiety in both patient and surgeon. A survey by Campbell and Ridler showed how little is known about the risk and prevention of this complication [24]. Less than 12% of surgeons use antithrombotic prophylaxis with heparin for all patients undergoing varicose vein surgery. Most employ selective heparin use based on other risk factors, such as previous deep vein thrombosis and contraceptive pill use.

Conclusions

Varicose vein surgery is common and mundane. It is often delegated to non-consultant staff and is frequently done reluctantly. As for so many conditions, a thoughtful and specialist approach can yield improved results. Much remains to be learned about the optimal approach. At a time of dramatic change in the non-invasive endovascular management of arterial disease it is astounding that varicose vein surgery has altered so little in the last 50 years. However, a new breed of enthusiast will ensure that venous research finally comes to the fore. Expect significant changes over the next decade.

Improving the results of varicose vein surgery

Sound evidence

- **Stripping the long saphenous vein reduces the rate of recurrence.**

- **Inversion stripping or sequential avulsion of the long saphenous vein reduces the risk of haematoma.**

Evidence needed

- **The pathophysiology of recurrent veins is not yet fully understood.**

- **It is unknown if stripping should be used for the short saphenous vein.**

- **It is uncertain if barrier methods are effective for primary or recurrent varicose veins.**

Chapter 21

References (randomised trials in bold)

1. Darke SG. The morphology of recurrent varicose veins. *Eur J Vasc Endovasc Surg* 1992; 6: 512-7.

2. Redwood NFW, Lambert D. Patterns of reflux in recurrent veins assessed by duplex scanning. *Br J Surg* 1994; 81: 1450-1.

3. Labropoulos N, Touloupakis E, Giannoukas AD, Leon M, Katsamouris A, Nicolaides AN. Recurrent varicose veins: investigation of the pattern and extent of reflux with colour flow duplex scanning. *Surgery* 1996; 119: 406-9.

4. **Jones L, Braithwaite BD, Selwyn D, Cooke S, Earnshaw JJ. Neovascularisation is the principal cause of varicose vein recurrence: results of a randomised trial of stripping the long saphenous vein. *Eur J Vasc Endovasc Surg* 1996; 12: 442-5.**

5. Nyamekye I, Shephard NA, Davies B, Heather BP, Earnshaw JJ. Clinicopathological evidence that neovascularisation is a cause of recurrent varicose veins. *Eur J Vasc Endovas Surg* 1998; 15: 412-5.

6. Earnshaw JJ, Davies B, Harradine K, Heather BP. Preliminary results of PTFE patch saphenoplasty to prevent neovascularisation leading to recurrent varicose veins. *Phlebology* 1998; 13: 10-13.

7. Turton EPL, Scott DJA, Richards SP et al. Duplex derived evidence of reflux after varicose vein surgery: neoreflux or neovascularisation. *Eur J Vasc Endovasc Surg* 1999; 17: 230-3.

8. **Jackobsen BH. The value of different forms of treatment for varicose veins. *Br J Surg* 1979; 66: 182-4.**

9. **Munn SR, Morton JB, Macbeth WAAG, McLeish AR. To strip or not to strip the long saphenous vein. A varicose vein trial. *Br J Surg* 1981; 68: 426-8.**

10. **Woodyer AB, Reddy PJ, Dormandy JA. Should we strip the long saphenous vein? *Phlebology* 1986; 1: 221-4.**

11. **Hammersten J, Pederson P, Cederlund C-G, Campanello M. Long saphenous vein saving surgery for varicose veins. A long term follow-up. *Eur J Vasc Surg* 1990; 4: 361-4.**

12. **Neglen P, Einarsson E, Eklof B. The functional long term value of different types of treatment for saphenous vein incompetence. *J Cardiovasc Surg (Torino)* 1993; 34: 295-301.**

13. **Rutgers PH, Kitslaar PJEHM. Randomised trial of stripping versus high ligation combined with sclerotherapy in the treatment of the incompetent greater saphenous vein. *Am J Surg* 1994; 168: 311-5.**

14. **Sarin S, Scurr JH, Coleridge-Smith PD. Stripping of the long saphenous vein in the treatment of primary varicose veins. *Br J Surg* 1994; 81: 1455-8.**

15. **Dwerryhouse S, Davies B, Harradine K, Earnshaw JJ. Stripping the long saphenous vein reduces the rate of reoperation for recurrent varicose veins: five year results of a randomized trial. *J Vasc Surg* 1999; 29: 589-92.**

16. **Durkin MT, Turton EPL, Scott DJA, Berridge DC. A prospective randomised trial of PIN versus conventional stripping in varicose vein surgery. *Ann R Coll Surg Engl* 1999; 81: 171-4.**

17. **Khan RBN, Khan SN, Greaney MG, Blair SD. Prospective randomized trial comparing sequential avulsions with stripping of the long saphenous vein. *Br J Surg* 1996; 83: 1559-62.**

18. Zamboni P, Marcellino MG, Capelli M et al. Saphenous vein sparing surgery: principles, techniques and results. *Cardiovasc Surg* 1998; 39: 151-62.

19. Glass GM. Prevention of recurrent saphenofemoral incompetence after surgery for varicose veins. *Br J Surg* 1989; 76: 1210.

20. Thomson WHF. Saphenous vein stripping and quality of outcome (letter). *Br J Surg* 1997; 84: 424-5.

21. **Gibbs P, Foy DMA, Darke SG. Recurrent varicose veins; to patch or not to patch. *Br J Surg* 1999; 86: suppl I: A112-3.**

22. **Sykes TCF, Brookes P, Hickey NC. A prospective randomized trial of tourniquet in varicose vein surgery. *Br J Surg* 1999; 86: suppl I: A44.**

23. **Raraty MGT, Greaney MG, Blair SD. There is no benefit from 6 weeks of compression after varicose vein surgery: a prospective randomized trial. *Br J Surg* 1997; 84: A574.**

24. Campbell WB, Ridler BM. Varicose vein surgery and deep vein thrombosis. *Br J Surg* 1995; 82: 1494-7.

Improving the results of varicose vein surgery

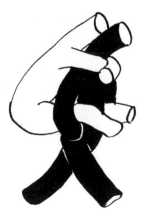

Chapter 22

The significance of perforating vein disease

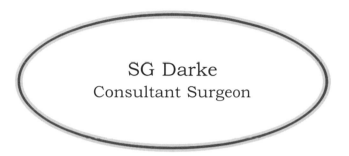

SG Darke
Consultant Surgeon

DEPARTMENT OF VASCULAR SURGERY,
ROYAL BOURNEMOUTH HOSPITAL, BOURNEMOUTH

Introduction

This chapter will focus exclusively on the role of ankle 'perforator disease' as a factor in the aetiology and management of venous ulceration. It is accepted that lower limb perforating veins are of significance in the pathogenesis of primary and, in particular, recurrent varicose veins.

Until relatively recently the almost universal view was that incompetent ankle perforating veins were a significant component of morphology leading to the development of venous ulceration. Thus their ligation should result in benefit to patients. This was mainly based on the views expressed over 40 years ago by Cockett in the United Kingdom [1] and Linton [2] in North America. Indeed, the principle that perforator ligation was an essential procedure in the management of venous ulcers remained unquestioned until relatively recently.

The evidence for this was based on the following observations:

- perforating veins can be shown to be 'incompetent' meaning that blood passes from the deep to the superficial system. Furthermore these veins are situated anatomically at the predominant sites of venous ulceration,
- incompetent perforating veins can be demonstrated in some patients with a venous ulcer,
- ligating these veins leads to ulcer healing.

Increasingly over the last 15 years, however, these views have been challenged because some ulcers heal with alternative surgery and without additional perforator ligation, irrespective of whether perforators are present and incompetent, and in certain groups of patients the results of perforator ligation are poor. There remains uncertainty as to the haemodynamic significance of incompetent ankle perforating veins.

Much of this scepticism has arisen following the introduction of duplex ultrasound imaging which is now established as the principle tool with which to investigate venous morphology. With this has increasingly developed the view that surgery should be tailored more precisely and appropriately to the specific venous abnormalities of an individual patient. This change in attitude now questions whether perforator ligation has any place in contemporary practice in the management of venous ulcers.

In contrast, however, is a rekindled enthusiasm for perforator ligation generated by the development of new and less invasive endoscopic techniques [3-7]. But even protagonists of the new technique seem to have no clear view about the clinical circumstances in which it is indicated [8].

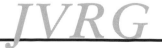

Anatomical and haemodynamic pathophysiology

Numerous anatomical, radiological and surgical studies have been undertaken that show a varying number and size of perforating veins in the calf that connect the superficial and deep venous systems [9]. They are present and incompetent in some clinically normal legs as well as in those with venous hypertension. Furthermore, it is of note that cadaveric dissection of ankle perforating veins reveals valves to be present in only the larger vessels (>1mm). Some of the valves are configured to direct blood from the deep to the superficial systems, i.e. in an 'incompetent' direction [10].

Nonetheless, in patients with leg ulceration due to chronic venous insufficiency, incompetent ankle perforators are found predominantly in the medial aspect of the middle third of the calf, becoming more prevalent with increasing clinical severity of venous insufficiency [11,12].

A particular difficulty with evaluation of the clinical significance of incompetent ankle perforating veins is the lack of a haemodynamic test to demonstrate their purported effect [13,14]. This makes it difficult to judge the significance of their presence and the effect of their ligation. Indeed the latter can only be estimated by the demonstration of clinical benefit.

Seminal work on the pathophysiology of perforating veins was conducted before the era of duplex ultrasound by Bjordal [15]. He undertook a series of classic studies employing simultaneous pressure measurements and electromagnetic flowmetry in patients undergoing primary varicose vein surgery under local anaesthetic. He confirmed outward ('incompetent') flow in ankle perforating veins but interestingly was among the first to conclude that in primary venous insufficiency the incompetence of the perforators was secondary to saphenous reflux.

There is recent evidence to support the concept that incompetence in the ankle perforating veins may be secondary to reflux in other systems. In a study from Edinburgh, patients were re-examined by duplex ultrasound a median of 14 weeks after saphenous ligation and stripping. In most instances previously incompetent ankle perforator veins became competent (and smaller) postoperatively, when coexistent reflux was confined to the superficial system. However, when all three systems were involved: perforators, deep and superficial veins, the perforators remained incompetent after saphenous ablation, as indeed did the deep veins [11].

So associated deep venous incompetence would seem to be a critical factor. This might be because deep incompetence inhibits perforator recovery. Alternatively, perforator incompetence under these circumstances may be an independent manifestation of widespread valvular malfunction. Recent important and detailed duplex studies revealed that perforator reflux becomes progressively more evident with the extent of coexistent superficial and, in particular, deep venous reflux [14].

The conclusions that might be drawn from this are that in the presence of a normal deep venous system, ankle perforators are incompetent as a consequence of saphenous reflux. If the long saphenous vein is ablated then the incompetence reverses. However, if the deep system is also incompetent, then this reversal no longer occurs.

As a compounding observation, however, it has been noted that, in time, deep incompetence too may recover after correction of superficial reflux. Walsh et al [16] reported the effect of saphenous ligation on coexistent reflux in the superficial femoral vein in 29 legs. Three of these also had popliteal reflux. In all but two legs the deep reflux was abolished following long saphenous surgery. The interval since the surgery was described as 'remote' but not specified. Similarly Sales et al [17] reported on the outcome of saphenous ligation in legs with combined saphenous and femoral reflux. In 16 legs competence was restored to the deep veins when the legs were re-examined 6 weeks after saphenous surgery. In the remaining patient the femoral reflux was reversed but popliteal incompetence remained.

These results, with conflicting implications, are clearly of relevance to the questions posed here. If deep incompetence usually recovers after superficial venous surgery, so too might ankle perforator reflux. Why then are these findings different from the Edinburgh experience regarding the status of the deep system after saphenous ligation and stripping? The time scales seem to be comparable - it would not seem to be a question of the time allowed for recovery to occur after saphenous surgery. It may be that the two series showing deep venous recovery principally evaluated the femoral veins as opposed to reflux in the popliteal veins. My own data, as yet unpublished, show no recovery of competence in the popliteal vein in patients undergoing saphenous surgery.

In conclusion, incompetent (flow from deep to superficial systems) ankle perforating veins can be demonstrated in clinically normal legs but become more evident with increasing clinical severity of both venous insufficiency and co-existent reflux in saphenous and deep veins. Incompetent ankle perforators are associated with, and possibly secondary to, saphenous incompetence. If the deep system is normal, perforating veins recover their valvular competence after saphenous ablation.

Where there is co-existent reflux in the superficial and deep systems the subsequent function of incompetent perforators after saphenous ligation and stripping remains uncertain. There is some evidence that the femoral veins (and possibly by implication the incompetent perforating veins) may recover valvular competence after saphenous surgery. This is less likely to be true of popliteal reflux. As yet it has not been possible to demonstrate any specific haemodynamic significance of incompetent ankle perforators using quantified tests.

Does ligation of incompetent ankle perforating veins heal venous ulcers?

The first step in attempting to address this question is to consider the underlying morphology demonstrable in patients with venous ulceration. Table 1 lists those series where this has been assessed systematically [18-26]. Important points will be apparent from this table. The first is that perforator incompetence as an isolated cause of venous ulceration without superficial or deep incompetence is so rare that it might be questioned whether this situation ever occurs at all. The significance of this is self-evident. Were there to be a significant proportion of patients with a venous ulcer and no demonstrable venous abnormality other than ankle perforator incompetence, this would be evidence to implicate ankle perforators as clinically significant. Where perforator incompetence does occur, it is invariably accompanied by either superficial or deep venous incompetence, or both. Most, though not all, legs with deep incompetence have coexistent superficial reflux. In assessing the clinical effect of perforator ligation, therefore, the picture is inevitably complicated by the influence of the correction of associated reflux, principally in the long saphenous system.

Additionally, the question of postoperative management in terms of the use of support stockings needs to be considered. There are no trials with a control group receiving best conservative care alone.

Early reports are particularly difficult to evaluate because they lack the general discipline of today's standards. They are invariably contaminated by synchronous saphenous ligation [1,2,27-32]. The first contemporary report was by Negus [33]. In a series of 109 ulcerated legs there was a 76 % healing rate at 3 years following open subfascial ligation of perforating veins. Half the patients had simultaneous saphenous ligation and nearly half wore support stockings postoperatively. There are no data as to the state of the deep system because this study antecedes duplex technology. There is no information as to the influence of synchronous saphenous ligation on ulcer healing.

Since then reports on perforator ligation have assessed new endoscopic procedures. Pierik and colleagues [5] described the outcome of subfascial endoscopic ligation in 40 legs of 38 patients; only 16 had active ulceration, the remainder had a healed ulcer. In only four legs was synchronous saphenous ligation undertaken. All patients wore support stockings

postoperatively. In 31 legs there was said to be associated deep venous incompetence, but the basis for this was not stated in the paper. No duplex examination was used. At mean follow-up of 3.9 years there was only one recurrent ulcer. Gloviczki and colleagues [6] reported the outcome of subfascial endoscopic perforator ligation in 11 legs, nine of which had active or recent venous ulceration. Six patients underwent synchronous saphenous ligation, all of whose ulcers remained healed. Interestingly ulcers in four of the five patients treated by subfascial ligation alone did not heal, even though all patients used compression stockings postoperatively.

In a subsequent report from the same unit [7] the haemodynamic consequences of perforator ligation were studied in 26 patients with active venous ulceration. Sixty-five per cent of patients underwent synchronous saphenous ablation. Statistically significant haemodynamic improvement could be demonstrated, but only in the patients who underwent synchronous saphenous ligation. Those having isolated perforator ligation did not improve significantly on haemodynamic testing, nor interestingly did a subgroup of patients with identified post-thrombotic disease (see below).

In a study by Bradbury et al [34], 43 patients were treated by saphenous and perforator ligation for recurrent venous ulceration . These were reviewed a median of 66 months after surgery with duplex imaging and foot volumetry. Thirty-four patients remained ulcer-free, of whom only one had popliteal incompetence. All nine patients that developed a further ulcer had popliteal incompetence. This finding was also reflected in the haemodynamic studies. Because all the patients underwent saphenous ligation synchronously the impact of perforator surgery was difficult to assess. No attempt was made to identify those with post thrombotic states.

This latter consideration brings us to another important piece of work by Burnand et al [35] who studied the influence of post-thrombotic obstructive damage, as demonstrated by ascending venography, on the outcome of 41 patients with venous ulceration. All underwent open subfascial ligation with saphenous ligation. Within 5 years recurrent ulceration occurred in all 23 patients who had evidence of previous deep vein thrombosis. In contrast, only one of those with normal deep veins had a recurrent ulcer (p<0.001).

In a subsequent study by Pierik et al [3] open and endoscopic ligation were compared. Thirty-nine patients with active medial venous ulceration were randomised to receive an open or an endoscopic procedure. The prime objective was to compare the incidence of wound sepsis and duration of hospital stay. What is of interest is the leg ulcer healing rate. At a mean follow-up of 21 months, 85% who had endoscopic and 90% who had open surgery had healed ulcers. However, 13 out of 19 in the open group and 14 out of 20 in the endoscopic group underwent synchronous saphenous ligation and stripping. No data are available in this respect as to which ulcers failed to heal. All the patients wore support stockings after

Table 1. Venous ulceration - morphology.

Author	Legs	Assessment	Ankle perforator incompetence alone	Superficial incompetence	Primary deep incompetence (Co-existing saphenous incompetence)	Post phlebitic disease
				CATEGORY %		
McEnroe [18]	118	Light Rheography		12	80 (14)	N/A
Hanrahan [19]	95	Duplex	8	36	49 (43)	N/A
Darke [20]	235	Venography/CWD	4	39	35 (28)	22
Shami [21]	59	Duplex		53	47 (32)	N/A
Lees [22]	25	Duplex		52	48 (12)	N/A
Weingarten [23]	148	Duplex		9	80 (55)	N/A
Van Rij [24]	120	Duplex/APG	2	67	31 (28)	N/A
Grabs [25]	111	Duplex		51	43 (38)	14
Scriven [26]	82	Duplex	2	57	41 (37)	50

CWD Continuous wave Doppler
APG Air Plethysmography
N/A Not available

operation indefinitely. The results of this second study are somewhat different from the first in that a much higher proportion of patients underwent synchronous saphenous ligation, which is more in keeping with others' experience.

There is a recent report from the North American Subfascial Endoscopic Perforator Surgery Registry [36]. In this multicentre study, the patient population, details and morphological evaluation were varied. One hundred and forty-six patients underwent endoscopic perforator ligation, with saphenous ligation at the same time in 87. One hundred and one patients had active and 21 had healed ulcers. It was possible to document the healing rate and the recurrent ulceration rate. In common with other series (Table 1) only 5% of legs had isolated perforator incompetence. The follow-up averaged 24 months and ulcer healing was achieved in 88% legs overall. Healing was improved in patients with synchronous saphenous surgery and no deep venous obstruction. Additionally, a significantly higher ulcer recurrence rate occurred in the 56 legs with post-thrombotic disease. This was diagnosed either from a definite previous history of deep vein thrombosis or from appearances on venography or duplex imaging at the time of preliminary evaluation. Primary deep incompetence did not seem to influence outcome. Although this study had limitations because the various patient groups and morphology were mixed, it also gave some data on isolated perforator surgery. The 2 year recurrence rate in the 38 legs undergoing perforator ligation alone was 45% compared with 25% where this was combined with saphenous stripping. The use of support stockings was not reported.

In conclusion, isolated ankle perforator incompetence is uncommon as a single morphological feature in patients with venous ulceration. There are few randomised trials and all reports have limitations, particularly regarding synchronous saphenous surgery and the use of support stockings postoperatively. There is little information on the benefit of perforator ligation alone without synchronous saphenous ligation. What evidence there is seems to suggest the advantage to be limited. There is more evidence of successful healing after combined saphenous and perforator ligation. Ulcer healing is less likely in patients with post-thrombotic disease or co-existing deep incompetence; this may of course be primary or secondary to previous thrombosis.

Does saphenous ligation alone heal venous ulceration?

The obvious question posed by the data analysed so far is whether venous ulcers heal just as well if the saphenofemoral junction alone is ligated and any incompetent perforators left untouched. A complicating factor from the evidence presented above, however, is the suggestion that certain patients will not do well even if both the saphenous and perforating veins are ligated. These are patients with post-thrombotic disease and

popliteal incompetence. It may well be, however, that popliteal incompetence is nothing more than a marker for the consequences of previous deep vein thrombosis. Patients who have a deep vein thrombosis are known to recanalise in about 90% of instances, but most go on to develop deep venous incompetence. This has been consistently shown by a number of prospective duplex follow-up studies [37-40].

Considering only patients with primary incompetence in the saphenous and perforating veins and a normal deep system, the first to report treatment by saphenous ligation alone was Recek [41]. In 1971 he described healing in 38 patients at 5 years treated by saphenous ligation alone. He concluded that the perforators were of no significance if the deep veins were normal. Subsequently, Hoare et al [42] reported a group of patients with normal deep veins, saphenous incompetence and associated perforator reflux in some. He speculated that superficial venous surgery alone should be sufficient to heal the ulcers.

Sethia and I [43] measured the dorsal foot vein pressures in a group of 12 patients with combined saphenous and perforator incompetence. They had normal deep veins on ascending and descending venography. Venous pressures were normalised by the use of an above knee tourniquet, simulating the anticipated effects of long saphenous ligation. After surgery the pressure studies were repeated and confirmed these predictions; all the patient's ulcers healed. On the basis of this finding, we reported a more extensive consecutive series of 213 patients referred with active venous ulceration. These patients were studied clinically, and by ascending and descending venography, and continuous wave Doppler ultrasound. It was possible to identify a group (39% of the total) with isolated saphenous and perforator incompetence and apparently normal deep veins. These patients underwent saphenous ligation alone . Healing was maintained over a mean 3.5 years in all but five of 54 legs. In the five with recurrent ulceration, other factors were shown in retrospect to account for the ulceration. The wearing of support stockings was left to the patients' discretion. Only one third did so, including three of the five patients with persistent ulceration [20].

A more contemporary but similar report by Bello et al [44] had the advantage that patients were assessed by duplex ultrasound. A total of 122 legs out of 325 studied were found to have normal deep veins. These patients were treated by saphenous surgery alone, many under local anaesthetic as a day case. Support stockings were only used to apply dressings until healing occurred which it did in a median of 18 weeks in all but 18 legs. Again, other factors were identified to account for the few that did not heal. Both of the above series contained a number of patients who also had saphenopopliteal ligation. A recent paper [45] specifically focused on a small group of patients with laterally placed ulcers healed by ligation of an incompetent short saphenous junction.

In conclusion, patients with combined saphenous and perforator incompetence and normal deep veins should be treated by saphenofemoral ligation alone. With these measures their ulcers heal without the ligation of perforating veins which often recover competence. Patients with saphenous, perforator and deep incompetence remain a special challenge and the role of surgery in these patients remains less certain.

Management of patients with a combination of superficial, perforator and deep incompetence

Patients with deep venous incompetence attributable to recognisable post-thrombotic disease, as already stated, seem to fare badly following surgery to the saphenous and perforating veins. They may be best managed with compression bandaging or skin grafting to achieve healing and then long term support stockings. It is important to note that the evidence to support this view is based on studies of patients with demonstrable post-thrombotic disease on imaging, either by venography or duplex. This is manifest as incomplete recanalisation. They may appear at one end of a spectrum of post-thombotic damage where there is a major residual obstructive component. These patients may depend on the superficial systems to act as collateral venous return [46].

What is less clear is the place of saphenous and perforator surgery in patients in whom the remaining identifiable consequence of deep vein thrombosis appears to be deep venous incompetence. These patients, of course, would be difficult to distinguish in a retrospective study from those with apparent 'primary'

deep incompetence. Most researchers have, understandably, left this area of morphology ill-defined (Table 1). My own experience in addressing this challenging group of patients was limited by the lack of duplex imaging at that time, although the evidence for post-thrombotic change was sought diligently with comprehensive ascending venography. Patients with an obstructive element were excluded, leaving information on 52 legs with apparently primary superficial, perforator and deep incompetence. In the first instance these patients were treated by saphenous ligation alone; at 4 year follow up only 21(40%) had healed. Nineteen of these subsequently underwent open perforator ligation of whom ten then healed [47].

In a detailed study of 11 legs with this morphology Padberg et al reported improved haemodynamic and clinical status in patients treated by saphenous and perforator ligation. There was no recurrent ulceration. Interestingly, in six legs the deep incompetence remained the same, in two it resolved and in the last two it progressed [48]. Akesson reported on a mixed group of 31 legs, of which 16 had post-thrombotic disease diagnosed by descending venography. However, after surgery to superficial and perforating veins, 70% remained ulcer-free after a median follow-up of 41 months [49].

From this limited information there is some evidence for saphenous and perforator ligation in these patients. Benefit seems most likely for patients with either primary deep incompetence or deep incompetence secondary to previous deep vein thrombosis where there are no obstructive sequelae. In contrast, patients with deep incompetence and remaining obstruction do badly with surgery.

The significance of perforating vein disease

Sound evidence

- Incompetent flow in ankle perforating veins can be reversed by surgical correction of superficial venous incompetence, when there is no associated deep venous insufficiency. Most patients in this group have healed ulcers after saphenous surgery alone.

Evidence needed

- There remains uncertainty as to the place of both saphenous and perforator surgery in patients with a combination of superficial, perforator and deep incompetence. Where there are no demonstrable post-thrombotic obstructive features on venography or duplex, the benefits of surgery directed towards these areas seems promising.

- But patients with clear evidence of post-thrombotic obstructive changes seem to do less well, and for them the value of surgical intervention is poor.

References (randomised trials in bold)

1. Cockett FB, Elgan Jones D. The ankle blow out syndrome; a new approach to the varicose ulcer problem. *Lancet* 1953; 1: 1-17.

2. Linton RR, Hardy JB. Post-thrombotic syndrome of the lower extremity - treatment by interruption of the superficial femoral vein and ligation and stripping of the long and short saphenous veins. *Surgery* 1948; 24: 452.

3. **Pierik EGJM, van Urk Hop WCJ, Wittens CHA. Endoscopic versus open subfascial division of incompetent perforating veins in the treatment of leg ulceration: randomised trial. *J Vasc Surg* 1997; 26: 1049-54.**

4. Wittens CHA, Pierik RGJ, Van Urk H. The surgical treatment of incompetent perforating veins. *Eur J Vasc Endovasc Surg* 1995; 9: 19-23.

5. Pierik EGJM, Wittens CHA, van Urk H. Subfascial endoscopic ligation in the treatment of incompetent perforating veins. *Eur J Vasc Endovasc Surg* 1995; 9: 38-41.

6. Gloviczki P, Cambria RA, Rhee RY, Canton LG, McKusick MA. Surgical technique and primary results of endoscopic subfascial division of perforating veins. *J Vasc Surg* 1996; 23: 517-23.

7. Rhodes JM, Gloviczki P, Canton L, Heaser TV, Rooke TW. Endoscopic perforator vein division with ablation of superficial reflux improves venous hemodynamics. *J Vasc Surg* 1998; 28: 839-847.

8. Whiteley MS, Galland RB, Smith JJ. Subfascial endoscopic perforator vein surgery (SEPS): current practice among British surgeons. *Ann R Coll Surg Engl* 1998; 80: 104-107.

9. Sarin S, Scurr JH, Coleridge-Smith PD. Medial calf perforators in venous disease; the significance of outward flow. *J Vasc Surg* 1992; 16: 40-46.

10. Barber RF, Shatara FI. The varicose disease. *NY State J Med* 1925; 25: 162-6.

11. Stuart WP, Adam DJ, Allan PL, Ruckley CV, Bradbury AW. Saphenous surgery does not correct perforator incompetence in the presence of deep venous reflux. *J Vasc Surg* 1998; 28: 834-838.

12. Delis KT, Ibgegbuna V, Nicolaides AN, Lauro A, Hafez H. Prevalence and distribution of incompetent perforating veins in chronic venous insufficiency. *J Vasc Surg* 1998; 28: 815-825.

13. Akesson H, Brudin L, Cwikiel W, Ohlin P, Plate G. Does the correction of insuficient superfifial and perforating veins improve venous function in patients with deep venous insufficiency? *Phlebology* 1990; 5: 113-123.

14. Zukowski AJ, Nicolaides AN, Szendro G, et al. Haemodynamic significance of incompetent calf perforating veins . *Br J Surg.* 1991; 78: 625-629.

15. Bjordal R Simultaneous pressure and flow recordings in varicose veins of the lower extremity. *Acta Chir Scand* 1970; 136: 309-317.

16. Walsh JC, Bergan JJ, Beeman S, Commen TP. Femoral venous reflux abolished by greater saphenous vein stripping. *Ann Vasc Surg* 1994; 8: 566-570.

17. Sales CM, Bilof ML, Petrillo KA, Luka NL. Correction of lower extremity deep venous incompetence by ablation of superficial venous reflux. *Ann Vasc Surg* 1996; 10: 186-189.

18. McEnroe CS, O'Donnell TF, Mackey WC. Correlation of clinical findings with venous haemodynamics in 386 patients with chronic venous insufficiency. *Am J Surg* 1988; 156: 148-152.

19. Hanrahan LM, Araki CT, Rodriguez AA, Kechejian GJ, Mamorte WW, Menzoian JO. Distribution of valvular incompetence in patients with venous stasis ulceration. *J Vasc Surg* 1991; 13: 805-812.

20. Darke SG, Penfold C. Venous ulceration and saphenous ligation. *Eur J Surg* 1992; 6: 4-9.

21. Shami SK, Sarin S, Cheatle TR, Coleridge-Smith PD. Venous ulcers and the superficial venous system. *J Vasc Surg* 1993; 17: 487-490.

22. Lees TA, Lambert D. Patterns of venous reflux in legs with skin changes associated with chronic venous insufficiency. *Br J Surg* 1993; 80: 725-728.

23. Weingarten MS, Branas CC, Czeredarczuk M, et al. Distribution and quantification of venous reflux in the lower extremity in chronic venous stasis with duplex scanning. *J Vasc Surg* 1993; 18: 753-9.

24. Van Rij AM, Solomon C, Christie R. Anatomic and physiological characteristics of venous ulceration. *J Vasc Surg* 1994; 20: 759-764.

25. Grabs AJ, Wakely MC, Nyamekye I, Ghauri ASK, Poskitt KR. Colour duplex ultrasonography in the rational management of chronic venous leg ulcers. *Br J Surg* 1996; 83: 1380-1382.

26. Sciven JM, Hartshorne T, Bell PRF, Naylor AR, London NJM. Single visit venous ulcer assessment clinic. the first year. *Br J Surg* 1997; 84: 334-336.

27. Dodd H, Calo AR, Mistry M, Rushford A. Ligation of ankle communicating veins in the treatment of the venous ulcer syndrome of the leg. *Lancet* 1957; 2: 1249.

28. Linton RR. The post thrombotic ulceration of the lower extremity, its etiology and surgical treatment. *Ann Surg* 1953; 138: 415.

29. Dodd H, Cockett FB. *The pathology and surgery of the veins of the lower limb.* Edinburgh: Livingstone, 1956.

30. Cockett FB. The pathology and treatment of venous ulcers of the leg. *Br J Surg.* 1955; 43: 260-278.

31. Cranley JJ, Krauss RJ, Strasser ES. Chronic venous insufficiency of the lower extremity. *Surgery* 1961; 49: 48-58.

32. De Palma RG. Surgical treatment for venous stasis. *Surgery* 1975; 76: 910.

33. Negus D, Friedgood A. The effective management of venous ulceration. *Br J Surg* 1983; 70: 623-627.

34. Bradbury AW, Stonebridge PA, Callam MJ, Ruckley CV, and Allan PL. Foot volumetry and duplex ultrasonography after saphenous and subfascial perforating vein ligation for recurrent venous ulceration. *Br J Surg* 1993; 80: 845-848.

35. Burnand KG, Lea Thomas M, O'Donnell TF, Browse NL. The relationship between postphlebitic changes in the deep veins and results of surgical treatment of venous ulcers. *Lancet* 1976; 1: 936-938.

36. Gloviczki PG, Bergan JJ, Rhodes JM, Canton LG, Harmsen S, Ilstrup DM. Mid term results of endoscopic perforator interruption for chronic venous insufficiency; lessons learned from the North American Subfascial Endoscopic Perforator Surgery registry. *J Vasc Surg* 1999; 29: 489-501.

37. Markel A, Manzo RA, Bergelin RO, Strandness DE. Valvular reflux after deep vein thrombosis: Incidence and time of occurrence. *J Vasc Surg* 1992; 15: 377-82.

38. Van Ramshorst B van Bemmelen PS Hoeneveld H Eikelboom BC. The development of venous incompetence after venous thrombosis: a follow-up study with duplex scanning. *J Vasc Surg* 1994; 19: 1059-66.

39. Caprini JA Arcelus JI Hoffman KN, et al. Venous duplex imaging follow-up of acute symptomatic deep vein thrombosis. *J Vasc Surg* 1995; 21: 472-6.

40. Johnson BF, Manzo RA, Bergelin RO, Strandness DE. Relationship between changes in the deep venous system and the development of the post thrombotic syndrome after an acute episode of lower limb deep vein thrombosis: a one to six year follow-up. *J Vasc Surg* 1995; 21:307-312.

41. Recek C. A critical appraisal of the role of ankle perforators for the genesis of venous ulcers in the lower leg. *J Cardiovasc Surg* 1971; 12: 45-49.

42. Hoare MC, Nicolaides AN, Miles CR, Shull K, Needham T, Dudley HAF. The role of primary varicose veins in venous ulceration. *Surgery* 1983; 92: 450-453.

43. Sethia KK, Darke SG. Long saphenous incompetence as a cause of venous ulceration. *Br J Surg* 1984; 71: 754-755.

44. Bello M, Scriven M, Hartshorne T, Bell PRF, Naylor AR, London NJM. Role of superficial venous surgery in the treatment of venous ulceration. *Br J Surg* 1999; 86: 755-759.

45. Bass A, Chayen D, Weimann EE, Ziss M. Lateral venous ulcer and short saphenous insufficiency. *J Vasc Surg* 1997; 25: 654-657.

46. Bello M, Scriven M, Hartshorne T, London NJM. Venous ulceration and continuous flow in the long saphenous vein. *Eur J Vasc Endovasc Surg* 1999; 17: 11-114.

47. Darke SG. Can we tailor surgery to the venous abnormality? In: Ruckley CV, Fowkes FGR, Bradbury AW, Eds. *Venous disease, epidemiology management and delivery of care.* Springer London, 1998: 139-42.

48. Padberg FT, Pappas PJ, Araki CT, Black TL, Hobson RW. Hemodynamic and clinical improvement after superficial vein ablation in primary combined venous insufficiency with ulceration. *J Vasc Surg* 1996; 24: 711-718.

49. Akesson H. Long-term clinical results following correction of incompetent superficial and perforationg veins in patients with deep venous incompetence and ulcers. *Phlebology* 1993; 81: 29-131.

Chapter 23

The case for endoscopic perforator surgery

G Stansby
Senior Lecturer and
Honorary Consultant Surgeon
K Delis
Senior Vascular Fellow

ACADEMIC SURGICAL AND VASCULAR UNITS,
ST. MARY'S HOSPITAL, LONDON

Introduction

Chronic venous disease and venous leg ulceration throw an enormous burden on health services. It is not surprising, therefore, that any new technique such as subfascial endoscopic perforator surgery (SEPS) that offers hope of improved results should excite great interest and debate. However, as with all new techniques, it is important that evidence of effectiveness is present before it is adopted widely.

The role of the calf perforating veins in leg ulceration

This is a controversial area and the exact pathophysiology of the skin changes found in chronic venous insufficiency remains poorly understood. However, it is agreed that the pathological changes are secondary to sustained venous hypertension in the microcirculation. One of the typical features of venous ulceration or its precursor skin changes is that it occurs on the medial side of the leg above the medial malleolus in the majority (>90%) of patients. Ulceration or changes on the foot or lateral calf are much rarer. This feature suggests that there must be some local factor involved, in addition to global changes in the venous system. For some time it has been suggested that this factor is the presence of incompetent perforating veins on the medial

aspect of the calf transmitting increased pressure from the deep veins to the skin above the medial malleolus. Large studies based on duplex ultrasonography have revealed, however, that isolated perforator incompetence is rare [1] and that it is reflux within the popliteal and crural veins that is associated with an especially high incidence of chronic venous ulceration, failure to respond to medical intervention and subsequent recurrence even if healing is initially achieved [2].

The introduction of SEPS and reports on its safety

Linton was the first to popularise the division of medial calf perforating veins in patients with chronic venous insufficiency and leg ulceration in an attempt to produce healing [3]. After initial enthusiasm, however, open operation fell out of favour because of problems with wound healing (up to 50% in some series) and a need for prolonged in-hospital stay. Subfascial endoscopic division of perforating veins was first reported by Hauer in 1985 [4]. Hauer's initial report of this technique, in the German language, was not widely disseminated until the first report in English by Fischer in 1989 [5]. Since then widespread interest has developed in this new technique for carrying out what is essentially the same operation as open perforator surgery, but more reliably and with a much smaller incision.

JVRG

Table 1. Complications of SEPS.

AUTHORS	COMPLICATIONS
Jugenheimer and Junginger 1992 [6]	saphenous neuralgia (10%) sural neuralgia (2%) haematomas (6%)
Pierik et al 1995 [7]	subfascial infection (5%) inflammatory reaction (2.5%)
Bergan et al 1996 [13]	atelectasis (3%) cellulitis (10%) wound haematoma (4.5%) wound seroma (3%)
Sparks et al 1997 [12]	wound infection (16%)
Kulbaski et al 1997 [15]	subfascial haematoma (5%) wound infection (5%)
Gloviczki et al 1999 [18]	saphenous neuralgia (6%) wound infection (6%) superficial vein thrombosis (3%) cellulitis (2.5%) deep vein thrombosis (1%) skin necrosis (1%)

Many thousands of SEPS procedures have now been described in published reports. Unfortunately most are case series and there have been few randomised studies. Data on safety and complications are, however, available from these studies (Table 1). The main complications of SEPS appear to be haematomas, wound infections and neuropraxias (usually sensory but occasionally motor). One of the largest studies included 103 legs in 72 patients undergoing the SEPS procedure [6]. Mean duration of the procedure was 27 minutes (range 20-36). There were no intraoperative complications. The mean number of perforating veins divided was four (range 2-11). In three patients (3% of legs) delayed healing at the insertion incision was noted. Sensory loss in the distribution of the sural nerve was found in two patients (2%), saphenous nerve distribution in ten patients (10%) and a significant haematoma in six patients (6%).

In 1997 the North American SEPS study (NASEPS) published its preliminary data [8]. This was a voluntary register set up to evaluate the feasibility and safety of the procedure. The authors reported data on 155 SEPS operations carried out on 148 patients. There were no early deaths or problems with deep venous thrombosis. Wound infection occurred in only 5% of the patients, most of whom had an open ulcer at the time of surgery. Stuart et al [9] subsequently compared 30 patients who had undergone a SEPS procedure with 37 retrospective controls who had the traditional open Linton's procedure. The two groups were well matched for age and indication for surgery. The open group had a significantly longer stay in hospital and a greater wound infection rate (9/37)

compared with none (0/30) in the SEPS group. Wittens and colleagues [10] published results from a prospective randomised trial comparing open to endoscopic perforator surgery for leg ulceration. The trial was stopped by the monitoring committee after 39 patients had been entered because of the much greater incidence of wound complications in the open group (10/19 versus 0/20, p<0.001). These data suggest that overall the complication rate for SEPS is much lower than for open perforator surgery.

Haemodynamic and long-term results of SEPS

The key question with regard to the SEPS operation is whether it imparts long-term benefit to the patient, particularly in terms of ulcer healing and prevention of recurrence. Wittens et al looked at 40 legs in 38 patients with recurrent or protracted venous ulcers in whom calf perforator veins were identified using duplex imaging [11]. The results were impressive with only one patient developing a recurrent leg ulcer at 3.9 years median follow-up. Of the 40 patients, 31 had associated deep venous incompetence. Bergan et al described 31 legs that underwent a SEPS procedure in 1996. Of these, 13 legs had a history of chronic (>6 months duration), recurrent ulceration and of these ulcers 11 of 13 (86%) healed within 8 weeks. Unfortunately no long-term follow-up was available. Sparks et al published results of SEPS for 19 legs treated as day-cases [12]. In this series 75%

(13/19) of legs had open ulceration. All active ulcers had healed at 90 days, and none had recurred at a mean follow-up of eight and a half months. In Sparks' study 12 of the 19 legs had additional procedures. However, no mention was made of how many patients had further surgery, only that any long saphenous incompetence was also dealt with at the time of operation.

NASEPS [8] published initial healing rates for 85 of the 106 patients included with open ulceration at time of surgery and showed a high success rate with 88% (75 patients) reportedly healed at follow-up. The probability of healing at 90 days was 67% (95% confidence interval 55% - 76%). There were, however, also four new or

dressings and strict elevation. Kulbaski et al [15] reported on 20 episodes of SEPS in 19 patients. Seventeen legs had active ulceration at the time of operation. On average, four perforating veins were divided in each case. At a mean follow-up of 8 months, initial complete healing occurred in 14 of 17 ulcers, three ulcers improved, and three healed ulcers at the time of SEPS remained healed subsequently.

Fitridge et al [16] have reported a study of 38 legs in 35 patients. All had uncomplicated varicose veins with both long saphenous and calf perforator incompetence on duplex ultrasonography. Patients were randomised to have incompetent calf perforators ligated or left intact, in

Table 2. Effectiveness of SEPS in healing ulceration.

AUTHORS	NUMBER OF SEPS PROCEDURES	% LSV Surgery	HEALING RATE	MEAN FOLLOW-UP (months)	RECURRENCE RATE
Pierik et al 1995 [7]	40	-	100%	34.8 (range 24-60)	2.5%
Bergan et al 1996 [13]	31	-	79%	> 2	0%
Pierik et al 1997 [11]	20	-	85%	12	0%
Sparks et al 1997 [12]	19	63%	100%	8.6 (range 3-16)	0%
Rhodes et al 1998 [17]	31	77%	100%	11	4%
Kulbaski et al 1997 [15]	20	-	82%	8	5%
Gloviczki et al 1999 [18]	158	55.7%	88%	12 24	16% 28%

LSV: long saphenous vein

recurrent ulcers out of the 120 total patients followed. In the NASEPS report from 1997, 88 patients (59%) had saphenofemoral junction (SFJ) ligation, whilst 38 patients (26%) had only the SEPS procedure performed and a further 16 only had additional calf avulsions or vein excisions.

There has been one recent study where SEPS was performed in isolation on a group of 40 patients who had all had previous stripping or high saphenous ligation [14]. Sixteen patients had active ulceration at time of surgery and nine of these healed (57%) within a median of 21 days, although there were no data on long-term follow-up. Although this is suggestive of benefit, there was no control group so it is difficult to tell if the benefit was greater than could have been obtained by intensive

addition to saphenofemoral junction ligation, stripping the long saphenous vein to the knee and stab avulsion of any visible varicosities in the leg. Patients were assessed with air plethysmography pre-operatively and 3 months postoperatively. No significant haemodynamic benefit was demonstrated in the SEPS group. However, none of the patients had chronic venous insufficiency.

Rhodes et al [17] also assessed the effect of SEPS on venous haemodynamics in 31 legs (26 patients) with significant chronic venous disease in a non-randomised study. Superficial reflux was present in 20 (65%) and deep venous reflux in 24 legs (77%). The 21 contralateral non-operated legs were used for comparison. Perforator incompetence was defined as outward flow longer than 0.3 secs in duration during the relaxation phase after calf compression. Simultaneous saphenous surgery was performed in 24 legs (77%). Haemodynamic assessment was carried out using strain-gauge plethysmography preoperatively and within 6 months of surgery. All active ulcers healed after surgery and only one recurred during a mean follow-up of 11.3 months. Improved calf muscle pump function was demonstrated by plethysmography but the number who had SEPS alone were too few to be certain that this improvement was due to perforator surgery. The authors concluded that SEPS resulted in improved calf muscle pump function but, in reality, the relative role of the SEPS procedure in producing the haemodynamic benefit remained unproven. They also pointed out that there were relatively few patients with post-thrombotic deep venous insufficiency and that results may also be worse for this group.

Finally, the NASEPS registry [18] has recently reported updated results with follow-up averaging 24 months (range 1 to 53 months). Cumulative ulcer healing at 1 year was 88% (median time to healing of 54 days); cumulative ulcer recurrence at 1 year was 16% and at 2 years 28%. Legs with post-thrombotic disease had a higher 2-year cumulative recurrence rate (46%) than did legs with primary valvular incompetence (20%). The authors concluded that interruption of perforators with ablation of superficial reflux was effective in decreasing the symptoms of chronic venous insufficiency and rapidly healing ulcers, but that surgery in patients with previous deep vein thrombosis was less successful.

Conclusions

SEPS appears to be safe and reliable at interrupting the medial calf perforating veins with relatively low complication rates. To become established as a recognised treatment, however, SEPS must not only show that it can consistently improve the symptoms of chronic venous insufficiency without significant morbidity, but also that any improvement is greater than could have been achieved by current accepted best practice. Unfortunately there has been no randomised controlled trial of SEPS against conservative treatment in the healing of leg ulcers; enthusiasts for evidence based medicine may quite rightly treat the procedure with some suspicion. In addition, SEPS development may still be in the steep part of the learning curve with regards to its technical effectiveness; results in studies published to date may not yet be optimal. Future controlled trials are therefore needed to define the role of this technique in the management of chronic venous insufficiency. There is no no proven role for SEPS in the management of uncomplicated varicose veins.

The case for endoscopic perforator surgery

Sound evidence

- SEPS is technically effective at eradicating calf perforators.

- SEPS produces significantly fewer complications than open surgery.

- SEPS and saphenous surgery combined produce good initial venous ulcer healing.

- Results are worse when there has been previous deep venous thrombosis.

- There is no justification for SEPS in uncomplicated varicose veins.

Evidence needed

- There is no evidence that SEPS alone improves long-term prognosis over conservative management or saphenous surgery alone.

References. (randomised trials in bold)

1. Labropoulos N, Leon M, Nicolaides AN, Giannoukas AD, Volteas N, Chan P. Superficial venous insufficiency: correlation of anatomic extent of reflux with clinical symptoms and signs. *J Vasc Surg* 1994; 20: 953-8.
2. Brittenden J, Bradbury AW, Allan PL, Prescott RJ, Harper DR, Ruckley CV. Popliteal vein reflux reduces the healing of chronic venous ulcer. *Br J Surg* 1998; 85: 60-2.
3. Linton RR. The communicating veins of the lower leg and the operative technique for their ligation. *Ann Surg* 1938; 107: 582-93.
4. Hauer G. Die endoscopische subfasciale diszision der perforansvenen-vorlaufige mitteilung. *VASA* 1985; 14: 59.
5. Fischer R. Surgical treatment of varicose veins; endoscopic treatment of incompetent Cockett veins. *Phlebology* 1989; 1040-1.
6. Jugenheimer M, Junginger T. Endoscopic subfascial sectioning of perforating veins in the treatment of primary varicositles. *World J Surg* 1992; 16: 971-5.
7. Pierik EG, Wittens CH, van Urk H. Subfascial endoscopic ligation in the treatment of incompetent perforating veins. *Eur J Vasc Endovasc Surg* 1995; 9: 38-41.
8. Gloviczki P, Bergan JJ, Menawat SS, et al. Safety, feasibility, and early efficacy of subfascial endoscopic perforator surgery: a preliminary report from the North American registry. *J Vasc Surg* 1997; 25: 94-105.
9. Stuart WP, Adam DJ, Bradbury AW, Ruckley CV. Subfascial endoscopic perforator surgery is associated with significantly less morbidity and shorter hospital stay than open operation (Linton's procedure). *Br J Surg* 1997; 84: 1364-5.
10. **Pierik EG, van UH, Hop WC, Wittens CH. Endoscopic versus open subfascial division of incompetent perforating veins in the treatment of venous leg ulceration: a randomized trial. *J Vasc Surg* 1997; 26: 1049-54.**
11. Pierik EG, van UH, Wittens CH. Efficacy of subfascial endoscopy in eradicating perforating veins of the lower leg and its relation with venous ulcer healing. *J Vasc Surg* 1997; 26: 255-9.
12. Sparks SR, Ballard JL, Bergan JJ, Killeen JD. Early benefits of subfascial endoscopic perforator surgery (SEPS) in healing venous ulcers. *Ann Vasc Surg* 1997; 11: 367-73.
13. Bergan JJ, Murray J, Greason K. Subfascial endoscopic perforator vein surgery: a preliminary report. *Ann Vasc Surg* 1996; 10: 211-9.
14. Proebstle TM, Weisel G, Paepcke U, Gass S, Weber L. Light reflection rheography and clinical course of patients with advanced venous disease before and after endoscopic subfascial division of perforating veins. *Dermatol Surg* 1998; 24: 771-6.
15. Kulbaski MJ, Eaves FF 3rd, Ofenloch JC, Lumsden AB. Subfascial endoscopic perforator surgery: new life for an old procedure? *J Soc Laparoendosc Surg* 1997; 1: 135-9.
16. **Fitridge RA, Dunlop C, Raptis S, Thompson MM, Leppard P, Quigley F. A prospective randomized trial evaluating the haemodynamic role of incompetent calf perforating veins. *Aust N Z J Surg* 1999; 69: 214-6.**
17. Rhodes JM, Gloviczki P, Canton L, Heaser TV, Rooke TW. Endoscopic perforator vein division with ablation of superficial reflux improves venous hemodynamics. *J Vasc Surg* 1998; 28: 839-47.
18. Gloviczki P, Bergan JJ, Rhodes JM, Canton LG, Harmsen S, Ilstrup DM. Mid-term results of endoscopic perforator vein interruption for chronic venous insufficiency: lessons learned from the North American subfascial endoscopic perforator surgery registry. The North American Study Group. *J Vasc Surg* 1999; 29: 489-502.

The case for endoscopic perforator surgery

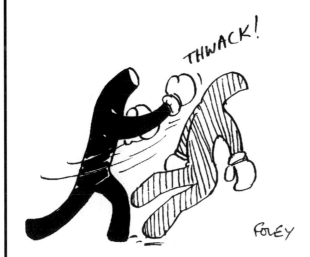

Chapter 24

The management of venous ulceration

RK MacKenzie
Research Fellow
AW Bradbury
Consultant Surgeon and
Senior Lecturer

DEPARTMENT OF VASCULAR SURGERY,
ROYAL INFIRMARY OF EDINBURGH, EDINBURGH

Introduction

Chronic venous insufficiency (CVI), culminating in chronic venous ulceration, is a common disease with a life-time risk of 1/100 and a point prevalence of 1/1000 in Northern Europe. Venous ulceration is estimated to consume 1-2% of United Kingdom National Health Service spending (about £600 million annually) [1]. Although limb loss and death are unusual, chronic venous ulceration is associated with a marked reduction in quality of life [2]. Despite this, venous disease has tended to receive a low priority in research funding and, as a result, there remains a lack of evidence regarding its management.

Evidence and guidelines

In recent years, three independent groups, the Royal College of Dermatologists (1995) [3], the Scottish Health Purchasing Information Centre (SHPIC) (1996) [4] and the Scottish Intercollegiate Guideline Network (SIGN) (1998) [5] have gathered evidence, assembled multi-disciplinary panels of 'experts', reached consensus and issued guidelines regarding the management of leg ulcers. The effect of implementing the SIGN guidelines is currently being assessed by the Scottish Leg Ulcer Project [6].

The quality of guidelines is reliant upon adhering to several important principles.

- A thorough and systematic review of the literature must be performed. The highly sensitive strategy developed by the UK Cochrane Collaboration was employed in the development of SIGN guidelines [7].
- The quality of evidence and the strength of the ensuing recommendation must be graded. SIGN used the US Agency for Health Care Policy and Research classification (Table 1) [8].
- The 'expert' panel must include representatives of all the medical and paramedical disciplines involved in the care of these patients; patients should have a voice too (Table 2).
- While evidenced-based guidelines are undoubtedly useful, their authors must not regard them as a panacea.

The SIGN development group specifically noted that their recommendations:

- should only be adopted after local discussion (local 'ownership' is crucial for successful implementation),
- should not be seen as a 'standard of care',
- do not guarantee a good outcome in every case, and
- are neither comprehensive nor exhaustive.

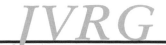

Table 1. Grading of evidence and recommendations.

Evidence

Ia Obtained from meta-analysis of randomised controlled trials.

Ib Obtained from at least one well-conducted randomised controlled trial.

IIa Obtained from at least one controlled study without randomisation.

IIb Obtained from at least one other well-designed quasi-experimental study.

III Obtained from expert committee reports and/or clinical experience of respected authorities.

Recommendation

A Requires at least one randomised controlled trial as part of a body of literature of overall good quality and consistency addressing the specific recommendation.

B Requires the availability of well conducted clinical studies but no randomised clinical trials on the topic of the recommendation.

C Requires evidence obtained from expert committee reports and/or clinical experiences of respected authorities. Indicates the absence of directly applicable clinical studies of good quality.

Nevertheless, guidelines do have some 'teeth'; the SIGN development group stated that 'significant departures from the local guidelines should be documented fully in the patient's care-notes at the time the relevant decision is taken' [9].

Clinical assessment

Definition of a venous ulcer

A breach in the skin between the knee and ankle joint, of presumed venous aetiology, that has been present for at least 4 weeks.

The patient

Before focusing on the ulcer, it is important to assess the whole patient. Many venous ulcers, particularly those that are refractory to treatment, are multifactorial in aetiology. Sustained healing will only be achieved once all the local and systemic aetiological factors have been treated; for example, diabetes mellitus (5%), rheumatoid arthritis (8%), peripheral arterial disease (20%), cardiac failure, anaemia, and renal disease. It is also apparent that certain life-style and socio-economic factors such as occupation, quality/type of housing, heating, nutrition and mobility have a bearing upon both aetiology and prognosis [10]. A change of housing and/or an increase in nursing and/or social support may be required.

The leg

The aetiology of a leg ulcer can usually be determined by a careful history and examination. Particular attention should be paid to the locomotor system, causes of oedema and, of course, the symptoms and signs of venous and arterial disease.

Locomotor It is important to assess the patient's mobility and helpful to watch them walk. Flat feet, a fixed ankle and reduced mobility at the knees/hips due to osteoarthritis will exacerbate venous hypertension. Features of rheumatoid arthritis should be noted.

Oedema This may be due to one or more of the following: venous disease, lymphoedema, cardiac failure, renal disease and hypoproteinaemia [11]. Oedema significantly impairs skin perfusion and ulcers will not heal until it is controlled by elevation, bandaging, or specific medical treatment.

Venous disease Skin changes of CVI are usually readily apparent. However, it is worth noting that in an obese, chronically ulcerated leg, significant and surgically correctable superficial venous reflux (particularly in the

Table 2. Composition of the SIGN development group on the management of chronic leg ulcers.

Vascular surgeon

District nurse

Pharmacist

Liaison district nurse and leg ulcer specialist

Physiotherapist

Dermatologist

Rheumatologist

General practitioner

Plastic surgeon

Practice nurse

Medical microbiologist

short saphenous distribution) may be missed on clinical examination alone. Hand-held Doppler (HHD) or preferably, duplex ultrasound imaging should be performed [12].

Arterial disease Up to 20% of patients with chronic venous ulceration have significant arterial disease which precludes the use of high grade compression and/or impairs wound healing [13].

> *Recommendation (grade B) Measurement of ankle brachial pressure index (ABPI) by HHD is essential in the assessment of chronic leg ulceration. Patients with an ABPI of < 0.8 should be assumed to have arterial disease and referred to a vascular surgeon.*

The ulcer

Description A full and structured description of the ulcer is important for both diagnosis and assessment of healing. The following specific features should be noted:

- position: gaiter area (medial, lateral, circumferential), foot (toes, pressure points), atypical,
- base: necrotic (black), sloughy (yellow/green), granulating (pink),
- margin: regular, irregular, epithelialising or not,
- surrounding tissue: infected, indurated, oedematous, friable,
- depth: shallow, deep and punched out, tendon or bone exposed (a grave prognostic sign).

Assessment of healing The total area of ulceration should be measured serially rather than simply the greatest dimension of the largest or 'index' ulcer. The taking of clinical photographs with a simple Polaroid Æ camera can be invaluable [14].

> *Recommendation (grade B) The surface area of the ulcer should be measured serially, either by tracing or photographic record.*

Investigations

Hand-held Doppler

As discussed above, this should be used in all patients to measure ABPI and define the pattern of venous reflux.

Duplex ultrasound imaging

This will provide physiological and anatomical information about reflux and/or obstruction in the deep and superficial veins. Duplex imaging also permits the non-invasive assessment of arterial disease and may allow the identification of patients suitable for endovascular treatment (angioplasty with, or without a stent). The presence of popliteal vein reflux appears to be an adverse prognostic sign in patients managed both medically [15] and operatively [16].

> *Recommendation (grade C) All patients with a chronic leg ulcer should undergo duplex ultrasonography.*

Angiography

Where non-invasive imaging is unavailable or inconclusive, angiography is required to assess arterial disease.

Venography

Venography is now little used, but may be required where duplex imaging is inconclusive.

Bacteriological examination

Most venous ulcers are colonised with bacteria rather than infected and routine swabbing is not indicated [17,18].

> *Recommendation (grade C) Bacteriological swabs should be obtained where there is clinical evidence of infection (excessive pain, cellulitis, pyrexia) or surgery (skin graft, insertion of a prosthetic bypass) is being considered.*

Biopsy

Up to 2% of chronic leg ulcers are malignant but the diagnosis is often missed [19].

> *Recommendation (grade C) Non-healing (12 weeks) and/or atypical ulcers should be biopsied under local anaesthetic. The tissue removed should include both the margin and the base.*

Patch testing

Many patients with a chronic venous ulcer have associated dermatitis which may be endogenous or exogenous due to irritants or contact allergy [20,21].

> *Recommendation (grade C) Leg ulcer patients with associated dermatitis should be referred for patch-testing with a leg ulcer series.*

Management

The patient

As discussed above, the patient should be treated in a 'holistic' manner with attention paid to medical and surgical co-morbidity, as well as socio-economic factors.

The leg

Compression therapy It is beyond doubt that compression heals venous ulcers [22,23]. In trials, multi-layer, graduated, high grade (40mmHg at the ankle) bandaging performs better than inelastic or short-stretch bandaging [24,25].

> *Recommendation (grade A) Multi-layer, graduated, elastic, high-grade compression should be used in all patients with uncomplicated venous ulcers.*

Pneumatic compression Two small prospective, randomised controlled trials have shown no statistically significant benefit [26,27].

The ulcer

Debridement and cleansing There have been no well conducted trials of chemical/mechanical debridement. A randomised study has suggested no advantage for sterile saline over ordinary tap water [28].

> *Recommendation (grade A) Venous ulcers should be cleansed with tap water and then carefully dried.*

Dressings There is evidence to suggest that the type of dressing applied has little bearing on ulcer healing [29-31]. A simple, inexpensive, non-adherent pad is satisfactory in most circumstances. Hydrocolloid [32] and/or foam dressings [33] may confer additional benefit in ulcers that are particularly painful.

> *Recommendation (grade A) Simple non-adherent dressings are recommended for most ulcers as no specific dressing has been shown to improve healing rates. Hydrocolloid or foam dressings should be considered in painful ulcers.*

Topical therapy No topical agent, including epidermal growth factor [34,35], has been shown to improve healing. Routine use of antibiotics does not improve healing [36,37]. Topical antibiotics are frequent sensitisers and should not be used [38].

> *Recommendation (grade B) Topical antibiotics should not be used in the treatment of venous ulcers.*

Systemic therapy No systemic drug therapy has been proved to improve ulcer healing (Table 3).

Table 3. Systemic pharmacotherapy for chronic leg ulceration.

Drug	Proposed mode of action	Comment
Stanozolol	enhances fibrinolysis to 'dissolve' fibrin cuff	reduces lipodermatosclerosis but no effect on healing rates [39]
Ergotamine	vein wall contraction leading to reduced vein diameter and reflux	may improve healing rates but narrow therapeutic index, not recommended [40]
Aspirin	reduces the thrombocytosis and increased platelet volume seen in venous hypertension	small studies have suggested an increase in healing rates [41,42]
Prostaglandin E1	inhibits platelet aggregation and neutrophil activation which may have an effect on 'white cell trapping'	may improve healing but only available as an expensive intra-venous preparation [43,44]
Pentoxifylline	inhibits cytokine mediated neutrophil activation and adhesion which may have an effect on 'white cell trapping'	improved healing in one small study [45] was not confirmed in a larger trial [46]
Hydroxyethylrutosides	decreases capillary permeability (mechanism unknown)	symptomatic improvement in CVI but no evidence of an effect on ulcer healing [47]

> *Recommendation (grade C) Systemic therapy is not recommended for the treatment of venous ulcers.*

Superficial venous surgery To date, no randomised controlled trial has compared the effects of 'best medical therapy', with and without venous surgery, on the healing and recurrence rates of venous ulceration. However, uncontrolled data suggest that, in the absence of deep venous disease, surgical eradication of superficial venous reflux is of benefit [48-51].

> *Recommendation (grade C) Patients with superficial venous reflux should be considered for surgery.*

Other surgery There is no proof that perforator surgery (open or endoscopic) alters the natural history of chronic venous ulceration [52]. Deep venous surgery remains an experimental procedure and there is no evidence that it affects the natural history of chronic venous ulceration. Similarly, there is no evidence that venous bypass affects the natural history.

Skin grafting Split skin grafting may augment healing and reduce recurrence, provided venous hypertension is controlled medically and/or surgically [53]. Pinch skin grafting has also been shown to improve early healing rates, but this does not appear to be sustained [54].

> *Recommendation (grade C) Patients with a venous ulcer should be considered for skin grafting providing venous hypertension can be controlled either by compression or superficial venous surgery.*

Arterial intervention In patients with significant arterial disease, vascular or endovascular reconstruction may augment healing rates by improving nutrition to the ulcer and allowing the use of compression. However, this has not been studied scientifically to date.

Reassessment

It is important to reassess the ulcer for signs of healing at regular intervals. Reassessment should follow the same format as the initial assessment. If the ulcer is not healing, consider:

- is the aetiology confirmed ?
- are there unrecognised, or new, co-morbidities ?
- should the ulcer be biopsied ?
- is the current management plan still appropriate ?
- is the patient compliant with treatment ?

> *Recommendation (grade C) The ulcer should be formally reassessed 12 weeks after the commencement of therapy and at intervals of 12 weeks thereafter until healed.*

Secondary prevention

Compression therapy

Compression hosiery has been demonstrated to reduce ulcer recurrence [55]. Class III stockings appear to be better than Class II [56]. The hazards of incorrectly fitted stockings are the same as for compression bandaging and, once again, the adequacy of arterial inflow must be formally assessed and documented.

> *Recommendation (grade C) Correctly fitted graduated compression should be prescribed to all patients with uncomplicated healed venous ulcers and worn for at least 5 years (probably for life).*

Surgery

The role of surgery in secondary prevention of venous ulceration remains unproved.

Drug therapy

No drug has been shown to reduce recurrence of venous ulcers.

Provision of care

Much has been written about a model of care for the provision of leg ulcer services. Uncontrolled data suggest that specialist leg ulcer clinics staffed by trained nurses obtain better healing rates than those that are commonly described in the normal community setting [57]. The effect of SIGN guidelines and specific nurse training on community healing rates is currently being investigated by the Scottish Leg Ulcer Project.

In practice, the provision of care will inevitably vary with location. However, the following are important components of any model.

- The overall treatment package should be delivered by an interdisciplinary team of interested doctors and nurses who communicate readily with each other and have easy access to the skills of other disciplines, such as physio- and occupational therapists.
- Carers should understand the multi-factorial aetiology of most leg ulcers and be capable of identifying, early in the course of the disease, patients who might benefit from surgical correction of underlying venous and arterial disease and/or other specialist input (Table 4).
- Patients are treated according to evidence-based guidelines derived from a systematic review of the available literature.
- The patients' treatment is viewed as a joint effort between primary and secondary care.

The benefits of a structured approach to leg ulcer have been clearly demonstrated by, amongst others, the Cheltenham and Gloucester [58,59] and the Leicester vascular groups [60,61].

Table 4. Suggested criteria for early specialist referral.

uncertain aetiology
atypical ulcer distribution
suspicion of malignancy
peripheral vascular disease (ABPI < 0.8)
surgically correctable superficial venous reflux
diabetes mellitus
rheumatoid arthritis or other suspected condition associated with vasculitis
dermatitis refractory to topical steroids
failure to respond to conventional therapy

Conclusions

The lack of evidence regarding the management of chronic leg ulceration is manifested by the SIGN guideline document where only seven references refer to grade Ia or Ib evidence, and few grade A recommendations are made. The lack of a randomised controlled trial investigating whether venous surgery confers additional benefit over best medical therapy in terms of the healing and recurrence of venous ulcers is particularly disappointing and needs to be addressed [62]. If surgeons are to persuade health-care funding bodies to support venous surgery such a trial will need to include a detailed health economic analysis. Research is also required into the epidemiology and natural history of the disease, models of care, primary prevention and pathogenesis. In the meantime, individuals involved in the care of patients with a leg ulcer should adopt evidence-based guidelines for local use, strive for a more structured and consistent approach to the disease, and carefully audit their results [63].

Summary of recommendations

(adapted from the 1998 SIGN Guideline report)

Grade A
- Graduated, multi-layer, high-grade compression bandaging is the treatment of choice for uncomplicated venous leg ulcers.

- Ulcerated legs should be washed in ordinary tap water.

- Simple non-adherent dressings are the first-line treatment of uncomplicated leg ulcers as no specific dressing has been shown to improve healing rates.

- Hydrocolloid or foam dressings may be of value in painful ulcers.

- Antibiotics should be reserved for evidence of frank infection and in patients being considered for arterial bypass surgery and/or skin grafting.

- Systemic therapy is not recommended in the treatment of leg ulcers.

- Correctly fitted, graduated compression hosiery should be prescribed for at least 5 years to all patients with a healed, uncomplicated venous leg ulcer.

Grade B
- Measurement of ABPI with hand-held Doppler is essential in all patients with leg ulceration.

- Patients with an ABPI < 0.8 should be assumed to have significant arterial disease.

- Ulcer surface area should be measured serially.

- Bacteriological swabs should only be taken where there is clinical evidence of infection, or prior to bypass surgery and/or skin grafting.

- Patients with associated dermatitis should be referred for patch testing with a leg ulcer series.

- Topical antibiotics should not be used as they are frequent sensitisers.

- Venous surgery should be considered in patients with superficial venous incompetence.

Grade C
- Ulcers should be reassessed formally every 12 weeks.

- An atypical or non-healing ulcer should be biopsied.

References (randomised trials in bold)

1. Laing W. *Chronic venous disease of the legs.* Office of Health Economics. London. 1992: 24-42.

2. Phillips T, Stanton B, Provan A, Lew R. A study of the impact of leg ulcers on quality of life: financial, social and psychological implications. *J Am Acad Dermatol* 1994; 31: 49-53.

3. Douglas WS, Simpson NB. Guidelines for the management of chronic venous leg ulceration. Report of a multi-disciplinary workshop. Royal College of Dermatologists and the Research Unit of the Royal College of Physicians. *Br J Dematol* 1995; 132: 446-52.

4. Scottish Health Purchasing Information Centre. *Leg ulcers.* Aberdeen. The centre; 1996.

5. Scottish Intercollegiate Guidelines Network. *The care of patients with chronic leg ulcer: a national clinical guideline.* SIGN publication number 26. Royal College of Physicians, Edinburgh, 1998.

6. Scottish Leg Ulcer Project. Professor C.V. Ruckley (personal communication).

7. Bradbury AW, Ruckley CV. Variations in vascular practice and the Cochrane Collaboration. *Eur J Vasc Endovasc Surg* 1996; 11: 125-6.

8. US Department of Health and Human Services. Agency for Health Care Policy and Research. The Agency; 1993. *Clinical practice guidelines.* AHCPR Publication No. 92-0023 p107.

9. Scottish Intercollegiate Guideline Network. *The legal implications of guidelines.* SIGN Secretariat, Royal College of Physicians, Edinburgh.

10. Callam MJ, Harper DR, Dale JJ, Ruckley, CV. Chronic leg ulceration: socio-economic aspects. *Scot Med J* 1988; 33: 358-60.

11. Diskin CJ, Stokes TJ, Dansby LM, Carter TB, Radcliff L, Thomas SB. Towards an understanding of oedema. *Br Med J* 1999; 318: 1610 13.

12. Stuart WP, Bradbury AW, Ruckley CV. When do we need duplex scanning to define venous reflux? *Scripta Phlebologica* 1998; 1: 12-5.

13. Callam MJ, Harper DR, Dale JJ, Ruckley CV. Arterial disease in chronic leg ulceration: an underestimated hazard? Lothian and Forth Valley leg ulcer study. *Br Med J* 1987; 294: 929-31.

14. Stacey MC, Burnand KG, Layer GT, Pattison M, Browse NL. Measurement of the healing of venous ulcers. *Aust N Z J Surg* 1991; 61: 844-8.

15. Brittenden J, Bradbury AW, Allan, PL, Prescott RJ, Harper DR, Ruckley CV. Popliteal vein reflux reduces the healing of chronic venous ulcer. *Br J Surg* 1998; 85: 60-2.

16. Bradbury AW, Stonebridge PA, Callam MJ, Ruckley CV, Allan PL. Foot volumetry and duplex ultrasonography after saphenous and subfascial perforator vein ligation for recurrent venous ulceration. *Br J Surg* 1993; 80: 845-8.

17. Hansson C, Hoborn J, Moller A, Swanbeck G. The microbial flora in venous leg ulcers without clinical signs of infection. Repeated culture using a validated standardised microbiological technique. *Acta Derm Venereol* 1995; 75: 24-30.

18. Gilliland EL, Dore CJ, Nathwani N, Lewis JD. Bacterial colonisation of leg ulcers and its effect on the success rate of skin grafting. *Ann R Coll Surg Eng* 1988; 70: 105-8.

19. Yang D, Morrison BD, Vandogen, YK, Singh A, Stacey MC. Malignancy in chronic leg ulcers. *Med J Aust* 1996; 164: 718-20.

20. Wilson CL, Cameron J, Powell SM, Cherry G, Ryan TG. High incidence of contact dermatitis in leg ulcer patients - implications for management. *Clin Exp Dermatol* 1991; 16: 250-3.

21. Kulozik M, Powell SM, Cherry G, Ryan TJ. Contact sensitivity in community-based leg ulcer patients. *Clin Exp Dermatol* 1988; 13: 82-4.

22. Fletcher A, Cullum N, Sheldon TA. A systematic review of compression treatment for venous leg ulcers. *Br Med J* 1997; 315: 576-80.

23. Palfreyman SJ, Lochiel R, Michaels JA. A systematic review of compression therapy for venous leg ulcers. *Vasc Med* 1998; 3: 301-13.

24. **Callam MJ, Harper DR, Dale JJ, et al. Lothian and Forth Valley leg ulcer healing trial, part 1: elastic vs. non-elastic bandaging in the treatment of chronic leg ulceration. *Phlebology* 1992; 7: 136-41.**

25. Thomas S. Bandages used in leg ulcer management. In: *Leg Ulcer Nursing Management - a Research-based Guide.* Eds: Cullum N, Roe B. Balliere Tindall, London, 1998: 63-74.

26. **Smith PC, Sarin S, Hasty J, Scurr JH. Sequential gradient pneumatic compression enhances venous ulcer healing in a randomised trial. *Surgery* 1990; 108: 871-5.**

27. **McCulloch JM, Marler KC, Neal MB, Phifer TJ. Intermittent pneumatic compression improves venous ulcer healing. *Adv Wound Care* 1994; 7: 22-6.**

28. **Hall Angeras M, Brandberg A, Falk A, Seeman T. Comparison between sterile saline and tap water for the cleaning of acute traumatic soft tissue wounds. *Eur J Surg* 1992; 158: 347-50.**

29. **Stacey MC, Jopp-Mackay AG, Rashid P, Hoskin SE, Thompson PJ. The influence of dressings on venous ulcer healing in a randomised trial. *Eur J Vasc Endovasc Surg* 1997; 13: 174-9.**

30. Thomas S. A guide to dressing selection. *J Wound care* 1997; 6: 479-81.

31. Cullum N. Topical applications in leg ulcer management. In: *Leg Ulcer Nursing Management - a Research-based Guide.* Eds: Cullum N, Roe B. Balliere Tindall, London, 1998: 35-62.

32. **Callam MJ, Harper DR, Dale JJ, et al. Lothian and Forth Valley leg ulcer healing trial, part 2: Knitted viscose dressing versus a hydrocolloid dressing in the treatment of chronic leg ulceration. *Phlebology* 1992; 7: 142-5.**

33. Blair SD. Do dressings influence the healing of chronic venous ulcers? *Phlebology* 1988; 3: 129-34.

34. Brown GL, Curtsinger L, Jurkiewicz MJ, Nahai F, Schultz G. Stimulation of healing of chronic wounds by epidermal growth factor. *Plast Reconstr Surg* 1991; 88: 89-94.

35. **Falanga V, Eaglstein WH, Bucal B, et al. Topical use of human recombinant epidermal growth factor in venous ulcers. *J Dermatol Surg Oncol* 1992; 18: 604-6.**

36. Alinovi A, Bassini P, Pini M. Systemic administration of antibiotics in the management of venous ulcers. *J Am Acad Dermatol* 1986; 15: 186-91.

37. Huovinen S, Kotilainen P, Jarvinen H, Malanin K, Sama S, Helander I. Comparison of ciprofloxacin or trimethoprim therapy for venous leg ulcers: results of a pilot study. *J Am Acad Dermatol* 1994; 31: 279-81.

38. Zaki I, Shall L, Dalziel KL. Bacitracin: a significant sensitizer in leg ulcer patients? *Contact Dermatitis* 1994; 31: 92-4.

39. **McMullin G, Watkin GT, Coleridge Smith PD. The efficacy of fibrinolytic enhancement with stanozolol in the treatment of venous insufficiency. *Phlebology* 1991; 6: 233-8.**

40. Bjerle P. Treatment of venous insufficiency with dihydroergotamine. *Vasa* 1979; 8: 158-62.

41. **Layton AM, Ibbotson SH, Davies JA, Goodfield MJD. The effect of oral aspirin in the treatment of chronic venous leg ulcers. *Lancet* 1994; 344: 164-5.**

42. **Ibbotson SH, Layton AM, Davies JA, Goodfield MJD. The effect of aspirin on haemostatic activity in the treatment of chronic venous leg ulceration. *Br J Dermatol* 1995; 132: 422-6.**

43. Beitner H, Hammar H, Olsson AG, Thyresson N. Prostaglandin E1 treatment of leg ulcers caused by venous or arterial incompetence. *Acta Dermatol* (Stockholm) 1980; 60: 425-30.

44. Rudofsky G. Intravenous prostaglandin E1 in the treatment of venous ulcers in a double-blind, placebo controlled trial. *VASA* 1989- Suppl.28, 39-43.

45. Colgan MP, Dormandy JA, Jones PW, et al. Pentoxifylline treatment of venous ulcers of the leg. *Br Med J* 1990; 300: 972-5.

46. Dale JJ, Ruckley CV, Harper DR, Gibson B, Nelson A, Prescott RJ. Randomised double blind placebo controlled trial of pentoxifylline in the treatment of venous leg ulcers. *Br Med J* 1999; 319: 875-8.

47. Wadworth AN, Faulds D. Hydroxyethylrutosides. A review of its pharmacology and therapeutic efficacy in venous insufficiency and related disorders. *Drugs* 1992; 44: 1013-32.

48. Darke SG, Penfold C. Venous ulceration and saphenous ligation. *Eur J Vasc Surg* 1992; 6: 4-9.

49. Scriven JM, Hartshorne T, Thrush AJ, Bell PR, Naylor AR, London NJ. Role of saphenous vein surgery in the treatment of venous ulceration. *Br J Surg* 1998; 85: 781-4.

50. Bello M, Scriven M, Hartshorne T, et al. Role of superficial venous surgery in the treatment of venous ulceration. *Br J Surg* 1999; 86: 755-9.

51. Burnand K, Thomas ML, O'Donnell T, Browse NL. Relationship between post-phlebitic changes in the deep veins and the results of surgical treatment of venous leg ulcers. *Br J Surg* 1998; 85: 781-4.

52. Stuart WP. Perforator Surgery; What is its role? In: *The epidemiology and management of venous disease.* Eds: Ruckley CV, Fowkes FGR, Bradbury, AW. Springer Verlag. London. 1998: 132-8.

53. Negus D. *Leg ulcers - a practical approach to managment.* Butterworth-Heinemann, London, 1991: 117-9.

54. Poskitt KR, James AH, Lloyd-Davies ER, Walton J, McCollum C. Pinch skin grafting or porcine dermis in venous ulcers: a randomised clinical trial. *Br Med J* 1987; 294: 674-6.

55. Moffat CJ, Dorman MC. Recurrence of leg ulcers within a community ulcer service. *J Wound Care* 1995; 4: 57-61.

56. Harper DR, Nelson, EA, Gibson B Prescott RJ, Ruckley CV. A prospective randomised trial of class II and III elastic compression in the prevention of venous ulceration. In: *Phlebology '95*. Eds: Negus D, Jantet G, Coleridge-Smith PD. Springer-Verlag. London, 1995: 872-3.

57. Moffatt CJ, Franks PJ, Oldroyd M, et al. Community clinics for leg ulcers and impact on healing. *Br Med J* 1992; 305: 1389-92.

58. Ghauri ASK, Nyamekye I, Grabs AJ, Farndon JR, Poskitt KR. The diagnosis and management of mixed venous/arterial ulcers in community based clinics. *Eur J Vasc Endovasc Surg* 1998; 16: 350-5.

59. Ghauri ASK, Nyameke I, Grabs AJ, Farndon JR, Whyman MR, Poskitt KR. Influence of a specialized leg ulcer service and venous surgery on the outcome of venous leg ulcers. *Eur J Vasc Endovasc Surg* 1998; 16: 238-44.

60. Scriven JM, Hartshorne T, Bell PR, Naylor AR, London NJ. Single-visit ulcer assessment clinic: the first year. *Br J Surg* 1997; 84: 334-6.

61. London NJM, Bello M, Scriven M. How to run an efficient venous service. In: *The epidemiology and management of venous disease.* Eds: Ruckley CV, Fowkes FGR., Bradbury AW. Springer-Verlag Ltd., London, 1998: pp 212-5.

62. Prescott RJ, Nelson EA, Dale JJ, Harper DR, Ruckley CV. Design of randomised controlled trials in the treatment of leg ulcers: more answers with fewer patients. *Phlebology* 1998; 13: 107-12.

63. Ruckley C.V. Caring for patients with chronic leg ulcer. *Br Med J* 1998; 316: 407-8.

Chapter 25

The Rare Diagnosis and Operations Register

A Cowan
Specialist Registrar
SD Parvin
Consultant Vascular Surgeon

DEPARTMENT OF VASCULAR SURGERY,
ROYAL BOURNEMOUTH HOSPITAL, BOURNEMOUTH

Introduction

The Rare Diagnosis and Operations Register is a collection of unusual vascular conditions seen, or operations performed, by members of the Joint Vascular Research Group (JVRG). Members contribute cases to one of the authors who stores them in a database, which is then available to any member of the group. It was set up in May 1995 following the spring meeting of the JVRG.

The database was started with the aim of creating a collection of unusual cases that could be analysed together. This would enable JVRG members to produce and publish collective reports of unusual vascular conditions, and thereby disseminate expertise and advice.

The database

At the beginning, members were asked to contribute any cases they thought unusual. In order to encourage as many members to include as many cases as possible, no preconditions were set. To facilitate data collection, a minimum of data were required on each patient. These included surgeon data (name, centre) and patient data (name, date of birth, hospital number) and included brief clinical details.

Each patient submitted was recorded with the date of submission. Initially there were a small number of categories that were particularly sought, though submissions were not confined to those groups. When more than three similar non-categorised patients were submitted, a new category was created.

At first there were six categories. These included popliteal entrapment, major vessel arteritis, carotid body tumour, mesenteric ischaemia, cystic degeneration and systemic lupus. This has expanded and at the time of writing there are 32 categories (Table 1).

The reports

Regular reports are produced that are circulated to the JVRG membership. Reports are in several parts (Table 2). Initially the cases were attributed to individual surgeons, but as the size of the group has increased, patients are now classified by referring centre. There are now 22 centres with approximately 30 contributing surgeons. Sent with the report are a newsletter and a proforma for completion during the next interval (usually 2-3 months). More recently submission directly by email to the author has been encouraged.

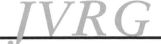

Table 1. Rare diagnosis categories with number collected.

Category	Total	Category	Total
Odd aortic aneurysms	30	Mesenteric ischaemia	122
Aortocaval fistula	16	Major vessel arteritis	24
Aorto-enteric fistula	27	Mycotic aneurysm	33
Arm ischaemia	48	Other odd aneurysms	39
Arteriovenous malformation	38	Paget-Schroetter syndrome	11
Brachial embolus	43	Popliteal entrapment	21
Leg ulcer calcification	4	Profunda femoris aneurysms	8
Carotid artery surgery	6	Right to left shunt (cardiac)	2
Carotid body tumour	111	Aortic aneurysm with renal abnormality	11
Cystic degeneration	6	Subclavian steal syndrome	23
Odd deep vein thrombosis	24	Thoracic outlet syndrome	23
Post radiotherapy arteritis	14	Trauma	56
Ehlers-Danlos syndrome	7	Visceral aneurysms	33
Klippel-Trenaunay syndrome	18	Vena caval obstruction	6
Lupus erythematosus	12	Young patients (<40 years old) with vascular disease	81
Midaortic syndrome	10	No category	102

Table 2. Structure of report circulated to the JVRG.

The Report

- A table of numbers submitted by category and by centre in total and since the last report

- A list of all new patients showing contributing surgeon, category and details of case

- A list of non-categorized cases with their details by centre

- A newsletter

- A proforma for subsequent case submissions

The results

The Rare Diagnosis and Operations Register has been running for 4 years. During that time 1009 patients have been submitted (Table 1). The number of submissions to the database, classified by centre is shown in Figure 1.

Future plans

It is our intention to use the Rare Diagnosis and Operations Register as the basis for a meeting that will look at the management of these unusual conditions using individual patients to illustrate presentations. In addition a compact disk of patient studies with illustrations is planned to coincide with the meeting. As an example of what might be achieved a brief description of one of the categories, cystic adventitial disease, follows. It includes a description of the condition together with five patients from the Register.

Cystic adventitial disease

First described in the external iliac artery over half a century ago [1], cystic adventitial disease (CAD) affects the popliteal artery in 85% of cases. The condition is rare,

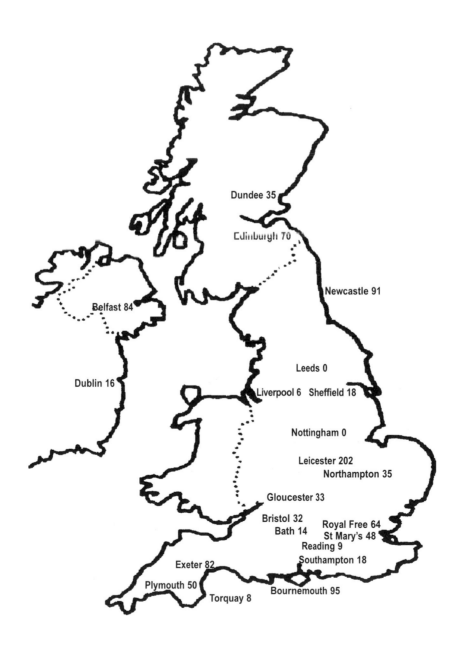

Dundee 35
Edinburgh 70
Newcastle 91
Belfast 84
Leeds 0
Dublin 16
Liverpool 6   Sheffield 18
Nottingham 0
Leicester 202
Northampton 35
Gloucester 33
Bristol 32
Bath 14   Royal Free 64
St Mary's 48
Reading 9
Southampton 18
Exeter 82
Plymouth 50   Bournemouth 95
Torquay 8

Figure 1. The number of submissions to the database, classified by centre.

with only 264 cases affecting the popliteal artery reported in the world literature up to 1995 [2]. Many names had been given to the condition in an attempt to describe the cystic mucinous appearance before there was agreement upon CAD [3].

The cysts are invariably multiple, containing amino acid laden mucinous or gelatinous material. Unlike atherosclerotic lesions, there is no calcium or cholesterol. These findings are suggestive of ectopic joint capsule or bursa, and may represent either true ganglion or a long-term response to trauma.

Otherwise healthy, young or middle aged men are most commonly affected, with rapid onset and deterioration of unilateral intermittent claudication, occasionally progressing to critical ischaemia. Symptoms can display periodicity with episodes of improvement between relapses [4]. Pedal pulses show no consistency in their presence or absence, though flexion of the knee causing obliteration of the pedal pulses has been suggested to be indicative of CAD [5,6]. In the absence of complete occlusion, a bruit may be heard over the popliteal artery. The cysts are rarely palpable. Popliteal entrapment syndrome is the main differential diagnosis in this age group

Although angiography elegantly demonstrates the scimitar or hourglass signs of CAD, occlusion of the popliteal artery, present in 30% of patients, makes this investigation less useful. The absence of collateral circulation or atherosclerotic change elsewhere, however, is useful. Duplex ultrasound imaging provides visualisation of the cysts, demonstrating a 'bright' rim, and also allows quantification of flow changes within the native vessel [7-9]. Computed tomography (CT) has gained favour for imaging, both for its ability to exclude popliteal entrapment and to allow therapeutic cyst drainage [10]. Magnetic resonance imaging (MRI), particularly T2-weighted images, seems to be particularly useful. No contrast or ionisation is required and the geometric flexibility of the available images is an advantage [11].

Spontaneous resolution is unusual and the mode of intervention is influenced by the presence of arterial occlusion. With complete occlusion, resection and interposition grafting provides 90-100% initial success according to graft type [12]. Long-term patency, as with surgery for atherosclerotic disease, seems better with vein grafting. A single case of thrombolysis followed by cyst excision has been reported.

When CAD causes arterial stenosis, a wide variety of approaches have been tried. Surgical evacuation of cyst contents with excision of the cyst walls provides excellent initial success (94%) [12]. There is, however, a 10% recurrence rate. Patching after evacuation alone is less successful (<75% success) and is not recommended. CT guided aspiration has been used in a small number of patients with limited success due to the viscous nature of the cyst contents.

The following patients are recorded on the database.

Patient 1

A 51-year-old woman presented with a 2-month history of unilateral claudication. Clinical examination revealed a weak femoral pulse with absent pulses beyond. Duplex ultrasound demonstrated echolucent material protruding into the common femoral artery (CFA)(Figure 2). Angiography also showed a filling defect in the CFA (Figure 3). Surgical exploration was performed revealing cysts in the anterior wall of the CFA. These were deroofed and evacuated without damage to the normal vessel. At 6 week follow-up there were normal pedal pulses and duplex imaging at 6 months showed no abnormality in the CFA (Figure 4).

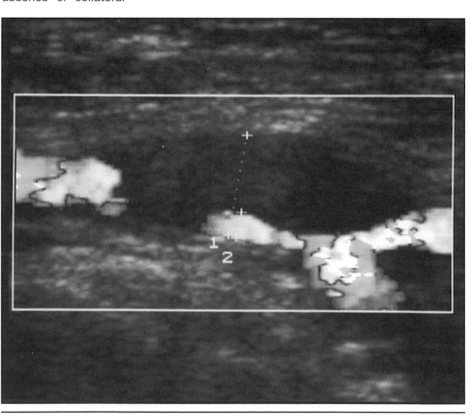

Figure 2. Common femoral bifurcation showing filling defect caused by cystic adventitial disease.

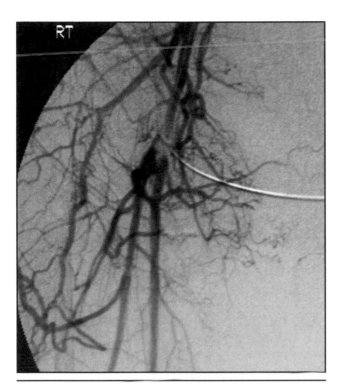

Figure 3. Preoperative angiogram showing filling defect at the common femoral bifurcation.

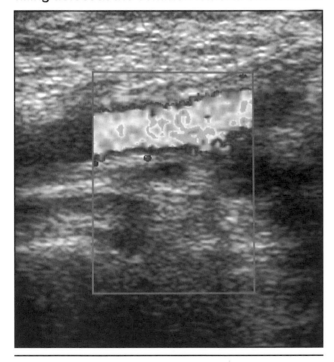

Figure 4. Common femoral bifurcation after surgery showing normal flow on duplex imaging.

Patient 2

A 53-year-old man presented with unilateral leg pain and numbness preventing his regular keep-fit activities. A provisional diagnosis of popliteal entrapment was made and popliteal stenosis was revealed by angiography. The presence of cysts was demonstrated using duplex imaging. Surgical exploration revealed a 2cm length of distal popliteal artery affected by CAD. The diseased segment was successfully bypassed using reversed saphenous vein. Duplex graft surveillance at 3 years was satisfactory.

Patient 3

A 46-year-old man was admitted electively for excision of a popliteal adventitial cyst causing unilateral claudication. At operation, gelatinous material was extruded restoring flow to the foot. Doppler pressures were normal at 3 months. The patient was readmitted 14 months later with recurrent cysts and a return of symptoms. At operation the cysts were found to have extended into the peroneal and anterior tibial compartments. Popliteal-distal bypass was performed with a good haemodynamic result. Three months later his symptoms recurred and MRI demonstrated residual cysts. These were aspirated under ultrasound control. One year after bypass grafting the vein graft was patent with normal Doppler ankle pressures.

Patient 4

A 29-year-old man presented with an acutely ischaemic leg with a short background of progressive claudication. For several years prior to this he had experienced recurrent episodes of subacute ischaemia with spontaneous resolution, allowing a return to marathon running. A previous fasciotomy had failed to relieve his symptoms. On examination his proximal popliteal pulse was satisfactory though becoming weak distally. Pedal pulses were absent and Doppler pressures virtually unrecordable. Angiography (Figure 5) revealed a smooth indentation in the proximal popliteal artery that was occluded at the level of the knee joint. Run-off reconstituted at the level of the anterior tibial origin

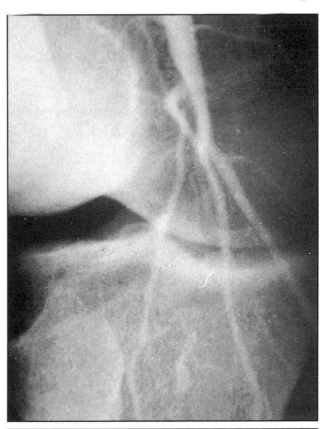

Figure 5. Angiogram showing popliteal artery indentation and occlusion.

Chapter 25

Chapter 25

though with proximal peroneal occlusion. At operation a 5cm long cyst was found encroaching on the popliteal and proximal anterior tibial arteries. There was thrombus in the tibioperoneal trunk. The diseased segment was excised and a reversed vein interposed between the popliteal artery and tibioperoneal bifurcation. Two years postoperatively the graft remains patent with good distal pulses.

Patient 5

A 43-year-old man presented with a short history of a cold, painful, pale leg and claudication after only a few metres. He gave a history of intermittent, though spontaneously resolving, episodes of calf claudication over the preceding months. Admission on two of these occasions had failed to reveal any abnormality. On examination, no pulses were palpable beyond the groin. The leg was critically ischaemic with no recordable ankle Doppler pressure. Angiography (Figure 6) demonstrated a short occlusion of the popliteal artery distal to a region of smooth medial indentation. At operation a 3cm smooth cyst was found encroaching on the popliteal artery with thrombus within the lumen distal to this. The affected segment was excised and replaced with a reversed vein graft. The cyst contained gelatinous material. At 4 years, the graft remains patent with normal peripheral perfusion.

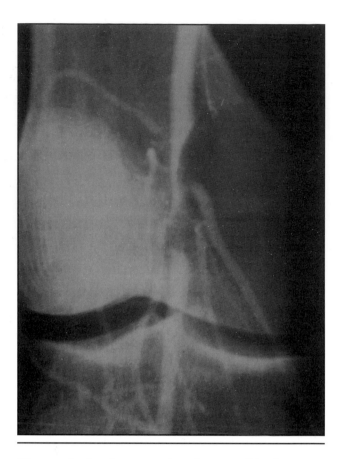

Figure 6. Angiogram showing popliteal artery indentation due to cystic adventitial disease.

References

1. Atkins HJB, Key JA. A case of myxomatous tumour arising in the adventitia of the left external iliac artery. *Br J Surg* 1947; 34: 246.
2. Tsolakis IA, Walvatne CS, Caldwell MD. Cystic adventitial disease of the popliteal artery: diagnosis and treatment. *Eur J Vasc Endovasc Surg* 1998; 15: 188-194.
3. Ishikawa K, Mishima Y, Kobayashi S. Cystic adventitial disease of the popliteal artery. *Angiology* 1961; 12: 357-366.
4. Parks RW, Barros D'Sa AAB. Critical ischaemia complicating cystic adventitial disease of the popliteal artery. *Eur J Vasc Endovasc Surg* 1994; 8: 508-513.
5. Ishikawa K. Cystic adventitial disease of the popliteal artery and of other stem vessels in the extremities. *Jap J Surg* 1987; 17: 221-229.
6. McAnespey D, Rosen RC, Cohen JM, Fried K, Elias S. Adventitial cystic disease. *J Foot Surg* 1991; 30 (Suppl. 2): 160-164.
7. Staff J, Zoller WG, Spengel FA. Image-directed Doppler ultrasound findings in adventitial cystic disease of the popliteal artery. *J Clin Ultrasound* 1989; 17: 689-691.
8. Kaufmann LS, Kupinski AM, Shah MD, Leather PR. The diagnosis of adventitial cystic disease of the popliteal artery by duplex scanning. *J Vasc Tech* 1987; 11: 132-135.
9. Inoue Y, Iwai T, Ohashi K, et al. A case of popliteal cystic degeneration with pathological considerations. *Ann Vasc Surg* 1992; 6: 525-529.
10. Deutsch A, Hyde J, Miller SM, Diamond CG, Schanche AF. Cystic adventitial degeneration of the popliteal artery: CT demonstration and directed percutaneous therapy. *AJR* 1985; 145: 117-118.
11. Chiche L, Baranger B, Cordoliani YS, Darrieus H, Guyon P, Vicq P. Two cases of cystic adventitial disease of the popliteal artery: new diagnosis considerations. *J Mal Vasc* 1994; 19: 57-61.
12. Flanigan DP, Burnham SJ, Goodreau JJ, Bergan JJ. Summary of cases of adventitial cystic disease of the popliteal artery. *Ann Surg* 1979; 189:165-175.

Chapter 26

Renal revascularisation

M Davis
Specialist Registrar
G Hamilton
Consultant Vascular Surgeon

DEPARTMENT OF SURGERY,
ROYAL FREE HOSPITAL, LONDON

Introduction

There are two main causes of renal artery disease: atherosclerotic renal artery stenosis and fibromuscular dysplasia. Over 80% of lesions are ostial and are a part of generalised atherosclerotic disease. The remainder involve the main stem of the renal artery or its branches. In children, renal artery stenosis, usually due to fibromuscular dysplasia, causes up to 25% of all cases of hypertension. Atherosclerotic renal artery disease is a major cause of renal disease in the elderly, resulting in hypertension and renal failure. The true incidence is unknown, due to its often undetected progression. Furthermore, significant renal artery disease is found in 40% of patients undergoing angiography for peripheral arterial occlusive or aneurysm disease and 30% of patients having coronary angiography [1].

A decision to intervene must be taken in the light of the poor prognosis of patients with atherosclerotic renal artery stenosis. Connolly et al [2] showed that patients' survival correlated with initial angiographic findings. Two year actuarial patient survival was 96% with unilateral renal artery stenosis, reducing to 74% for bilateral renal artery stenosis and only 47% for unilateral occlusion with an occlusion or stenosis on the contralateral side. Mailloux et al [3] showed that once on dialysis as a result of atherosclerotic renal artery stenosis, patients had a 5 year survival of only 12%.

Atherosclerotic renal artery stenosis is a progressive disease [4] with hypertension and deteriorating renal function. Accurate assessment of the progression has been made using duplex ultrasonography. An average progression of renal artery stenosis in all severities of disease occurs at a rate of 7% per year; whilst in stenoses greater than or equal to 60%, progression was 30% at 1 year, 44% at 2 years and 48% at 3 years [5]. Despite antihypertensive medication, atherosclerotic renal artery stenosis tends to progress, resulting in renal ischaemia and loss of renal mass [5]. Restoring renal artery patency can reduce the need for antihypertensive medication [6] and may slow the progression of renal failure [7]. A multidisciplinary approach including renal physician, vascular surgeon and radiologist is important for the assessment and treatment of patients with renal artery disease.

Treatment

Indications for further investigation with a view to intervention include:

- deteriorating renal function,
- poorly controlled hypertension despite best medical therapy in patients with >70% stenosis of either renal artery,
- acute renal failure following angiotensin converting enzyme inhibitors,
- flash pulmonary oedema or refractory congestive cardiac failure,
- incidental stenoses (see below).

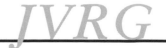

Based on the fact that such lesions are at a high risk of occlusion, it has been suggested that normotensive patients with normal renal function who are found to have an incidental renal artery stenosis should undergo percutaneous transluminal angioplasty or stent placement (PTRA/Stent PTRA) if the lesion is >75%. The benefit of this practice, however, needs to be established by randomised clinical trials.

In most units only symptomatic patients are currently offered intervention, however, each patient needs to be considered individually by a multidisciplinary team. Options for intervention include angioplasty with or without stenting, surgical revascularisation or nephrectomy.

Renal revascularisation is deemed successful if:

Hypertension
- Cure: diastolic blood pressure 90 mmHg or less and no medication.
- Improvement: 15% reduction in diastolic blood pressure or same blood pressure with less medication.

Renal function
- Success if creatinine improved or stabilised.

Radiological
- If there is a residual stenosis of less than 20% and a pressure gradient of less than 10mmHg.

Methods of renal revascularisation

Endovascular revascularisation - percutaneous transluminal renal angioplasty

There is a paucity of randomised controlled trials relating to the efficacy of renal angioplasty. Most studies involve only a small number of patients, but when data from 12 of these were combined, meaningful results were obtained [8-19]. In 1031 patients who had PTRA for atherosclerotic renal artery stenosis in whom a satisfactory technical result was achieved, 17% of patients were cured and 47% of patients were improved. However, in 35% the procedure failed to achieve a clinical improvement. In addition, 73% of the patients who benefited (i.e. cured or improved) continued to require antihypertensive medication.

Better results can be obtained with fibromuscular dysplasia. In 314 patients with fibromuscular renal artery stenosis [8-16], 43% were cured, 42% improved and in only 15% did the procedure fail. More than 50% of patients who benefited did not require further antihypertensive medication and recurrence was rare.

Many radiologists now favour stenting in addition to PTRA (Figure 1). Most experience has been gained using balloon expandable stents such as the Palmaz stent (Johnson and Johnson Interventional Systems) and the AVE stent (Arterial Vascular Engineering Inc.). Self-expanding stents are available such as the Wallstent (Schneider) and the Memotherm stent (Bard).

Stent PTRA is technically more demanding due to severe aortic atheroma, renal artery angulation and the occasional need for a brachial approach to position the stent accurately. The use of these prostheses is still relatively novel and needs to be considered with caution as, despite initial good results, restenosis rates determined by angiography have been reported to range from 3-39% [20,21]. Furthermore, subsequent surgery following occlusion of a metallic stent is technically more challenging. It is therefore important that stents should not be used in distal lesions where surgical rescue may be rendered impossible.

The use of stents at present is reserved for the following reasons:

- failure of initial angioplasty,
- renal artery dissection after PTRA,
- restenosis at a previous PTRA site,
- ostial lesions,
- patients not fit for surgery.

Stents are usually not indicated for fibromuscular dysplasia.

Results of PTRA
Most studies quote a technical success rate for PTRA of 90%. The number of technical failures can now be reduced by the use of stents, however, long-term results are awaited.

The effects of PTRA on blood pressure and on renal function are difficult to predict. Farmer et al [22] followed-up 16 patients after renal angioplasty with single kidney glomerular filtration rate measurements. They concluded that there was no significant difference between mean glomerular filtration rates before and after angioplasty (i.e. angioplasty did not improve renal function in the short term).

There is a lack of data from randomised trials on the value of percutaneous techniques in the management of atheromatous renal artery disease. The Scottish and Newcastle Renal Artery Stenosis group [23] compared angioplasty versus medical therapy in hypertensive patients with both unilateral and bilateral disease. They concluded that angioplasty resulted in a statistically significant improvement in systolic blood pressure in hypertensive patients compared with medical treatment alone, but this benefit was only seen in patients with bilateral disease. There was no significant difference in

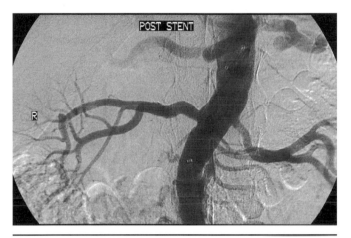

Figure 1. Angiograms demonstrating the result of renal artery stent insertion. (Reproduced with the kind permission of Dr. A. Watkinson, Consultant Radiologist, Royal Free Hospital, London).

renal function as assessed by serum creatinine between the two groups. Major outcome events (such as death, cardiovascular or cerebrovascular event, or dialysis) were similar in both groups; there was, however, a complication rate of 27.5% following intervention. The difficulty of performing randomised controlled trials in this disease is highlighted by the above study which recruited only 55 patients from such a large population.

The efficacy and outcome following angioplasty or medical therapy in atherosclerotic renal artery stenosis was studied in Essai Multicentrique Medicaments vs Angioplastie (EMMA) [24]. Patients were randomised to antihypertensive treatment (n=26) or angioplasty (n=23). Ambulatory blood pressure measurements were taken at baseline and 6 months after randomisation. In those allocated to angioplasty, medication was stopped after the procedure, but was recommended if hypertension recurred. Mean ambulatory pressure did not differ between control and angioplasty groups at the end of the study, although antihypertensive medication had been restarted in 17 of 23 patients who had an angioplasty

(74%). It was concluded that angioplasty did result in a reduction in antihypertensive therapy although it was associated with a morbidity rate of 17%.

In the Dutch randomised trial of arterial stenting (n=43) versus balloon angioplasty (n=42) for ostial atherosclerotic renovascular lesions, the primary success rate for PTRA was 57% compared with 88% for stents. Angiography 6 months later showed restenosis rates of 48% and 14% for PTRA and stent PTRA respectively. Multivariate linear regression analysis showed no difference in clinical results between PTRA and stent PTRA with respect to creatinine concentration, mean blood pressure and median number of antihypertensive drugs taken [25]. As yet, there is insufficient long-term follow-up of stent PTRA to demonstrate any clinical benefit over PTRA.

Percutaneous techniques are not without significant mortality and morbidity. In a retrospective analysis of 108 patients who underwent stent deployment for renal artery stenosis [26], complications occurred in 7.2% and there was a 30 day mortality rate of 3.2%, reflecting the comorbid condition of these patients.

Placement of renal artery stents in a solitary kidney has not been the subject of a randomised trial. In a retrospective analysis [27] of 21 patients with a solitary functioning kidney who underwent stenting, renal function had improved or stabilised in 71% (n=15) at follow-up (range 6-25 months). Major complications occurred in four patients (19%) and included one death within 30 days of stenting. In this high risk group, stenting appears to be a relatively safe procedure to salvage a solitary kidney.

Conclusions

Percutaneous renal artery revascularisation is an established and reliable procedure in capable hands. In most instances PTRA should be considered the primary treatment of choice in renal artery stenosis, particularly in fibromuscular dysplasia, but now also in ostial atherosclerotic lesions. The excellent, anatomically superior, results with stent PTRA have made this the current favoured intervention. The clinical evidence for the superiority of stent PTRA, however, does not exist. Stent placement should be reserved for primary or secondary PTRA failure, either due to recoil, dissection or restenosis.

Further randomised controlled trials are required in this field. A comparison of PTRA and best medical therapy is about to commence - the ASTRAL study (Angioplasty and Stent for Renal Arterial Lesions). The use of stent PTRA will be at the discretion of participating centres. Randomised comparisons of stent PTRA and surgery in suitable patients are surely needed.

In the light of the above evidence, the new practice of 'drive by' angioplasty (treating incidental stenoses found on angiography performed for other reasons, mainly cardiological) is to be deplored.

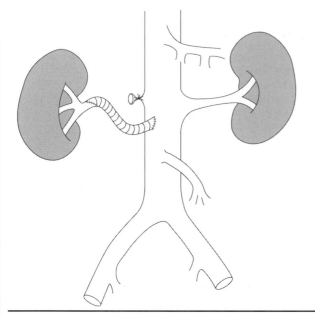

Figure 2. Aorto-renal bypass is performed using either long saphenous vein, PTFE, Dacron or occasionally internal iliac artery.

Surgical revascularisation

The indications for renal artery surgery are listed below, however, each individual patient needs to be considered according to the extent of vascular disease and their risk factors.

- Significant aortic aneurysm or aortic occlusive disease with concomitant renal artery stenosis.
- Grossly atheromatous, hostile aorta thereby precluding percutaneous approach.
- Occlusion of a renal artery origin with preservation of the kidney by collaterals.
- Young fit patient.
- Solitary kidney in patient fit for general anaesthetic.

There are no randomised controlled trials of the various surgical procedures available for renal revascularisation. A number of surgical options are available: aorto-renal bypass (Figure 2), renal endarterectomy (Figure 3), aortic resection and renal bypass (Figure 4), and extra-anatomical bypasses - hepatorenal, splenorenal and supracoeliac (Figures 5a and 5b).

Results of Surgery

Since the advent of percutaneous techniques, surgery for renal artery stenosis is less common. A randomised trial comparing PTRA and surgical reconstruction as initial therapy was conducted in 58 patients with atherosclerotic unilateral renal artery stenosis [28]. Technically successful PTRA was achieved in 83%, whilst surgical success was recorded in 97% of patients. The primary patency rate after 2 years was 75% after PTRA and 96% after surgery. There was no significant difference between the two groups with regard to hypertension, renal function or to secondary results.

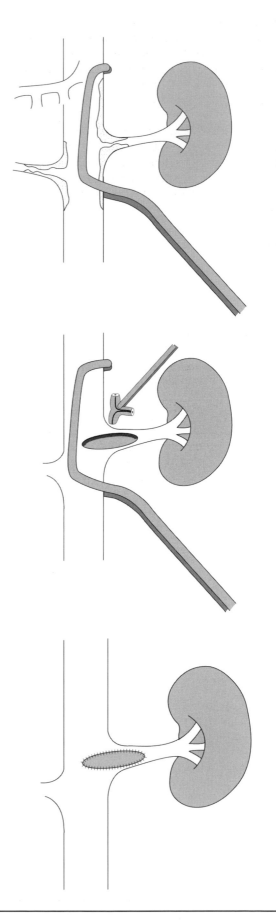

Figure 3. Renal endarterectomy with patch closure.

Complications were categorised into major, minor and radiological technical problems. After PTRA there were 17% major complications as compared with 31% after surgery. There were 48% minor complications after PTRA compared with 31% following surgery. The frequency of major and minor complications, however, did not differ statistically between the groups. Some 17% of the PTRA group required subsequent surgical reconstruction to achieve these results. It was concluded that PTRA could be recommended as the first choice therapy for atherosclerotic renal artery stenosis, provided it was combined with intensive follow-up and aggressive reintervention.

Surgery in the young fit patient may be a better, more cost effective option than angioplasty, especially in the light of a very low long-term restenosis rate of 3-4% [29,30]. The results of surgical revascularisation are shown in Table 1.

The management of asymptomatic renal artery stenosis in patients requiring infrarenal aortic surgery remains controversial. Some do not support incidental renal artery reconstruction [37]. At late follow-up (mean of 6.3 years) high grade renal artery stenosis was associated with increased systolic blood pressure and the need for increased antihypertensive medication. However, surgery had a favourable outcome as it was not associated with decreased survival, dialysis dependence or worsening creatinine levels.

Reoperation for the complications of renal artery reconstructive surgery undertaken for treatment of

Table 1. Reported results of surgical revascularisation

Treatment of hypertension (cure/improvement)	63-91% [31,32]
Treatment of renal failure (cure/improvement)	33-91% [31,33]
Primary patency rates	93-97% [34,35]
Restenosis rate	3-4% [29,30]
Morbidity	6-43% [35,33]
Mortality	2-8% [34,36]

renovascular hypertension is reported from a series of 373 patients [38]; secondary operations were required in 58 patients, representing a reoperation rate of 15.5%. Reoperation followed persistent or recurrent hypertension secondary to graft thrombosis, perianastomotic graft narrowing or progressive non-anastomotic graft stenoses. Procedures performed included nephrectomy (n=31), bypass with vein (n=15) or prosthetic graft (n=8). It was concluded that reoperation is technically challenging; early diagnosis with prompt surgery was advocated to optimise results. This scenario may become more of a problem to the vascular surgeon in the future if the use of stents in high risk patients continues to escalate.

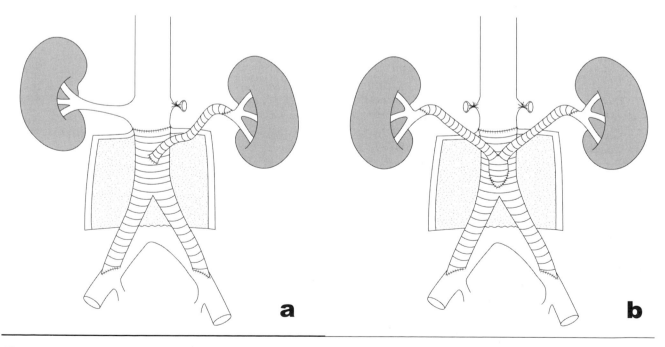

Figure 4. Simultaneous aortic and renal reconstruction (a) Renal bypass performed using 6-8mm PTFE or Dacron. The graft is sutured onto the aortic graft with an end-to-end renal anastomosis. (b) In bilateral renal artery disease an inverted bifurcated graft is used.

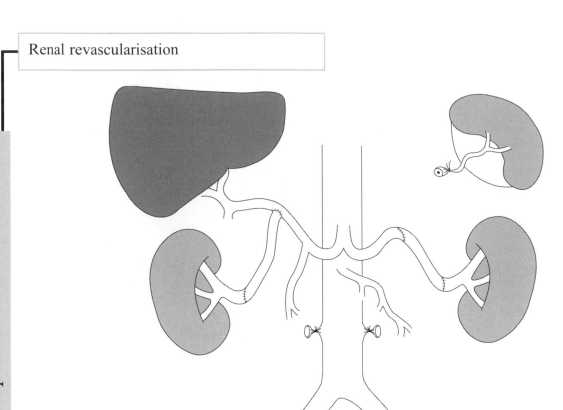

Figure 5a. Extra-anatomic bypass grafts. The right kidney can be revascularised from the common hepatic artery. In approximately 40% of cases this can be via the gastroduodenal branch; alternatively an interposition saphenous vein graft is used. The left kidney can be revascularised using the splenic artery. The spleen remains *in situ* receiving blood from splenic collaterals and the short gastric arteries.

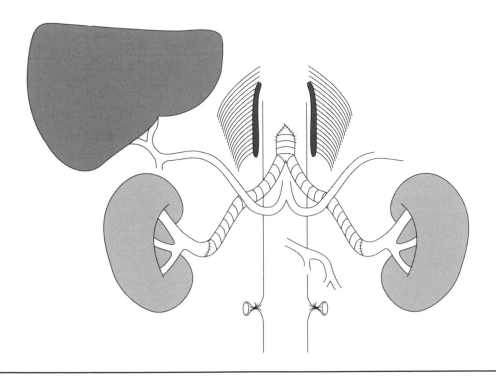

Figure 5b. Extra-anatomic bypass grafts. Supracoeliac approach.

Nephrectomy

Nephrectomy is the oldest surgical procedure for the treatment of renovascular hypertension. It continues to be an appropriate option when there is a normal contralateral kidney, but the ipsilateral kidney is shrunken (<8cm) and producing renin. Contralateral nephrectomy may also be performed as part of revascularisation of a viable ipsilateral kidney. Such an operation is indicated when the renal vein renin ratio is greater than 1.5.

Conclusions

There is a lack of randomised trials available to determine the patients that would benefit from best medical therapy alone, angioplasty, stent placement or surgery.

The ASTRAL trial started in October 1999 in patients for whom there is uncertainty regarding intervention or best medical treatment. Patients are randomised to either best medical therapy alone, or best medical therapy with revascularisation by angioplasty and/or stent. This trial promises to define the role of intervention. Randomised studies comparing endovascular and surgical revascularisation are needed but are fraught with difficulty.

At present, best care is delivered using a multi-disciplinary team approach of physicians, radiologists and vascular surgeons, ideally in a centre involved in clinical trials. Clinical evidence is sparse in this area, a situation that should be resolved by interested clinicians.

Chapter 26

Renal revascularisation

Sound evidence

- **Angioplasty is the treatment of choice for renal artery fibromuscular dysplasia.**

Evidence needed

- **The long-term results of angioplasty versus stent in atherosclerotic renal arterial lesions.**

- **The role of percutaneous techniques versus surgery in preserving renal function.**

- **The role of percutaneous techniques versus surgery in refractory hypertension.**

- **The best surgical approach for atherosclerotic renal arterial lesions.**

References (randomised trials in bold)

1. Harding MB, Smith LR, Himmelstein SI, et al. Renal artery stenosis: prevalence and associated risk factors in patients undergoing routine cardiac catheterization. *J Am Soc Nephrol* 1992; 2: 1608-16.

2. Connolly JO, Higgins RM, Mackie AD, Drury PL, Hendry BM, Scoble JE. Presentation, clinical features and outcome in different patterns of atherosclerotic renovascular disease. *QJM* 1994; 87: 413-21.

3. Mailloux LU, Bellucci AG, Mossey RT, et al. Predictors of survival in patients undergoing dialysis. *Am J Med* 1988; 84: 855-62.

4. Wollenweber J, Sheps SG, Davis GD. Clinical course of atherosclerotic renovascular disease. *Am J Cardiol* 1968; 21: 60-71.

5. Zierler RE, Bergelin RO, Davidson RC, Cantwell-Gab K, Polissar NL, Strandness DE, Jr. A prospective study of disease progression in patients with atherosclerotic renal artery stenosis. *Am J Hypertens* 1996; 9: 1055-61.

6. Ramsey LEWPC. Blood pressure response to percutaneous angioplasty for renovascular hypertension: an overview of published series. *Br Med J* 1990; 300: 569-72.

7. Harden PN, MacLeod MJ, Rodger RS, et al. Effect of renal-artery stenting on progression of renovascular renal failure. *Lancet* 1997; 349: 1133-6.

8. Tegtmeyer CJ, Kellum CD, Kron IL, Mentzer RM, Jr. Percutaneous transluminal angioplasty in the region of the aortic bifurcation. The two-balloon technique with results and long-term follow-up study. *Radiology* 1985; 157: 661-5.

9. Miller GA, Ford KK, Braun SD, et al. Percutaneous transluminal angioplasty vs. surgery for renovascular hypertension. *Am J Roentgenol* 1985; 144: 447-50.

10. Geyskes GG, Puylaert CB, Oei HY, Mees EJ. Follow-up study of 70 patients with renal artery stenosis treated by percutaneous transluminal dilatation. *Br Med J* 1983; 287: 333-6.

11. Greminger P, Steiner A, Schneider E, et al. Cure and improvement of renovascular hypertension after percutaneous transluminal angioplasty of renal artery stenosis. *Nephron* 1989; 51: 362-6.

12. Klinge J, Mali WP, Puijlaert CB, Geyskes GG, Becking WB, Feldberg MA. Percutaneous transluminal renal angioplasty: initial and long-term results. *Radiology* 1989; 171 : 501-6.

13. Colapinto RF, Stronell RD, Harries-Jones EP, et al. Percutaneous transluminal dilatation of the renal artery: follow-up studies on renovascular hypertension. *Am J Roentgenol* 1982; 139: 727-32.

14. Sos TA, Pickering TG, Sniderman K, et al. Percutaneous transluminal renal angioplasty in renovascular hypertension due to atheroma or fibromuscular dysplasia. *N Engl J Med* 1983; 309: 274-9.

15. Baert AL, Wilms G, Amery A, Vermylen J, Suy R. Percutaneous transluminal renal angioplasty: initial results and long-term follow-up in 202 patients. *Cardiovasc Intervent Radiol* 1990; 13: 22-8.

16. Martin LG, Price RB, Casarella WJ, et al. Percutaneous angioplasty in clinical management of renovascular hypertension: initial and long-term results. *Radiology* 1985; 155: 629-33.

17. Schwarten DE. Percutaneous transluminal renal angioplasty. *Urol Radiol* 1981; 2: 193-200.

18. Canzanello VJ, Millan VG, Spiegel JE, Ponce PS, Kopelman RI, Madias NE. Percutaneous transluminal renal angioplasty in management of atherosclerotic renovascular hypertension: results in 100 patients. *Hypertension* 1989; 13: 163-72.

19. Grim CE, Yune HY, Donohue JP, Weinberger MH, Dilley R, Klatte EC. Renal vascular hypertension. Surgery vs. dilation. *Nephron* 1986; 44 Suppl 1: 96-100.

20. Rees CR, Palmaz JC, Becker GJ, et al. Palmaz stent in atherosclerotic stenoses involving the ostia of the renal arteries: preliminary report of a multicenter study. *Radiology* 1991; 181: 507-14.

21. Hennequin LM, Joffre FG, Rousseau HP, et al. Renal artery stent placement: long-term results with the Wallstent endoprosthesis. *Radiology* 1994; 191: 713-9.

22. Farmer CKT, Reidy J, Kaira PA, Cook GJR, Scoble J. Individual kidney function before and after renal angioplasty. *Lancet* 1998; 352: 288-9.

23. **Webster J, Marshall F, Abdalla M, et al. Randomised comparison of percutaneous angioplasty vs continued medical therapy for hypertensive patients with atheromatous renal artery stenosis. Scottish and Newcastle Renal Artery Stenosis Collaborative Group.** *J Hum Hypertens* **1998; 12: 329-35.**

24. **Plouin PF, Chatellier G, Darne B, Raynaud A. Blood pressure outcome of angioplasty in atherosclerotic renal artery stenosis: a randomized trial. Essai Multicentrique Medicaments vs Angioplastie (EMMA) Study Group.** *Hypertension* **1998; 31: 823-9.**

25. **van de Ven PJG, Kaatee R, Beutler JJ, et al. Arterial stenting and balloon angioplasty in ostial atherosclerotic renovascular disease: a randomised trial.** *Lancet* **1999; 353: 282-6.**

26. Rodriguez-Lopez JA, Werner A, Ray LI, et al. Renal artery stenosis treated with stent deployment: indications, technique, and outcome for 108 patients. *J Vasc Surg* 1999; 29: 617-24.

27. Shannon HM, Gillespie IN, Moss JG. Salvage of the solitary kidney by insertion of a renal artery stent. *Am J Roentgenol* 1998; 171: 217-22.

29. Novick AC, Ziegelbaum M, Vidt DG, Gifford RW, Jr., Pohl MA, Goormastic M. Trends in surgical revascularization for renal artery disease. Ten years' experience. *JAMA* 1987; 257: 498-501.

30. **Weibull H, Bergqvist MD, Bergentz S-E, Jonsson K, Hulthen L, Manhem P. Percutaneous transluminal renal angioplasty versus surgical reconstruction of atherosclerotic renal artery stenosis: a prospective randomized study.** *J Vasc Surg* **1993; 18: 841-52.**

31. Benjamin ME, Hansen KJ, Craven TE, et al. Combined aortic and renal artery surgery. A contemporary experience. *Ann Surg* 1996; 223: 555-65.

32. Dean RH. Surgical reconstruction of atherosclerotic renal artery disease. In: Branchereau A, Jacobes M, Eds. *Long term results of arterial interventions.* Armonk, New York: Futura Publishing Company, 1997: 205-16.

33. Reilly JM, Rubin BG, Thompson RW, et al. Revascularization of the solitary kidney: a challenging problem in a high risk population. *Surgery* 1996; 120: 732-6.

34. Steinbach F, Novick AC, Campbell S, Dykstra D. Long-term survival after surgical revascularization for atherosclerotic renal artery disease. *J Urol* 1997; 158: 38-41.

35. Darling RC, III, Shah DM, Chang BB, Leather RP. Does concomitant aortic bypass and renal artery revascularization using the retroperitoneal approach increase perioperative risk? *Cardiovasc Surg* 1995; 3: 421-3.

36. Cambria RP, Brewster DC, L'Italien G, et al. Renal artery reconstruction for the preservation of renal function. *J Vasc Surg* 1996; 24: 371-82.

37. Williamson WK, Abou-Zamzam AM, Jr., Moneta GL, et al. Prophylactic repair of renal artery stenosis is not justified in patients who require infrarenal aortic reconstruction. *J Vasc Surg* 1998; 28: 14-22.

38. Stanley JC, Whitehouse WM, Jr., Zelenock GB, Graham LM, Cronenwett JL, Lindenauer SM. Reoperation for complications of renal artery reconstructive surgery undertaken for treatment of renovascular hypertension. *J Vasc Surg* 1985; 2: 133-44.

Chapter 27

New initiatives in the prevention and treatment of graft infection

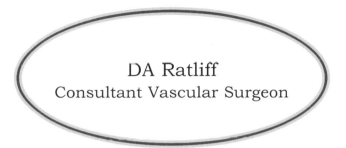

DA Ratliff
Consultant Vascular Surgeon

DEPARTMENT OF SURGERY,
NORTHAMPTON GENERAL HOSPITAL, NORTHAMPTON

Graft infection is a very serious complication of arterial reconstructive surgery with high associated rates of amputation and mortality. Fortunately it is relatively uncommon, but problems in diagnosis and treatment create one of the most formidable surgical challenges. The true incidence is uncertain but lies within the range 0.5 to 2.6% of vascular reconstructions [1-4]. There are many differing approaches to management.

The main new initiative in the prevention of graft infection involves the use of antibiotic-bonded grafts. There is continuing interest in their use for conservative treatment of graft infection by graft excision and *in situ* replacement, as an alternative to conventional surgical management in selected cases. Other new approaches to treatment include the replacement of infected aortic prostheses with autogenous deep lower extremity veins and arterial allografts.

Pathogenesis

Graft infection may be divided into early (<4 months) and late infection [5], although there is no accepted definition and its aetiology is complex. Micro-organisms can infect the prosthesis through direct implantation at the time of surgery, through the wound if there is a complication of healing, or through haematogenous or lymphatic routes from remote sites of infection. It is thought that the majority of graft infections, both early and late, result from implantation at the time of initial surgery.

At operation, a graft is placed in a closed system. An acute inflammatory reaction occurs initially, followed by a chronic inflammatory response which is associated with fibroblast infiltration of the perigraft space and graft interstices [6]. This is important for initial healing and subsequent graft incorporation as the fibrosis matures. A concept termed 'the race for the surface' has been used to describe the events that arise at the interface after implantation of a prosthesis [7]. A contest between tissue cell integration and bacterial adhesion to the surface takes place. If human cells are the first to attach to the graft ahead of micro-organisms, it is likely that no prosthesis-related infection will occur. If bacteria adhere and form a nidus, however, a biofilm may develop which protects the bacteria from host defences and antibiotics. Some bacterial strains are known to produce a slime layer in culture. *Staphylococcus aureus* produces an extracellular glycocalyx (mucin), which promotes its adherence to the graft, in addition to coagulase and a wide variety of toxic proteolytic enzymes. *Staphylococcus epidermidis* also produces a mucin which binds itself to the prosthetic material and has a protective action by reducing the penetration of antibiotics and inhibiting the action of antibodies and phagocytes [8].

The pathological consequences of graft infection depend on the virulence of the organism, the host response and its site. Early graft infections are relatively uncommon and are usually associated with virulent pathogens such as *Staphylococcus aureus* and the

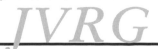

Gram-negative bacteria, *Streptococcus faecalis*, *Escherichia coli*, *Klebsiella*, *Pseudomonas aeruginosa* and *Proteus*. Multiple organisms may be present. They tend to be associated with serious complications such as systemic sepsis, infected false aneurysm, external drainage through wound infection and erosion into bowel. In contrast, late graft infections are commonly the result of less virulent bacteria, such as *Staphylococcus epidermidis*, and are typically more difficult to diagnose. Clinical signs are usually absent but local signs develop as the infection progresses. These include tenderness and erythema of the skin overlying the graft, a perigraft mass or a discharging sinus [9].

The clinical manifestations of graft infection are the result of the balance between the pathogenicity of the organism and the host immunological defences. Bacteria such as *Staphylococcus epidermidis* have been found frequently in prosthetic grafts removed for reasons other than sepsis [10], and it is possible that only a small proportion of grafts contaminated with this organism develop overt signs of infection [11]. The physiological status of bacterial cells living in biofilms is heterogeneous and determined by the location of each individual cell within the multiple layers of cells forming the biofilm [12]. Cells located in the external layers are metabolically active and frequently reproducing, but they are highly susceptible to antibacterial agents and host defences. Cells located in the deeper layers of the biofilm have scarce access to nutrients and oxygen and show reduced or no reproductive activity. Their metabolism is differentiated towards the synthesis of glycocalyx and, because these cells are almost dormant, they are resistant to antibacterial agents and host defences. When the biofilm approaches its critical mass, the cells in the outer layer may be released to cause acute episodes in the course of an otherwise almost silent infection. The degree of this cellular differentiation is proportional to the age of the biofilm and is an additional factor responsible for the complexity of the clinical syndrome of graft infection.

Identification of the infective organism

The causative organism may be difficult to identify. During acute episodes of systemic infection, blood cultures can be useful and these should be repeated at short intervals [12]. Samples may also be obtained from wounds, perigraft fluid aspirated under ultrasound or computed tomographic control, or directly from the explanted graft. They must be transported to the microbiology laboratory in an adequate liquid medium to be processed immediately. Sections of graft should be extensively vortexed or sonicated by ultrasound to detach bacterial cells from the biomaterial and disperse them in the medium [12]. Adequate volumes of the suspension and sequential dilutions should be plated on appropriate solid media. The graft itself should be incubated with vigorous

shaking for up to 10 days or until evident bacterial growth is observed. An equally long incubation period should be adopted for inoculated plates. Antibiotic treatment should be based on the bactericidal activity of antibiotics rather than on their inhibitory activity; the former is more relevant for biofilm bacteria [13]. Although an improvement in culture techniques may be a factor in the recent change in the observed pattern of graft infection, such techniques still cannot be considered ideal because they do not generally allow an accurate microbiological diagnosis before graft removal.

Predisposing factors

Graft infections are commonly associated with operative events leading to bacterial contamination of the graft, or with patient risk factors that predispose to infection due to impaired host defences (Table 1). The important association of graft infection with the use of groin incisions has been well documented and the development of complications in a groin wound is frequently the precursor of an infected prosthesis [3]. The incidence of graft infection is increased with emergency surgery, early revision surgery, long operations and those associated with substantial blood loss. Simultaneous gastrointestinal, biliary and urological procedures also increase the risk of graft contamination during the procedure but more commonly colonisation results from a postoperative complication such as an anastomotic or biliary leak.

Table 1. Risk factors for graft infection.

Bacterial contamination of the graft

- **Faulty aseptic technique**
- **Groin incision(s)**
- **Emergency surgery**
- **Early revision surgery**
- **Long operations**
- **Operations with substantial blood loss**
- **Simultaneous gastrointestinal and other procedures**
- **Prolonged preoperative hospital stay**
- **Severity of arterial ischaemia (gangrene)**
- **Intercurrent remote infection**
- **Postoperative superficial wound infection**

Impaired host defences

- **Malnutrition**
- **Diabetes mellitus**
- **Chronic renal failure**
- **Autoimmune disease**
- **Obesity**
- **Malignancy**
- **Corticosteroid therapy**
- **Leucopenia**

Patients who are at increased risk of graft infection include those with malnutrition, diabetes mellitus, chronic renal failure, autoimmune disease, obesity and those who are immunocompromised due to malignancy, corticosteroid therapy or leucopenia. Infected or gangrenous lesions on the feet are associated with infection of groin wounds and grafts. The severity of the arterial ischaemia is an important risk factor; Earnshaw et al have shown the risk of wound infection in patients undergoing lower limb vascular reconstruction is significantly increased in those with rest pain and skin necrosis or rest pain alone compared to claudication or aneurysm [14]. In this study *Staphylococcus aureus* and *Escherichia coli* were most common and over one half of the patients with wound infection had a similar organism isolated from the skin before their operation.

The type of graft is also important. Graft infection is predominantly a problem of prosthetic grafts. Autogenous vein has inherent resistance to infection. Bacterial adherence to Dacron is 10-100 times greater than to polytetrafluoroethylene (PTFE) and varies with the bacterial species [15]. No clinical difference in the incidence of graft infection between these two types of prosthetic material has, however, been found [1,3].

Prevention

Preoperative measures

Antibiotic prophylaxis reduces wound infections in vascular surgery and is mandatory, although opinion varies as to its optimal duration [28]. There are no hard data from clinical trials that antibiotic prophylaxis prevents graft infection; this may largely be due to the small incidence of infection and so the large size of study that would be necessary [28]. Prophylaxis should commence before operation. It is common practice to give the first dose of antibiotic on induction of anaesthesia, followed by two postoperative doses to provide cover for the first 24 hours. There is no evidence of significant benefit from more prolonged courses of antibiotics, a practice that may be associated with the proliferation of resistant organisms [16]. Therapeutic serum and tissue levels must be maintained throughout the operation to ensure adequate protection and intraoperative redosing is recommended if there is substantial blood loss, the procedure is prolonged or other circumstances occur which might increase the risk of infection (e.g. opening the bowel, synchronous procedures) [16]. There are no standard recommendations for prophylaxis in other situations where the risk is increased, such as active lower limb infection or tissue loss, emergency surgery or reoperation. It is justified to give a full course of antibiotics in this situation (5 days), although this is not of proven benefit.

The choice of antibiotic will be determined by the sensitivities of the organisms most frequently encountered. Broad spectrum cover with Augmentin (amoxycillin with clavulanate), or cefuroxime plus metronidazole is popular. Vancomycin or teicoplanin may be used in hospitals with methicillin-resistant *Staphylococcus aureus* (MRSA). One of these agents and/or gentamicin may be used when the presence of resistant organisms is suspected, for example after prolonged preoperative hospital admission.

Preparation of the skin before surgery may reduce skin contamination and consequently the risk of graft infection. Antiseptic baths with chlorhexidine have not, however, been shown to be beneficial [17]. Removal of hair by shaving should be carried out as close to the time of surgery as possible. Skin preparation with povidone-iodine or chlorhexidine is carried out immediately before surgery. There is no evidence to suggest that any one solution is superior [5]. Sterile plastic adhesive drapes are widely used to separate the operative field from the pubic area and perineum. Their use has not been shown to reduce the incidence of wound infection, even in the groin [18], but they do serve to prevent contact of the graft with the skin.

Intraoperative measures

Meticulous surgical and aseptic technique is of paramount importance in reducing the incidence of wound infection and the risk of graft infection [3,33]. Tissues should be handled carefully with attention to haemostasis to prevent haematoma formation. Groin incisions should be avoided whenever possible. When these are necessary, minimal dissection of the lymphatics should be carried out, divided channels should be ligated and the incisions closed in at least two layers with accurate approximation of the skin edges to eliminate the dead space, reduce seroma formation and promote primary healing. Avoidance of undercutting the skin edge is important in the exposure of the femoral artery in the groin and the long saphenous vein in the thigh. This can result in skin flap necrosis and hence threaten the graft. Oblique groin incisions and preoperative vein marking by duplex may help to reduce flap necrosis. Wound healing in the thigh is also improved by the use of three or four incisions with short intervening skin bridges rather than one long continuous incision. Routine vacuum drainage of groin wounds does not prevent either lymphocoele or wound infection [19].

With regard to aortic grafts, simultaneous gastrointestinal procedures should be avoided to prevent graft contamination with enteric organisms. If the bowel is inadvertently entered during division of adhesions or exposure of the aorta, the incision should be closed and the arterial reconstruction rescheduled for a second occasion a few days later. If a bowel resection is necessary, the reconstruction may often be delayed in cases of occlusive disease but, if surgery is urgent, an extra-anatomic bypass may be considered as an alternative. Elective repair of aortic aneurysm is probably best delayed for a short interval until the patient has recovered from the bowel resection. An exception to this may occur in large aneurysms when it may be preferable to carry out both procedures together. In this instance it is probably best to repair the aneurysm first and close the retroperitoneum, before carrying out the bowel resection. Where symptomatic coincidental pathology of the 'clean contaminated' category is present, such as gallstones, a combined procedure may be appropriate. In this situation cholecystectomy should be performed only after the aortic graft has been implanted and the retroperitoneum completely closed. Most asymptomatic gallstones, however, can safely be left untreated at the initial operation.

After insertion of an aortic graft it is essential that the duodenum and remaining bowel are separated from the graft to prevent the development of a secondary aortoenteric fistula. This requires complete closure of the retroperitoneum with interposition of greater omentum between the duodenum and the graft if necessary.

Rifampicin-bonded Dacron grafts

The inclusion of antibiotic in graft material is one potential way to reduce graft infection in the immediate perioperative period when it is most at risk. Rifampicin becomes attached to the surface of gelatin-coated Dacron through ionic bonding [20,21] and has excellent activity against both *Staphylococcus aureus* and methicillin-resistant staphylococci (MRSA) [20,22]. Animal experiments have shown that the rifampicin remains bound to these grafts in an active concentration for at least 72 hours [21].

There are three ongoing randomized trials of rifampicin bonding, the Italian [23], European [24] and Joint Vascular Research Group (JVRG) studies [25]. In the Italian study 600 patients undergoing aortic reconstruction were randomly allocated into two groups; the rifampicin-bonded group received a Gelseal graft (Vascutek, UK) which had been soaked for 15 minutes in a solution of rifampicin (1 mg/ml saline) and the control group received the same untreated graft. All patients received systemic antibiotic prophylaxis. Clinical follow-up was performed at 1, 6, 12 and 24 months after surgery. The incidence of graft infection was 2% at 2 years (12 cases). There was no significant difference between the two groups (1.7% rifampicin-bonded vs. 2.3% controls). All graft infections originated in the groin and *Staphylococcus aureus* was isolated in 50%. There was a significant prevalence of lymphatic complications and early revisional surgery in patients with graft infection [23].

In the European study the efficacy of rifampicin bonding in the prevention of early postoperative wound and graft infection was examined in 2,522 patients undergoing aortic reconstruction using the same protocol as the Italian study [24]. A significant reduction in superficial and deep wound infections (Szilagyi grades I and II) was found in patients receiving rifampicin-bonded grafts (2.9% vs. 4.4% controls) [26]. A positive trend was found for graft infection (0.3% vs. 0.6% controls) but this was not statistically significant [24].

In the JVRG study, extra-anatomic grafts were chosen as they have the highest risk of infection [25]. A total of 257 patients were randomized to rifampicin bonding (1 mg/ml rifampicin soak for 15 minutes before graft insertion) or a control group. The rate of early graft infection (within 1 month of surgery) was very low (0.4%). Only one patient in the control group developed a graft infection and this proved fatal. The rate of infective complications was similar in both groups (15% rifampicin-bonded vs. 21% controls). The total number of infective wound complications was greater in patients with one or more preoperative risk factor for infection (26%) than in patients with none (10%). When the 125 patients with preoperative risk factors were evaluated, however, the rate of infective wound complications remained similar (23% rifampicin-bonded vs. 30% controls) and this was not statistically significant. In contrast to the European study, the early results showed no advantage from the routine use of rifampicin bonding. The late results of this study with follow-up to 2 years have not yet been reported.

There is debate about the concentration of rifampicin that should be used. Increasing the concentration of rifampicin of 10 mg/ml significantly reduced the incidence of prosthetic graft infection, compared to 1 mg/ml, following a challenge of *Staphylococcus epidermidis* or MRSA in sheep [27]. A much higher concentration of 60 mg/ml is recommended for treatment of infected grafts by *in situ* replacement [28].

Although rifampicin has a wide spectrum of activity it is not effective against some Gram-negative organisms and this may be a limitation. Other antibiotics may be investigated for use either alone, or in combination. Fluoroquinolones, for example, have shown promise in eradicating biofilms and a method has been developed to bind ciprofloxacin to Dacron and then release the drug upon application of heat [29,30]. Rifampicin combinations with vancomycin, teicoplanin or ciprofloxacin have been shown to be significantly more bactericidal against biofilms than other antibiotic combinations in animal studies [31].

Definitive recommendations about the role of antibiotic bonding in the prevention of graft infection may be made only when the late results of the above three randomized trials are known. Even then, the studies are unlikely to have sufficient power to show a statistically significant advantage for rifampicin soaking. Until then, the policy of using a rifampicin-bonded gelatin-coated graft in patients known to be at high risk of infection seems reasonable. The method is simple and no disadvantages have been identified.

Postoperative measures

Early recognition and aggressive treatment of any wound infection is essential to avoid potential infection of the underlying graft. It is mandatory that graft coverage is maintained at all times. Exposure of a graft section will inevitably lead to infection unless urgent action is taken to restore healthy overlying tissue. In the groin the simplest way to achieve this is by debridement and resuture but sartorius myoplasty is an excellent alternative when this is not possible [32]. If there is any doubt clinically about the depth or extent of wound infection, simple palpation of the defect with a sterile glove and aseptic technique will rapidly clarify the situation; not uncommonly a cavity may be detected with a pulsating graft in its base that was not evident initially.

Failure of prosthetic grafts to develop a protective endothelial lining renders them susceptible to late colonisation and infection through bacteraemia. After graft insertion, patients should be informed of this potential risk. Interventional urological procedures, colonoscopy and dental treatment are important and antibiotic prophylaxis has been recommended in these circumstances [33-36]. The risk is very low, however, and other studies have shown no benefit from dental-type antibiotic prophylaxis [37]. The current balance of opinion is that prophylaxis should probably be recommended for patients with vascular grafts, although it is not of proven benefit.

Treatment

The management of graft infection is controversial and depends on the site and extent of the infection, the virulence of the infecting organism, the need for distal revascularisation and involvement of anastomoses. There are many differing approaches, each of which may be appropriate in certain circumstances; each patient should be considered individually. The effectiveness of new treatment initiatives should be compared against conventional surgical management.

Total graft excision and extra-anatomic bypass

Standard treatment of aortic graft infection has involved an aggressive surgical approach with total excision of the graft including some adjacent artery, debridement of infected perigraft tissue, extra-anatomic

bypass to uninvolved arterial segments and the administration of culture-specific antibiotics. This has been associated historically with high mortality and amputation rates [38,39] and a significant risk of secondary haemorrhage from the aortic stump, which is usually fatal [1]. Revascularisation may be immediate or can be staged. The extra-anatomic bypass may be inserted 48-72 hours before graft excision without increasing the risk of recurrent infection. This approach has been recommended whenever possible, providing the patient's condition is stable [40,41]. Not surprisingly, mortality in unstable patients requiring emergency surgery is higher than those in whom urgent or elective repair is possible [42].

Considerable improvement in results with the traditional approach has been reported, particularly in the last decade [41-44]. Kuestner et al [44] reported an extensive review of current treatment for secondary aorto-enteric fistula in 33 patients, the group with prosthetic graft infection at highest risk [2,39]. Perioperative mortality, amputation and aortic stump disruption rates were 18%, 6% and 6% respectively. Cumulative cure was 70% at 3 years, with 90% secondary patency of the extra-anatomic bypass at 4 years. The improved survival rate was attributed to the following factors: dramatic and ongoing improvement in preoperative preparation, intraoperative anaesthetic management and postoperative care, thorough debridement of the infected retroperitoneum, perigraft tissue and of the infected artery (aorta), and the routine performance of the extra-anatomic revascularisation before the transabdominal removal of the infected graft which avoids lower body ischaemia with all of its adverse metabolic consequences [44]. Complete excision of the graft with extra-anatomic bypass provides a satisfactory long-term outcome and remains the standard with which other approaches must be compared [41].

Total graft excision and in situ graft replacement

Previous dissatisfaction with the results of conventional surgical treatment and reports of success with various methods of conservative management led to the development of in situ graft replacement as an alternative option in selected cases. Patients most suitable are those with negative bacterial cultures, no signs of systemic sepsis and minimal contamination at surgery: especially those with late graft infections due to *Staphylococcus epidermidis*. Several techniques are available.

Prosthetic replacement
The first large series treated with in situ replacement was reported by Walker et al in patients with secondary aorto-enteric fistula [45]. The proximal part of the graft was removed and replaced with a new section of Dacron

covered by an omentoplasty to separate it from the duodenum. Good results have been reported recently from Italy with *in situ* replacement by a standard PTFE graft in clinically and bacteriologically selected patients [46]. Before placement, the surrounding necrotic tissues were debrided as thoroughly as possible and the field washed repeatedly with antiseptic solution containing 2% povidone iodine. An omental wrap was subsequently carried out. All patients received intravenous antibiotics for 6 weeks after operation, followed by a 2 month course of oral therapy.

Antibiotic-bonded graft

The concept of using an antibiotic-bonded graft is logical and attractive. *In situ* replacement with a rifampicin-bonded graft (10-15 min soak with 60 mg/ml) has been used with good initial results [20,47,48]. No large series with a long follow-up has yet been reported. The technology of bonding antibiotics to vascular grafts continues to develop [28]. The antibiotic-bonded graft may have an important place in the treatment of this problem in the future.

Autogenous vein for aortic graft infection

The use of autogenous superficial femoral and popliteal veins (SFPV) to create a neo-aortoiliac system in the treatment of graft infection was first reported in 1993 by Clagett et al [49] and has subsequently been adopted by others [50,51]. This approach has the advantages that it avoids extra-anatomic revascularisation and uses autogenous vein with its attendant bacterial resistance. Clagett's group has recently reported excellent results in 41 patients treated by this technique since 1990 [52] (Fig. 1). Perioperative mortality was 7.3% and 5% required amputation. The problem of aortic stump disruption was avoided and no patient developed haemorrhage or a false aneurysm in relation to the proximal aortic anastomosis. At 5 years the cumulative secondary patency rate of the grafts was 100%. Four patients developed permanent oedema which was controlled by compression stockings; none had venous ulceration. No aneurysmal dilatation of the SFPV grafts occurred. Six patients were of interest because their grafts became bathed in pus postoperatively due to major gastrointestinal

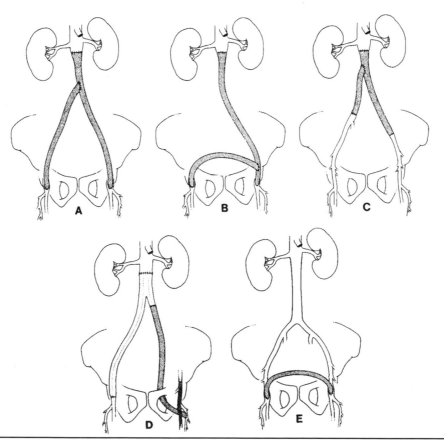

Figure 1. Aortoiliac/femoral reconstructions using SFPV in 41 patients (31 with graft infection, 10 with regional infection, recurrent failure of standard vascular prostheses or young patients with small vessels). (A) 14 (34%) patients underwent SFPV aortounilateral bypass with a limb also fashioned from SFPV anastomosed end-to-side. (B) 13 (32%) patients underwent SFPV aortofemoral bypass with a SFPV femoral crossover bypass. (C) 3 (7%) patients underwent SFPV aortoiliac reconstructions. (D) 6 (15%) underwent aortofemoral bypass single-limb replacement or iliofemoral bypass with SFPV grafts. (E) 5 (12%) patients had femoral crossover bypass alone performed with SFPV grafts. (With permission from the Journal of Vascular Surgery. Clagett G P, Valentine R J, Hagino R T. Autogenous aortoiliac-femoral reconstruction from superficial-femoral popliteal veins: feasibility and durability. *J Vasc Surg* 1997; 25: 255-270).

complications or femoral wound infections; on re-exploration for treatment of these, all the grafts were found to be intact and there were no subsequent acute disruptions or vein blow-outs. The principal disadvantage was that the procedures were long and arduous with a mean operative time of 7.9 hours. The mean blood transfusion requirement was six units. A two-team approach is preferable, although in this series the majority of the operations were performed by a single surgical team. The other limitation was that poor results were obtained in patients with secondary aorto-enteric fistula. A conventional surgical approach of total graft excision and extra-anatomic bypass remained the authors' preference for the treatment of this condition. Nevertheless aortoiliac-femoral reconstruction with SFPV grafts is a successful and durable option for graft infection and other complex aortic problems.

Alternative autografting techniques include the use of long saphenous vein and endarterectomised superficial femoral artery. The long saphenous vein can be used when it is large (>8mm diameter) but in general it is not suitable for aortoiliac replacement. Previous experience with such grafts has been disappointing with frequent failures as a result of focal and generalised neointimal hyperplasia. They are also prone to kinking. The proximal end of a SFPV graft is 1.0-1.5 cm in diameter, however, which allows comfortable anastomosis to the aorta [52].

Arterial allografts

Another approach is the use of allografts for *in situ* replacement of infected aortic prostheses as described by Kieffer et al and other groups [53-55]. Availability is dependent on arterial allograft tissue banks such as have been developed in France and Italy [53,54]. Perioperative mortality of *in situ* aortic replacement with this technique is high (24% in 100 patients) and the resistance of the allograft to infection is incomplete [53]. This may lead to persistent septic complications, including aortic rupture. An additional cause for concern is the long-term results; there is a 25% incidence of vessel occlusion at 2 years due to chronic rejection and the grafts are prone to secondary late deterioration [53]. Fresh or preserved vessels were used as arterial conduits in the 1940s but poor long-term results, with increased thrombogenicity and late atheromatous degeneration and aneurysm formation led to their abandonment and a search for alternative prostheses [56]. Immunosuppressive treatment is now available and may improve the long-term patency of arterial allografts, but it is obviously contraindicated in infected patients. This technique is unlikely to be adopted widely for these reasons.

Additional techniques

Partial graft excision is effective for infection limited to one limb of an aortic graft [57]. The affected graft limb is excised, usually through a retroperitoneal approach, with revascularisation via an obturator foramen bypass. There are other specific situations in which subtotal graft preservation may be reasonable [58].

Some surgeons have adopted a conservative approach [59] with antibiotic irrigation in selected cases [60] (Fig. 2). Despite successful results in a small number of patients, methods which involve leaving infected aortic grafts in place are unlikely to be adopted widely due to concern about persistent infection and death [4].

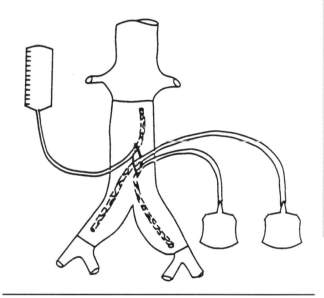

Figure 2. Technique for antibiotic irrigation of an infected graft. Three 5mm silicone drainage tubes are placed to lie between the native aneurysm sac and the prosthesis, each directed toward the anastomosis. For nonbifurcated prostheses, two tubes are used. Each tube has several side holes cut in the part that lies inside the sac. (With permission from Journal of Vascular Surgery. Morris G E, Friend P J, Vassallo D J, Farrington M, Leapman S, Quick C R G. Antibiotic irrigation and conservative surgery for major aortic graft infection. *J Vasc Surg* 1994; 20: 88-95).

Antibiotic irrigation may also be used as adjunctive treatment, such as to sterilise the graft bed and aortic stump after graft excision or in combination with *in situ* replacement.

Gentamicin bead insertion has been described in small series, in combination with graft excision, to lower the risk of aortic stump rupture, and as a conservative method of treating localised prosthetic infections in the groin [61]. Collagen mesh impregnated with gentamicin offers a newer alternative and has the advantage that it does not require removal [62], but its value in graft sepsis needs to be substantiated.

Parenteral antibiotics are universally used in the management of graft infection but the optimal duration of treatment is unknown. Many surgeons continue oral antibiotics after a course of parenteral therapy for months, or even years.

Conclusions

The best way to handle the problem of graft infection is to avoid it in the first place. The importance of prevention, and of meticulous surgical and aseptic technique cannot be overemphasised. The use of antibiotic-bonded grafts to prevent contamination at the time of initial operation is likely to become more widely adopted, particularly in patients at high risk of infection. When infection does occur each individual case requires careful consideration. There is unlikely ever to be a single 'best' treatment option. Total graft excision with extra-anatomic bypass should be employed when there is gross contamination with obvious sepsis. A conservative approach such as *in situ* replacement with an antibiotic-bonded graft may be justified when there is minimal contamination. Experience to date with autogenous vein is limited but the results are impressive.

Individual vascular surgeons have limited experience of graft infection. Improved results may be achieved by transfer of patients to large vascular centres whenever possible, where there may be greater experience of these complex problems and where several surgeons may be available to operate simultaneously.

Finally, this whole subject may change substantially with endovascular repair of abdominal aortic aneurysms. No infection was reported in 190 patients undergoing endoluminal repair with straight and bifurcated grafts [63]. Three (2.2%) of 136 patients who underwent endovascular repair with an aorto-uni-iliac device developed infection in the femorofemoral crossover bypass and one of them died [64]. It is too early to draw any conclusions about the risk of graft infection with this new technique or its treatment.

Prevention and treatment of graft infection

Sound evidence

- Antibiotic prophylaxis reduces wound (but not graft) infections.

- Overt sepsis, positive blood culture, extensive retroperitoneal infection and secondary aorto-enteric fistula are associated with a poor prognosis.

- Total graft excision and extra-anatomic bypass remains the standard treatment for aortic graft infection. Results have improved in the last decade.

- *In situ* graft replacement with an antibiotic-bonded graft is an acceptable alternative in selected patients with minimal contamination.

- *In situ* graft replacement with autogenous vein is a successful and durable treatment option.

Evidence needed

- Antibiotic-bonded grafts have not been shown to reduce the incidence of graft infection.

- Long-term results of *in situ* graft replacement with antibiotic-bonded grafts are unknown.

References (randomised trials in bold)

1. Calligaro KD, Veith FJ. Diagnosis and management of infected prosthetic aortic grafts. *Surgery* 1991; 110: 805-813.

2. Yeager RA, Porter JM. Arterial and prosthetic graft infection. *Ann Vasc Surg* 1992; 6: 485-491.

3. Lorentzen JE, Nielsen OM, Arendrup H, et al. Vascular graft infection: an analysis of sixty-two graft infections in 2411 consecutively implanted synthetic vascular grafts. *Surgery* 1985; 98:81-86.

4. O'Hara PJ, Hertzer NR, Beven EG, Krajewski LP. Surgical management of infected abdominal aortic grafts: review of a 25-year experience. *J Vasc Surg* 1986; 3: 725-731.

5. Hicks RCJ, Greenhalgh RM. Pathogenesis of vascular graft infection. *Eur J Vasc Endovasc Surg* 1997; 14 (Suppl A): 5-9.

6. Olofsson P, Rabahie GN, Matsumoto K, et al. Histopathological characterlstlcs of explanted human prosthetic arterial grafts: implications for the prevention and management of graft infection. *Eur J Vasc Endovasc Surg* 1995; 9: 143-151.

7. Gristina AG. Biomaterial-centred infection: microbial adhesion versus tissue integration. *Science* 1987; 237: 1588-1595.

8. Levy MF, Schmitt DD, Edmiston CE, et al. Sequential analysis of staphylococcal colonisation of body surfaces of patients undergoing vascular surgery. *J Clin Microbiol* 1990; 28: 664-669.

9. Bandyk DF, Esses GE. Prosthetic graft infection. *Surg Clin North Am* 1994; 74: 571-590.

10. Vinard E, Eloy R, Descotes JR, et al. Human vascular graft failure and frequency of infection. *J Biomed Material Research* 1991; 25: 499-513.

11. Wooster DL, Louch RE, Kradjen S. Intraoperative bacterial contamination of vascular grafts: a prospective study. *Can J Surg* 1985; 28: 407-409.

12. Selan L, Passariello C. Microbiological diagnosis of aortofemoral graft infection. *Eur J Endovasc Surg* 1997; 14 (Suppl A): 10-12.

13. Anwar H, Dasgupta MK, Costerton JW. Testing the susceptibility of bacteria in biofilms to antibacterial agents. *Antimicrob Agents Chemother* 1990; 34: 2043-2046.

14. **Earnshaw JJ, Slack RCB, Hopkinson BR, Makin GS. Risk factors in vascular surgical sepsis. *Ann Roy Coll Surg Engl* 1988; 70: 139-143.**

15. Schmitt DD, Bandyk DF, Pequet AJ, Towne JB. Bacterial adherence to vascular prostheses. *J Vasc Surg* 1986; 3: 732-740.

16. Santini C, Baiocchi P, Serra P. Perioperative antibiotic prophylaxis in vascular surgery. *Eur J Vasc Endovasc Surg* 1997; 14: (Suppl A): 13-14.

17. **Earnshaw JJ, Berridge DC, Slack RCB, Makin GS, Hopkinson BR. Do preoperative chlorhexidine baths reduce the risk of infection after vascular reconstruction? *Eur J Vasc Surg* 1989; 3: 323-326.**

18. Cruse PJE, Foord R. The epidemiology of wound infection. A 10-year prospective study of 62,939 wounds. *Surg Clin North Am* 1980; 60: 27-40.

19. **Dunlop MG, Fox JN, Stonebridge PA, Clason AE, Ruckley CV. Vacuum drainage of groin wounds after vascular surgery: a controlled trial. *Br J Surg* 1990; 77: 562-563.**

20. Strachan CJL, Newsom SWV, Ashton TR. The clinical use of an antibiotic-bonded graft. *Eur J Vasc Surg* 1991; 5: 627-632.

21. Lachapelle K, Graham AM, Symes JF. Antibacterial activity, antibiotic retention, and infection resistance of a rifampicin-impregnated gelatin-sealed Dacron graft. *J Vasc Surg* 1994; 19: 675-682.

22. Zavasky DM, Sande MA. Reconsideration of rifampicin. A unique drug for a unique infection. *JAMA* 1998; 279: 1575-1577.

23. **D'Addato M, Curti T, Freyrie A and Italian Investigators Group. Prophylaxis of graft infection with rifamcipin-bonded Gelseal graft: 2-year follow-up of a prospective clinical trial. *Cardiovasc Surg.* 1996; 4: 200-204.**

24. **D'Addato M, Curti T and Freyrie A. The rifampicin-bonded Gelseal graft. *Eur J Vasc Endovasc Surg* 1997; 14 (Suppl A): 15-17.**

25. **Braithwaite BD, Davies B, Heather BP, Earnshaw JJ on behalf of the Joint Vascular Research Group. Early results of a randomized trial of rifampicin-bonded Dacron grafts for extra-anatomic vascular reconstruction. *Br J Surg* 1998; 85: 1378-1381.**

26. Szilagyi DE, Smith RF, Elliott JP, Vrandecic MP. Infection in arterial reconstruction with synthetic grafts. *Ann Surg* 1972; 176: 321-333.

27. Vicaretti M, Hawthorne WJ, Ao PY, Fletcher JP. An increased concentration of rifampicin bonded to gelatin-sealed Dacron reduces the incidence of subsequent graft infections following a staphylococcal challenge. *Cardiovasc Surg* 1998; 6: 268-273.

28. Strachan CJL. Antibacterial prophylaxis in peripheral vascular and orthopaedic prosthetic surgery. *J Antimicrob Chemother* 1993; 31 (Suppl B): 65-78.

29. Reid G. Bacterial colonization of prosthetic devices and measures to prevent infection. *New Horizons* 1998; 6 (Suppl 2): 58-63.

30. Ozaki CK, Phaneuf MD, Bide MJ, Quist WC, Alessi JM, LoGerfo FW. In vivo testing of an infection-resistant vascular graft material. *J Surg Res* 1993; 55: 543-547.

31. Blaser J, Vergers P, Widmer AF, Zimmerli W. In vivo verification of in vitro model of antibiotic treatment of device-related infection. *Antimicrob Agents Chemother* 1995; 39: 1134-1139.

32. Maser B, Vedder N, Rodriguez D, Johansen K. Sartorius myoplasty for infected vascular grafts in the groin. Safe, durable and effective. *Arch Surg* 1997; 132: 522-526.

33. Bandyk DF, Bergamini TM. Infection in prosthetic vascular grafts. In *Vascular Surgery*, Ed. Rutherford R B, 4th Ed, 1995, 588-604.

34. Stansby G, Byrne MTL, Hamilton G. Dental infection in vascular surgical patients. *Br J Surg* 1994; 81: 1119-1120.

35. Wooster DL, Krajden S. Selection of antibiotic coverage in vascular patients undergoing cystoscopy. *J Cardiovasc Surg* 1990; 31: 469-473.

36. Earnshaw JJ. Prevention of infection after vascular reconstruction. *J Antimicrob Chemother* 1989; 23: 480-483.

37. Jones L, Braithwaite BD, Heather BP, Earnshaw JJ. Mechanism of late prosthetic vascular graft infection. *Cardiovasc Surg* 1997; 5: 486-489.

38. Bunt TJ. Synthetic vascular graft infections. I. Graft infections. *Surgery* 1983; 93: 733-746.

39. Bunt TJ. Synthetic vascular graft infections. II. Graft-enteric erosions and graft-enteric fistulas. *Surgery* 1983; 94: 1-9.

40. Calligaro KD, DeLaurentis DA, Veith FJ. An overview of the treatment of infected prosthetic vascular grafts. *Adv Surg* 1996; 29: 3-16.

41. Sharp WJ, Hoballa JJ, Mohan CR, et al. The management of the infected aortic prosthesis: a current decade of experience. *J Vasc Surg* 1994; 19: 844-850.

42. Menawat SS, Glovisczki P, Serry RD, Cherry KJ Jnr, Bower TC, Hallett JWJnr. Management of aortic graft-enteric fistulae. *Eur J Vasc Endovasc Surg* 1997; 14 (Suppl A): 74-81.

43. Yeager RA, Porter JM. The case against the conservative nonresectional management of infected prosthetic grafts. *Adv Surg* 1996; 29: 33-39.

Chapter 27

44. Kuestner LM, Reilly LM, Jicha DL, Ehrenfeld WK, Goldstone J, Stoney RJ. Secondary aorto-enteric fistula: contemporary outcome with use of extra-anatomic bypass and infected graft excision. *J Vasc Surg* 1995; 21: 184-196.

45. Walker WE, Cooley DA, Duncan JM, Hallman GL, Ott DA, Reul GJ. The management of aortoduodenal fistula by *in situ* replacement of the infected abdominal aortic graft. *Ann Surg* 1987; 205: 727-732.

46. Fiorani P, Speziale F, Rizzo L, Taurino M, Giannoni MF, Lauri D. Long-term follow-up after *in situ* graft replacement in patients with aortofemoral graft infections. *Eur J Vasc Endovasc Surg* 1997; 14 (Suppl A): 111-114.

47. Naylor AR, Clark S, London MJM, et al. Treatment of major aortic graft infection: preliminary experience with total graft excision and *in situ* replacement with a rifampicin bonded prosthesis. *Eur J Vasc Endovasc Surg* 1995; 9: 252-256.

48. Torsello G, Sandmann W. Use of antibiotic-bonded grafts in vascular graft infection. *Eur J Vasc Endovasc Surg* 1997; 14 (Suppl A): 84-87.

49. Clagett GP, Bowers BL, Lopez-Viego MA, et al. Creaton of a neo-aortoiliac system from lower extremity deep and superficial veins. *Ann Surg* 1993; 218: 239-249.

50. Nevelsteen A, Lacroix H, Suy R. Infrarenal aortic graft infection: *in situ* aortoiliofemoral reconstruction with the lower extremity deep veins. *Eur J Vasc Endovasc Surg* 1997; 14 (Suppl A): 88-92.

51. Sicard GA, Reilly JM, Doblas M, et al. Autologous vein reconstruction in prosthetic graft infection. *Eur J Vasc Endovasc Surg* 1997; 14 (Suppl A): 93-98.

52. Clagett GP, Valentine RJ, Hagino RT. Autogenous aortoiliac-femoral reconstruction from superficial-femoral popliteal veins: feasibility and durability. *J Vasc Surg* 1997; 25: 255-270.

53. Ruotolo C, Plissonnier D, Bahnini A, Koskas F, Kieffer E. *In situ* arterial allografts: a new treatment for aortic prosthetic infection. *Eur J Vasc Endovasc Surg* 1997; 14 (Suppl A): 102-107.

54. Chiesa R, Astore D, Piccolo G, et al. Fresh and cryopreserved arterial homografts in the treatment of prosthetic graft infections: experience of the Italian Collaborative Vascular Homograft Group. *Ann Vasc Surg* 1998; 12: 457-462.

55. Desgranges P, Beaujan F, Brunet S, et al. Cryopreserved arterial allografts used for the treatment of infected vascular grafts. *Ann Vasc Surg* 1998; 12: 583-588.

56. Meade JW, Linton RR, Darling RC, Menendez CV. Arterial homografts: a long-term clinical follow-up. *Arch Surg* 1966; 93: 392-9.

57. Miller JH. Partial replacement of an infected arterial graft by a new prosthetic polytetrafluoroethylene segment: a new therapeutic option. *J Vasc Surg* 1993; 17: 546-558.

58. Calligaro KD, Veith FJ. Graft preserving methods for managing aortofemoral prosthetic graft infection. *Eur J Vasc Endovasc Surg* 1997; 14 (Suppl A): 38-42.

59. Gordon A, Conlon C, Collin J, et al. An 8-year experience of conservative management for aortic graft sepsis. *Eur J Vasc Surg* 1994; 8: 611-16.

60. Morris GE, Friend PJ, Vassallo DJ, Farrington M, Leapman S, Quick CRG. Antibiotic irrigation and conservative surgery for major aortic graft infection. *J Vasc Surg* 1994; 20: 88-95.

61. Nielsen OM, Noer HH, Jorgensen LG, Lorentzen JE. Gentamicin beads in the treatment of localised vascular graft infection - long-term results in 17 cases. *Eur J Vasc Surg* 1991; 5: 283-5.

62. Jensen LP, Nielsen OM, Jorgensen LG, Lorentzen JE. Conservative treatment of vascular graft infections in the groin. *Eur J Vasc Endovasc Surg* 1977; 14 (Suppl A): 43-46.

63. May J, White GH, Waugh R, et al. Adverse events after endoluminal repair of abdominal aortic aneurysms: a comparison during two successive periods of time. *J Vasc Surg* 1999; 29:32-9.

64. Walker SR, Braithwaite B, Tennant WG, MacSweeney S T, Wenham PW, Hopkinson BR. Early complications of femorofemoral crossover bypass grafts after aorto uni-iliac endovascular repair of abdominal aortic aneurysms. *J Vasc Surg* 1998; 28: 647-50.

Chapter 28

Management of methicillin-resistant
Staphylococcus aureus infection in vascular patients

NJM London
Professor of Surgery
A Nasim
Specialist Registrar

DEPARTMENT OF SURGERY,
LEICESTER ROYAL INFIRMARY, LEICESTER

Introduction

Staphylococcus aureus is the most common cause of nosocomial infection recognised in the USA National Nosocomial Surveillance System [1] and it is the leading cause of surgical site infection. The number of UK patients with *S. aureus* bacteraemia is increasing yearly [2], with 5978 cases reported in 1994 and 10137 in 1998. More than 95% of patients worldwide with *S. aureus* infection do not respond to first-line antibiotics such as penicillin. Additionally [3], methicillin-resistant strains of *S. aureus* (MRSA) were first described in England in 1961, shortly after methicillin became available for clinical use [4]. They have subsequently spread throughout the world and are now a major cause of nosocomial infection. The prevalence of MRSA in hospitals varies considerably from one region to another; this is also the case among hospitals in the same city. In some hospitals MRSA accounts for less than 10% of all *S. aureus* isolates, whereas in others it accounts for up to 65%. In Trent in 1998, 20% of *S. aureus* causing bacteraemia were methicillin resistant, whereas the overall figure for England and Wales [2] was 32%.

Epidemiology of MRSA

The main reservoir of MRSA in hospitals is patients colonised or infected with MRSA. Although colonised patients have no signs or symptoms of infection, they serve as a source from which transmission may occur. Colonised personnel and contaminated environmental surfaces may also serve as reservoirs but are not as important as infected patients. There are no UK studies examining the prevalence of MRSA in the community, but a study of ten nursing homes in the West Midlands [5] found that 17% of elderly residents were colonised with such bacteria. Hospital admission within the previous year, especially for surgery, significantly increased the risk of carriage.

MRSA is most frequently transmitted from one patient to another by a person who has not washed his or her hands between examining patients [6]. Health care personnel who have persistent nasal colonisation may transmit the organism to those in their care, especially if they develop a concurrent viral upper respiratory infection or MRSA sinusitis. Transmission via contaminated articles or environmental surfaces may occur but is a less important source.

MRSA colonisation

Like other strains of *S. aureus*, the site most commonly colonised with MRSA is the anterior nares. Other body sites that may be colonised include open wounds, the respiratory tract, perineum, upper extremities, urinary tract and axillae. Some patients remain colonised for only a few weeks and then become culture-negative without any specific therapy, but others may remain colonised for over 3 years.

JVRG

Preventing spread of MRSA

It is vital that hospitals apply scrupulous infection control policies, coordinated and monitored by an adequate infection control team. In particular, hand-washing, aseptic technique and ward cleaning are essential and, where appropriate, patients with MRSA need to be isolated. There is little doubt, however, that prolonged isolation may lead to profound depression and seriously compromise care, particularly if there is a shortage of nursing staff on the ward.

MRSA infections

Between 40% and 60% of hospitalised patients colonised with MRSA develop an overt infection. The most common problems caused by MRSA are surgical infection (28%), bacteraemia (21%), skin and soft tissue infection (21%) and lower respiratory tract infection (15%). MRSA infection is associated with prolonged hospital stay and increased hospital cost. One study from the United States has shown that patients with serious MRSA infection stayed in hospital an average of 12 days longer and had an average hospital cost £3,200 greater than comparable patients with methicillin-susceptible *S. aureus* infection. A study [7] from New York has shown that the mortality attributable to MRSA infection was 2.5 times higher than that attributable to methicillin-sensitive *S. aureus* infection (21% versus 8%). Some of the mortality difference may have been related to the poorer condition of those who became infected with MRSA, but it was also due to the lack of effectiveness of vancomycin in curing MRSA. Vancomycin has a narrow therapeutic index that allows little room for increasing blood concentration without incurring a substantial loss of tolerance [8].

MRSA in the Leicester Royal Infirmary vascular unit

During the period 1993 to 1998, a total of 115 patients had MRSA infection. This represented 4% of the total patients passing through the vascular unit during that time. Of the 115 patients, 67 were colonised and 48 were infected by MRSA. The number of MRSA positive patients has increased yearly: in 1994 six (1%) patients were positive, whereas in 1998 35 (5%) were positive. Each year, roughly 50% of those who have been MRSA positive have developed a clinical infection (Figure 1). The proportion of wound or graft infections caused by MRSA has increased from 1 of 28 (2%) in 1994 to 11 of 28 (40%) in 1998 (Figure 2). The risks of MRSA colonisation and infection during the period 1993 to 1998 for aortic procedures, carotid endarterectomy and infrainguinal reconstructions are shown in Table 1.

The rest of this report will examine the 48 MRSA infections. One was a brachial embolectomy wound infection that eventually resolved. Two patients had infection after carotid endarterectomy; both had a Dacron patch inserted. In one patient, the common carotid artery, internal carotid artery and external carotid artery were excised and ligated under transcranial Doppler monitoring; the patient survived, stroke-free. In the other patient the infected carotid artery was excised and a vein graft was inserted; this patient survived but developed a hemiparesis.

Eleven patients with elective aortic aneurysm repairs developed an infection. Five developed pneumonia, two developed septicaemia and two developed wound infections; all of these nine patients survived. One patient developed a false aneurysm at the site of insertion of an endovascular stent; this was repaired and the patient survived. One patient developed a crossover graft infection after endovascular aortic aneurysm repair and died. One patient developed intra-abdominal sepsis after an aortobifemoral graft and died.

With respect to ruptured aortic aneurysms, five patients developed MRSA infection. Two developed pneumonia and one developed a wound infection; all three patients survived. Two patients developed graft infections and both died. With respect to aortic reconstruction for occlusive disease, two patients developed a wound infection and survived while two developed graft infection involving the femoral arteries and died.

Table 1. Incidence (%) of MRSA carriage, infection and graft infection during 1993-1998.

	Carotid Endarterectomy	Aortic procedure	Lower limb arterial procedure
MRSA carriage	0.5	5	7
MRSA infection	0.25	3	3
MRSA graft infection	0.25	0.7	0.7

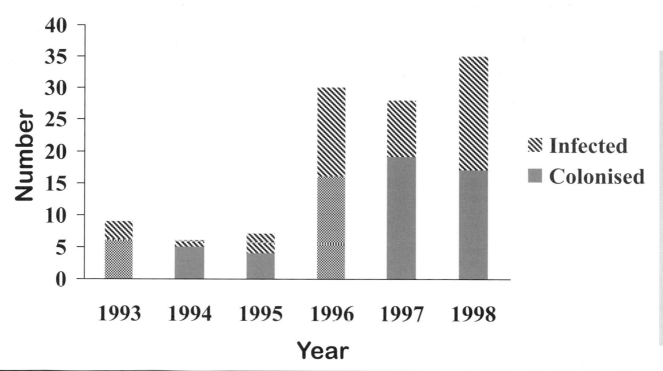

Figure 1. Number of MRSA colonised and infected patients in the Leicester Royal Infirmary vascular unit by year from 1993 to 1998.

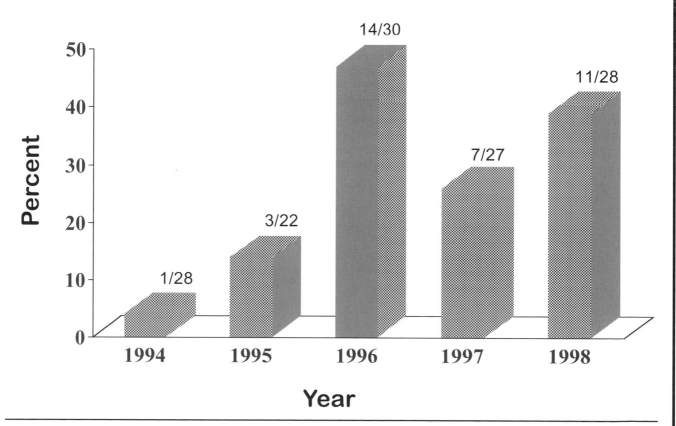

Figure 2. Proportion (%) of graft infections caused by MRSA during 1994-1998.

Considering lower limb procedures, 25 patients developed clinical MRSA infection. Nineteen of these were wound infections and four of these patients died from unrelated causes. One patient developed a primary arterial infection after a femoral embolectomy which resulted in arterial rupture and haemorrhage that was repaired with a vein patch. Five days later the vein patch ruptured and an obturator bypass was performed; the limb was salvaged and the patient survived. Five patients developed graft infections, one of which was in a Dacron iliofemoral crossover; the patient required an above knee amputation and survived. Four vein grafts became infected; three resulted in amputation (one patient died) and one patient did not undergo amputation but died of MRSA sepsis.

In summary, the two patients with carotid infection both survived (one had a stroke). All of the patients with an infected aortic graft died. Two of the five patients with lower limb graft infections died while the remaining three had amputations. The most striking aspect of the lower limb infections was the ability of MRSA to destroy native artery and the susceptibility of vein grafts to MRSA infection. Whether this represents a genuinely increased pathogenicity of MRSA compared to methicillin-sensitive *S. aureus* or simply reflects the relatively poor activity of vancomycin against MRSA is uncertain.

Treatment of MRSA infection

Vancomycin is the drug of choice for treating MRSA infection caused by multi-drug resistant strains. Some strains are susceptible to rifampicin and adding this to vancomycin may improve outcome. Rifampicin should not be used alone to treat MRSA infection because *S. aureus* strains easily develop resistance to this agent. An alternative to vancomycin is teicoplanin; both drugs are glycopeptides and the pros and cons of each are listed in Table 2. There are no published studies that have

addressed the duration of vancomycin therapy in patients with MRSA infection. It has been our policy to treat patients with vascular graft infection for a minimum of 6 weeks and for other infections (wound infection, pneumonia) to continue vancomycin for a week after clinical resolution of the infection. In order to minimise the psychological sequelae of prolonged patient isolation, some patients have been managed at home after an initial period of hospital treatment. This can be achieved by inserting a Hickman line and arranging for the district nursing service to administer once daily teicoplanin. It is of great concern that there are now reports from the United States, Japan and France of *S. aureus* with intermediate level resistance to vancomycin (VISA). It is thus very important that vancomycin is used only when essential, both to prevent the spread of VISA strains and to lessen the selection pressure for the eventual emergence of MRSA with transferable high-level glycopeptide resistance [9].

Managing patients with MRSA who need vascular reconstruction

Patients who are known to be MRSA positive are presumably at a higher risk of developing an MRSA infection if they require surgery. The management of such patients should start with a reconsideration of the risk/benefit ratio of reconstructive surgery; in the case of lower limb arterial occlusive disease, angioplasty, if possible, may be a lower risk alternative. If surgery is unavoidable, it seems sensible to attempt eradication of MRSA before operation and the methods of doing this are shown in Table 3. The issue of vancomycin prophylaxis and its duration should be discussed by the clinician in charge of the patient and a consultant in communicable diseases. The main concern about uncontrolled vancomycin prophylaxis is, of course, the emergence of VISA.

Table 2. Comparison of vancomycin with teicoplanin.

	Vancomycin	Teicoplanin
Toxicity	High. Nephrotoxic and ototoxic	Low. Nausea, diarrhoea and rash
Administration	Intravenous infusion over 60-100 minutes	Intravenous or intramuscular injection
Frequency	Twice daily	Once daily
Cost	£30/day	£50/day

Table 3. Treatment of MRSA carriers. Treatment should be guided by an infection control physician.

Nasal carriage

·   Apply mupirocin 2% in a paraffin base (Bactroban Nasal) to each nostril three times daily for 5 days.

·   Culture nasal swab 2 days after treatment; if positive, repeat the treatment once and check also for throat carriage.

·   If nasal swab remains positive, or the strain shows mupirocin resistance, consider alternative topical treatment (e.g. 0.5% neomycin + 0.1% chlorhexidine cream (Naseptin) or 1% chlorhexidine cream).

·   Avoid repeated courses of mupirocin and the topical use of antibiotics that may be required for systemic use (e.g. fusidic acid, gentamicin).

Skin carriage

·   Daily antiseptic bathing for 5 days (repeated if necessary) e.g. with 4% chlorhexidine, 2% triclosan, or 7.5% povidone-iodine.

·   Wash hair twice weekly with an antiseptic shampoo/detergent.

·   Hexachlorophane 0.33% powder for axillary or groin carriage.

Throat carriage

·   Significance in relation to spread is unclear. May be difficult to eradicate.

·   If there is clear evidence of transmission, consider a single 5-day course of oral treatment with either rifampicin plus fusidic acid or, for susceptible organisms, ciprofloxacin.

Future prospects

There are currently two antimicrobials under clinical development that have activity against MRSA. Quinupristin/daflopristin (Synercid) is a synergistic combination of two streptogramins. However, it is only bacteriostatic and has to be given intravenously. The oxazolidones are a new class of antimicrobials with activity against MRSA. One of this group, oxazolidone (Linezolid) is orally active against enterococci, pneumococci and *S. aureus*, including MRSA. Both of these antibiotics are broad spectrum and this in itself may encourage the development of opportunistic resistance; for this reason future research must focus on targeted therapy.

Conclusions

MRSA infection has emerged as a major problem in many hospitals throughout the world and when it occurs in vascular patients it poses a considerable therapeutic challenge. We have noted that MRSA can lead to disruption of both native artery and vein grafts and, in our experience, MRSA infection of aortic grafts is uniformly fatal. There is little doubt that prevention of MRSA infection is better than attempted cure. The most important elements of this approach are scrupulous hand washing, and effective communication and interaction with the hospital infection control team.

References

1. Centers for Disease Control and Prevention. *National Nosocomial Infection Surveillance System report: data summary from October 1986-April 1996*. Atlanta (GA): U.S. Department of Health and Human Services, 1996.
2. Standing Medical Advisory Committee (Department of Health). *The path of least resistance*. Main report. London: Department of Health, 1998.
3. Neu HC. The crisis in antibiotic resistance. *Science* 1992; 257: 1064-72.
4. Michel M, Gutmann L. Methicillin-resistant *Staphylococcus aureus* and vancomycin-resistant enterococci: therapeutic realities and possibilities. *Lancet* 1997; 349: 1901-6.
5. Fraise AP, Mitchell K, O'Brien SJ, Oldfield K, Wise R. Methicillin-resistant *Staphylococcus aureus* (MRSA) in nursing homes in a major UK city; an anonymised point prevalence survey. *Epidemiol Infect* 1997; 118: 1-5.
6. Tackling antimicrobial resistance. *Drug Ther Bull 1999*; 37: 9-16.
7. Rubin RJ, Harrington CA, Poon A, Dietrich K, Greene JA, Moiduddin A. The economic impact of *Staphylococcus aureus* infection in New York Hospitals. *Emerg Inf Dis* 1999; 5: 9-17.
8. McEvoy GK, editor. *American hospital formulary service drug information* 1997. Bethesda (MD): American Society of Health-System Pharmacists; 1997.
9. Johnson AP. Intermediate vancomycin resistance in *Staphylococcus aureus*; a major threat or a minor inconvenience? *J Antimicrob Chemother* 1998; 42: 289-91.

Chapter 29

The value of shunting in complex vascular trauma of the lower limb

AAB Barros D'Sa
Consultant Vascular Surgeon

VASCULAR SURGERY UNIT,
THE ROYAL VICTORIA HOSPITAL, BELFAST, NORTHERN IRELAND

Introduction

Complex vascular injuries of the lower limb, once almost exclusively encountered on the battlefield, were starkly witnessed during major wars of this millennium. During this period, progressive industrialisation, the global proliferation of motor vehicles, a plague of urban violence and, worse still, indiscriminate assault by terrorists using sophisticated weaponry have all contributed to such injuries in civilian life.

The nature and severity of penetrating lower limb vascular trauma reflects the energy dissipated on impact by wounding agents such as bullets or shrapnel from bombs, mines, shells and rockets [1,2]. The wounding energy dictates the degree of disruption of blood vessels and surrounding tissues. The transient 'cavitational effect' from a high velocity bullet damages structures perpendicular to its actual trajectory and in the process fragments of bone become secondary missiles. A shot-gun discharge at close range produces a concentrated cluster of severe injuries. In a road accident the wounding energy of a suddenly decelerating vehicle results in violent and precipitate angulation and fracture of long bones, generating immense shearing forces which damage all soft tissue structures. The avulsive forces involved in posterior dislocations of the knee will tear apart the popliteal artery and surrounding tissues.

Regardless of aetiology, therefore, features meriting the description of 'complex' are concurrent injury to artery, vein and collateral vessels, comminuted fractures with periosteal stripping, joint dislocation, disruption of muscle and soft tissue, nerve injury and varying degrees of wound contamination. Injuries of the head, chest and abdomen are frequently present and it is from these that the casualty may succumb at the scene of the trauma, or in transit, through exsanguination or vital organ injury. Others in hypovolemic shock may survive as a result of speedy and optimal resuscitation, and timely operative intervention in a trauma centre.

Pathophysiology of complex injury

Typically, both in wartime and in civilian life, the patient tends to be young and male, with lower limb injuries involving the main vessels adjacent to a fracture; classic examples are comminuted fracture of the femur, open tibial fracture and fracture dislocations of the knee. The vascular injuries per se are considered to be 'severe' because artery and vein are transected or avulsed, long segments are crushed or multiply damaged, the vessels may be denuded of viable muscle and soft tissue, atherosclerosis may be present and, to compound matters, the wound may be massively contaminated. The scenario can be further complicated by delay in admission or treatment or, indeed, failure to recognise vascular injury.

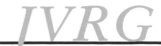

The value of shunting in complex vascular trauma of the lower limb

Arrest of distal inflow and tissue hypoperfusion and hypoxia is compounded by hypovolaemic shock and general vasoconstriction. Striated muscle, deprived of its main blood supply, may tolerate 'warm ischaemia' for about 6 - 8 hours depending on the level of injury and the availability of collateral flow. If unrelieved by fresh arterial inflow, myonecrosis and amputation will follow in the majority of cases. In complex limb trauma 10 - 48% of patients have vascular injuries and, not surprisingly, the amputation rates reported can be as high as 85% [3-11].

Paradoxically, restoration of flow leads to ischaemia-reperfusion injury (IR) directly proportional to the duration of preceding ischaemia [12]. It represents a further assault on cell membranes, increasing their permeability and causing both interstitial and cellular oedema of muscle (Fig 1). Only in recent years has there been an appreciation of the complex biochemical and cellular pathophysiology of IR, mediated by the generation of oxygen-derived free radicals, activation of neutrophils and the production of arachidonic acid metabolites. These complex interactions produce exudation, muscle oedema and rising pressure within muscle compartments confined within inelastic fascial envelopes. Fractured bone, disrupted soft tissues and haematoma further aggravate the swelling. In this ensuing compartment syndrome, tissue perfusion is further reduced, followed by microvascular stasis and thrombosis, aseptic muscle necrosis, ischaemic nerve palsy, Volkmann's contracture with fixed plantar flexion and finally amputation. The

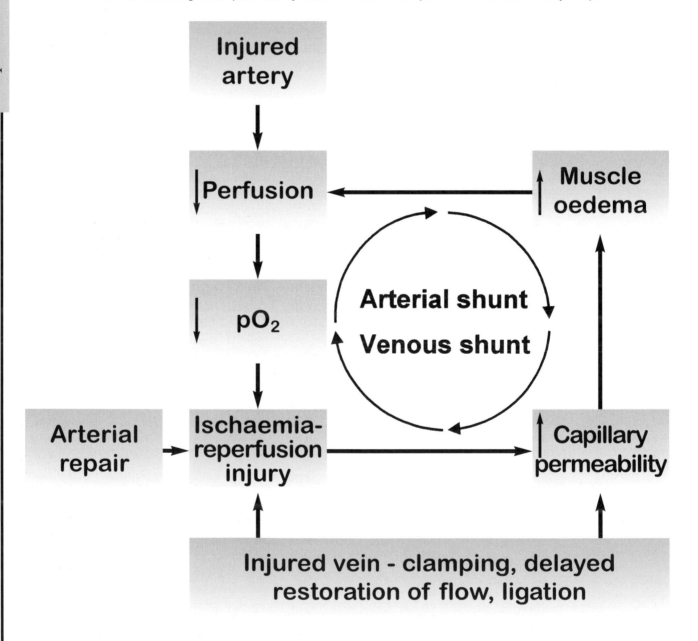

Figure 1. Diagram depicts the pathophysiological sequelae of arterial injury and repair, and the influence of clamping/ligating a concomitantly injured vein. The beneficial effect of early arterial and venous shunting in countering that process is illustrated.

remote injurious effects of IR on the heart, lungs, brain and bowel may bring about multisystem failure and death [13,14].

When the main vein is also injured, venous drainage is impaired and clamping raises venous pressure; ligation of such a vein markedly raises venous pressure for a prolonged period. In either case, resistance is offered to arterial inflow thereby promoting tissue hypoxia. Experimental work at my own centre [15] has now proven that delay, or failure to ensure outflow through the injured vein, exacerbates the IR which follows repair of an injured adjacent artery. This study has also shown that delayed restoration of venous drainage in combined arterial and venous injury not only leads to significantly more lipid peroxidation and tissue oedema in the limb concerned, but also causes remote lung injury characterised by non-cardiogenic pulmonary oedema.

Contamination at the time of wounding will compound the adverse effects of IR. Acting synergistically, Gram-positive cocci, Gram-negative cocci and Gram-negative bacilli cause cellulitis and even necrotising fasciitis. The anaerobic environment of ischaemic tissue facilitates the regeneration of clostridial spores, some species of which cause gas gangrene, an outcome promoted by delayed diagnosis, defective wound care, main vessel ligation and unrelieved compartment hypertension. Admittedly, fasciotomy alleviates the effects of IR but superinfection by *Pseudomonas aeruginosa* may prolong morbidity and threaten the limb.

The vital importance of time

Complex lower limb vascular injuries demand the cooperative endeavours of the vascular and orthopaedic surgeon, and sometimes too, the plastic surgeon. In the multiply injured patient, injuries of the head, chest and abdomen take precedence over limb vascular trauma and ischaemia time is necessarily prolonged. In order to abbreviate that period of ischaemia and therefore minimise IR, control of bleeding, resuscitation and definitive surgery should be overlapping rather than sequential stages of management. Even when those measures are executed expeditiously, a finite, and sometimes unacceptably long, period of time is required for exposure, wound care, bone fixation and repair of vessels.

A keen awareness of the passage of time and the understandable wish to intervene quickly may induce lapses in operative principles and surgical technique. If wound care is cursory, sepsis and other complications may presage amputation. The desirable objective of restoring flow urgently before even stabilising a fracture is often achieved at the cost of less than ideal techniques of repair. For example 'hour-glass' constriction often follows lateral suture, stenosis complicates end-to-end anastomosis under tension, an interposed vein graft which is too short disrupts and one far too slack kinks - all these sequelae result in thrombotic occlusion. In aiming to save time an important venous channel may be ligated causing compartment hypertension, compounding IR and even compromising an adjacent arterial repair. The later robust attentions of the orthopaedic surgeon manipulating bone fragments for reduction and fixation of the fracture may well disrupt a delicately executed vascular repair.

However, if fracture fixation precedes vascular repair the damage to soft tissue and vessels by bone fragments is averted. When vessels are then repaired ideal lengths of vein will be employed to reconstruct both artery and the vein. This sequence of procedures prolongs ischaemia time and the orthopaedic surgeon, conscious of that constraint, might conceivably resort to hurried, less than optimal and even defective fixation, which in turn is likely to compromise bony union.

The case for shunting artery and vein

Any measure which promotes the efficient use of the crucial commodity of time and which will influence limb survival is a welcome bonus. The placement of intravascular shunts in both artery and vein (Fig 2) at the earliest opportunity ensures time is used profitably from the outset. This policy, which has been in force at my own centre for two decades, offers the best solution to some of the dilemmas in operative treatment described above [16-19]. An indwelling shunt rejoining the ends of a severed artery immediately halts the noxious effects of ischaemic hypoxia, revitalising the limb and lowering the degree of IR. Equally, intraluminal shunting of an injured main vein re-establishes drainage of the distal limb and is of particular importance as other vein and lymphatic channels are also usually damaged. The act of shunting immediately imposes a disciplined and logical sequence on subsequent manoeuvres, and fosters interdisciplinary co-operation and harmony in the operating theatre. Having been relieved of the burden of maintaining an anxious eye on the clock, the vascular surgeon may now follow a sequence of steps (Fig 3) the dividends of which are better technique, less sepsis, reduced need for fasciotomy and a lower incidence of compartment syndrome, ischaemic nerve palsy and amputation, all of which facilitate early discharge from hospital[20].

Having observed the benefits of intravascular shunting of both artery and vein over a period of time, a shunt specifically intended for limb vascular trauma has been conceived [21]. That in turn stimulated experimental studies at HM Defence Medical Establishments with the aim of developing a temporary shunt [22].

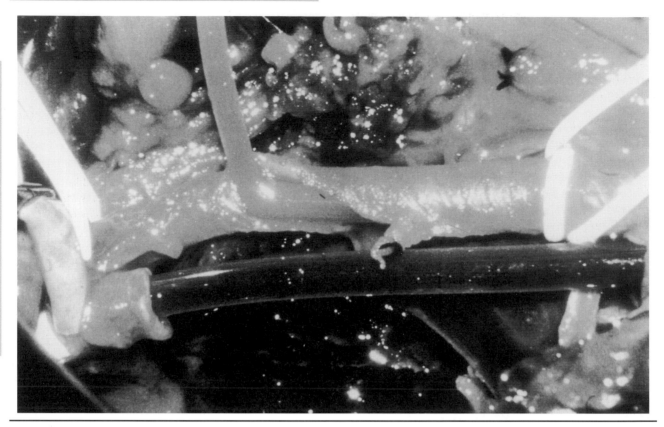

Figure 2. Intra-vascular shunts: Brener shunt in a torn popliteal artery above and a Javid shunt in a transected popliteal vein below, preparatory to vein graft replacement of each vessel. (With permission from Barros D'Sa, A.A.B. (1998) In: Limb Salvage and Amputation in Vascular Disease (eds R.M. Greenhalgh, C.W. Jamieson and A.N. Nicolaides), p.143. W.B. Saunders).

Diagnosis and early management

Control of external bleeding and standard resuscitation measures to secure an airway, maintain ventilation and correct hypovolemic shock are vital. In principle, the use of tourniquets or arterial forceps in wounds is ill-advised. Tetanus toxoid, and prophylactic cefuroxime and metronidazole, should be administered routinely. Once the patient is stable, the nature of vascular injury can be assessed. Bleeding, an expansile haematoma, an audible bruit, absent pulses, pallor, mottling, coolness

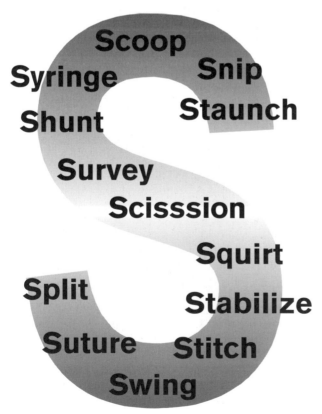

Figure 3. Aide-mémoire for the sequence of steps in the operative management of complex limb vascular injury: staunch the bleeding, snip damaged ends of vessels, scoop out clot, syringe in heparinized saline, shunt both artery and vein, survey the wound and identify nerve injury, perform scission of non-viable soft tissue, squirt saline to irrigate wound, stabilize fractured bone, stitch or repair both artery and vein, swing tissue for cover, suture the wound (delayed primary if contaminated) and, if necessary, split fasciae (fasciotomy). (With permission from Barros D'Sa, A.A.B. Complex vascular and orthopaedic limb injuries. _Journal of Bone and Joint Surgery_ 1992; 74B: 178).

and numbness distally are commonly observed. If after general resuscitation the limb circulation fails to improve, arterial injury should be suspected. Notoriously, a dislocated knee tends to reduce spontaneously and the clinician must remain alert to the possibility of vascular injury when examining a leg which may look normal.

Pulse waveform and ankle pressure measurements are of far greater significance than audible Doppler signals. Although duplex imaging is being employed increasingly to locate vascular injury, its impracticality in open limb injuries simply underlines the importance of angiography [23]. A surgeon who has no access to angiography is compelled to rely on clinical acumen and inevitably some explorations will be unproductive.

The benefits of surgery centred on the use of intravascular shunts should not lead to unreasonable optimism in dealing with the very mutilated leg. Over-zealousness in treating an irreparably damaged leg commits the patient, and of course the surgeon, to a protracted series of operations and anaesthetics, prolonged hospital stay and eventually the disappointment of amputation, often of a septic insensate leg, and of course, rehabilitation is delayed. Therefore primary amputation may well be in the patient's best interest; scoring systems [24] can assist objective appraisal in the difficult case, but the decision to amputate a young person's leg is best made after consultation with experienced colleagues.

Operative management

Access is gained through standard incisions, bleeding from damaged vessels is controlled and their ends trimmed back to pristine wall. The proximal arterial clamp is simply released to allow clot to be washed out; thrombus from the distal artery is retrieved by a balloon catheter after which heparinized saline (20 units/ml) is perfused distally.

One of the many commercially available shunts is used to restore arterial flow by joining the ends of an artery and similarly to re-establish venous outflow (Figs 2 and 4). Silicone elastomer or similar tubing of suitable consistency, length and calibre, the ends of which have been tailored carefully to prevent intimal damage, are acceptable alternatives. Venous blood should first be flushed out to protect the myocardium from a sudden bolus rich in potassium and the products of ischaemia-reperfusion. The side arm of a Brener shunt (Fig 2) is ideal for this purpose and is also a convenient portal for blood gas estimation, injecting heparinized saline or contrast agent for on-table angiography [21]. By attenuating IR compartment pressures are maintained within a safe range and there is time for a precise operative approach. If life-saving surgery of the head or torso is time-consuming, shunts reconnecting vessels of the lower limb buy time for their later definitive repair.

Chapter 29

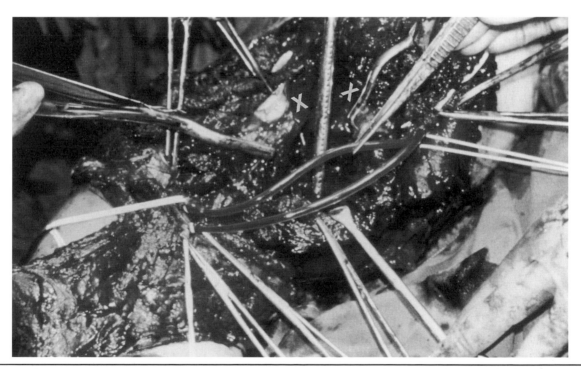

Figure 4. A virtually dismembered leg at mid-thigh: Javid shunt bridging lengthy gap in femoral artery and perfusing distal limb; another shunt bridging adjoining femoral vein and draining the leg. Ends of a fractured femur (XX) being manipulated prior to fixation. (With permission from Barros D'Sa AAB and Moorehead RJ. *European Journal of Vascular Surgery* **1989; 3:579).**

The value of shunting in complex vascular trauma of the lower limb

With shunts in place the surgeon has ample time to inspect the wound, identify nerve injury, remove debris, bone fragments and foreign bodies, and irrigate the tissues copiously to lower the concentration of the bacterial innoculum. Reperfusion will have sharpened the distinction between viable and dead tissue enabling precise debridement and good haemostasis. After careful wound care, the orthopaedic surgeon proceeds to reduce the fracture [25]. Long intravascular shunts (Fig 4) may be helpful in providing the necessary slack for manipulating bone prior to restoration of skeletal integrity, either by internal or external fixation [26].

When artery and vein are injured concurrently, and shunts have not been used, the artery should be repaired first. With shunts in place, however, neither artery nor vein deserves preferential attention and the order of repair is immaterial. The ample availability of time eliminates the use of expedient and flawed techniques of repair; instead, vein graft of adequate calibre, usually harvested from the contralateral limb, is interposed. The shunt over which the vein graft is drawn acts as a stent and prevents 'purse-stringing' at the anastomosis by enhancing precise technique. If donor vein is of inadequate calibre, a compound vein graft of suitable diameter can be constructed affording better prospects for long term patency. A well tried method is to use two, and if necessary three, equal segments of vein of suitable length, opened longitudinally to form panels whose valves have been excised; these are then sewn together side by side to create a panelled compound graft. This graft may either be fashioned over a shunted vessel or prepared 'on the bench' and slipped over the shunt. Alternatively, the same objective is achieved using a longitudinally slit length of vein bereft of valves, wound spirally over a bridging shunt; the adjoining margins of vein are sutured to produce a spiral compound vein graft. In situations of severe soft tissue damage an extra-anatomic vein bypass graft tunnelled through clean tissues is prudent.

Reports of the success of polytetrafluoroethylene grafts in potentially infected wounds should not induce complacency or obscure the risks of infection. Unlike a vein graft which is liable to break down under the action of bacterial collagenases, some argue that a prosthetic graft will remain immune, except at its anastomoses with the host vessel.

Vein repair restores venous outflow, reduces the impact of IR and enhances patency of an adjacent arterial repair. As the vein is usually a conduit of larger calibre than its companion artery, it is better able to tolerate lateral suture but, by the same token, its replacement by a small calibre interposition graft is futile. A compound vein graft ought to be fashioned and sutured into place over a shunt (Fig 5) even in an attempt to remedy the effects of recent injudicious ligation.

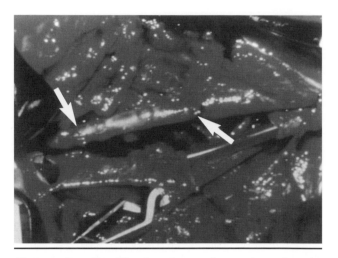

Figure 5a. Popliteal artery above (previously shunted) repaired using reversed interposition vein graft (between arrows). Popliteal vein below (also previously shunted) being repaired by a panelled compound vein graft.

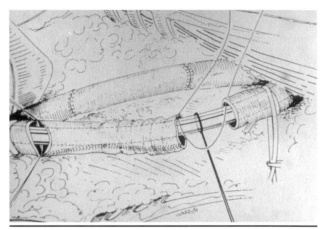

Figure 5b. Diagramatic representation of Figure 5a. (With permission from Barros D'Sa, A.A.B. (1996) In: Emergency Vascular Practice (eds A.D.B. Chant & A.A.B. Barros D'Sa). Arnold, London, UK).

Final steps

Intravascular shunting of both artery and its adjacent vein has limited the need for fasciotomy. A mannitol infusion within the first 12 - 24 hours is helpful in accelerating the inactivation of oxygen-derived free radicals and in reducing IR as long as the patient is haemodynamically stable. Rises in compartment pressure in complex leg injuries leave the muscles vulnerable, especially within the anterior compartment which is bounded by rigid osseous and fascial confines. As a rule, fasciotomy is indicated when admission is delayed 4 - 6 hours, significant bone and soft tissue injury exists, the muscle is oedematous and does not contract, compartment pressure exceeds 40 mm Hg or the foot is plantar flexed at completion of vascular repair. The standard double-incision approach decompressing all four compartments is both simple and effective [27].

Shunting of severed vessels will have provided sufficient time for proper wound care, so that at closure the quality and viability of tissues can be relied upon. The elimination of dead space and satisfactory vessel cover using healthy adjacent soft tissue and muscle will strongly influence the success of vascular repair. If a vein graft is exposed to desiccation, particularly in a contaminated field, breakdown and secondary haemorrhage are probable. Superficial muscles, such as the sartorius and gracilis, with their blood supply intact, can be used to ensheath a graft; in extreme cases a free vascularised musculocutaneous flap is required to cover the vascular repair and, perhaps, exposed bone. It is fairly safe to proceed to primary closure of incisions employed in closed injuries but contaminated wounds demand delayed primary suture after 5 - 7 days, or when deemed safe after one or more inspections.

The injured limb is nursed in a horizontal position. Antibiotics, anticoagulation and maintenance of good fluid balance are important therapeutic measures. Low molecular weight heparin not only aids graft patency but also discourages deep vein thrombosis; mature judgement should be exercised in the multiply injured patient. Close monitoring of pulse, capillary refill time, Doppler pulse waveforms and pressures will alert the clinician to a fall in distal blood flow. Thrombotic occlusion of a vessel repair usually reflects the use of suboptimal reconstructive methods, often employed in a hurried attempt to restore flow. Suspicion of graft failure should be confirmed by immediate angiography and followed, if necessary, by swift revision of the repair. With the introduction of a routine policy of shunting the incidence of re-exploration and revision of grafts fell sharply in my own hospital.

Complex vascular trauma to the leg

The problem

- Vessels are injured in 10%-48% of cases of complex limb trauma.

- 85% of these limbs are amputated and fatality is not uncommon.

- Treatment of damaged artery, vein, bone and soft tissue takes time.

- Prolonged ischaemia, increasing venous hypertension and the effects of ischaemia-reperfusion injury adversely affect outcome.

- The climate of urgency induces lapses and flaws in operative care further compounding the problem.

The solution

- Early shunting of both injured artery and vein.

- Immediate restoration of arterial inflow and of venous outflow.

- Tissue hypoxia is reversed, venous hypertension is relieved and the effects of ischaemia-reperfusion injury are minimized.

- A logical and disciplined sequence of operative steps is introduced.

- Morbidity is reduced and the chances of limb salvage and survival are improved.

References

1. Rich NM, Baugh JH, Hughes CW. Acute arterial injuries in Viet Nam. *J Trauma* 1970; 10: 359-69.

2. Barros D'Sa AAB, Hassard TH, Livingston RH, Irwin JWS. Missile-induced vascular trauma. *Injury* 1980; 12: 13-20.

3. Smith RF, Szilagyi DE, Elliott JP. Fracture of long bones with arterial injury due to blunt trauma. *Arch Surg* 1969; 99: 315-24.

4. Hewitt RL, Smyth AD, Drapanas T. Acute traumatic arterial venous fistulas. *J Trauma* 1973; 13: 901-906.

5. McNamara JJ, Brief DK, Stremple JF, et al. Management of fractures with associated arterial injury in combat casualties. *J Trauma* 1973; 13: 17-19.

6. Rosenthal JJ, Gaspar MR, Gjerdrum TC. Vascular injuries associated with the femur. *Arch Surg* 1975; 110: 494-497.

7. Weaver FA, Rosenthal RE, Waterhouse G, Adkins RB. Combined skeletal and vascular injuries of the lower extremities. *Am J Surg* 1984; 50: 189-97.

8. Allen MJ, Nash JR, Ioannidies TT, Bell PRF. Major vascular injuries associated with orthopaedic injuries to the lower limb. *Ann R Coll Surg Engl* 1984; 66: 101-104.

9. Lange RH, Bach AW, Hansen ST, Johansen KH. Open tibial fractures with associated vascular injuries: prognosis for limb salvage. *J Trauma* 1985; 25: 203-8.

10. Menzoian JO, Doyle JE, Cantelmo NL, LoGerfo FW, Hirsch E. A comprehensive approach to extremity vascular trauma. *Arch Surg* 1985; 120: 801-5.

11. Bishara RA, Pasch AR, Lim LT, et al. Improved results in the treatment of civilian vascular injuries associated with fracture and dislocations. *J Vasc Surg* 1986; 3: 707-11.

12. Granger DN, Höllwarth ME, Parks DA. Ischaemia-reperfusion injury: role of oxygen-derived free radicals. *Acta Physiol Scand [Suppl]* 1986; 548: 47-63.

13. Yassin MMI, Barros D'Sa AAB, Parks TG, et al. Mortality following lower limb ischaemia-reperfusion: systemic inflammatory response? *World J Surg* 1996; 20: 961-967.

14. Yassin MMI, Barros D'Sa AAB, Parks TG, et al. Lower limb ischaemia reperfusion alters gastrointestinal structure and function. *Br J Surg* 1997; 84: 1425-29.

15. Harkin DW, Barros D'Sa AAB, Yassin MMI, et al. Reperfusion injury is greater with delayed restoration of venous outflow in concurrent arterial and venous limb injury. *Br J Surg* 1999 (in press).

16. Barros D'Sa AAB. How do we manage acute limb ischaemia due to trauma. In: Greenhalgh RM, Jamieson CW, Nicolaides AN, Eds. *Limb salvage and amputation for vascular disease*. London: Saunders, 1988: 135-50.

17. Barros D'Sa AAB. Upper and lower limb vascular trauma. In: Greenhalgh RM, Ed. *Vascular surgical techniques*. London: Ballière Tindall, 1989: 47-65.

18. Barros D'Sa AAB. 25 years of vascular trauma in Northern Ireland. *Br Med J* 1995; 310: 1-2.

19. Barros D'Sa AAB. Adjunctive use of intravascular shunts in management of arterial and venous injuries. In: Yao ST, Pearce WH, Eds. *Progress in Vascular Surgery*. Stamford, Connecticut: Appleton & Lange 1997; 28: 353.

20. Barros D'Sa AAB. Complex vascular and orthopaedic limb injuries. Editorial. *J Bone Joint Surg (Br)* 1992; 74: 176-78.

21. Barros D'Sa AAB. The rationale for arterial and venous shunting in the management of limb vascular injuries. *Eur J Vasc Surg* 1989; 3: 471-4.

22. Walker AJ, Mellor SG, Cooper GJ. Experimental experience with a temporary intraluminal heparin-bonded polyurethane arterial shunt. *Br J Surg* 1994; 81: 195-198.

23. Rose SC, Moore EE. Trauma angiography: the use of clinical findings to improve patient selection and case preparation. *J Trauma* 1988; 28: 240-5.

24. Gregory RT, Gould RJ, Peclet M, et al. The mangled extremity syndrome (MES): a severity grading system for multisystem injury of the extremity. *J Trauma* 1985; 25: 1147-50.

25. Elliott JRM, Templeton J, Barros D'Sa AAB. Combined bony and vascular limb trauma: a new approach to treatment. *J Bone Joint Surg [Br]* 1984; 66-B: 281.

26. Barros D'Sa AAB, Moorehead RJ. Combined arterial and venous intraluminal shunting in major trauma of the lower limb. *Eur J Vasc Surg* 1989; 3: 577-81.

27. Mubarak SJ, Owen CA. Double-incision fasciotomy of the leg for decompression in compartment syndromes. *J Bone Joint Surg [Am]* 1977; 59-A: 184-7.

Chapter 30

Non-surgical factors that affect surgical outcome

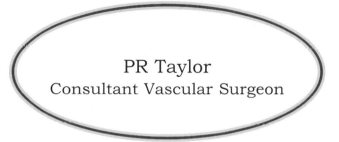

PR Taylor
Consultant Vascular Surgeon

DEPARTMENT OF SURGERY,
GUY'S HOSPITAL, LONDON

Introduction

The well publicised problem at the paediatric cardiac surgical unit in Bristol served to highlight outcome following surgical procedures. The adverse publicity resulted in two surgeons being physically attacked in the street by distressed relatives following the unfavourable verdict by the General Medical Council. This unfortunate episode has turned the spotlight on the whole of British surgery. Arterial surgery is, in the main, performed on relatively elderly patients who have a poor prognosis compared to the general population due to the widespread nature of atherosclerosis affecting the carotid and coronary arteries. This discipline can expect to be examined very thoroughly, as the results in terms of death, stroke and limb loss can be readily audited. Vascular problems after surgery tend to declare themselves early, and in-hospital morbidity and mortality will give a good guide to the outcome of surgical care. However, surgeons work as part of a team that includes a large number of other disciplines. The purpose of this chapter is to investigate factors other than the surgeon which may affect outcome following vascular operations.

Patient physiology may have the most influence on outcome, together with the degree of urgency of the surgery. The way in which audit of results is performed undoubtedly alters outcome. The hospital to which a patient is admitted is important. The anaesthetist, adjuvant techniques used during surgery, the intensive care unit, nursing and physiotherapy also play an important role in determining outcome.

Patient physiology

POSSUM refers to the Physiological and Operative Severity Score for enUmeration of Morbidity and mortality. It was originally devised for general surgical patients and, when applied to vascular patients, seemed to overpredict death. The Portsmouth group developed P-POSSUM which seemed more accurately to predict death in a prospective study [1]. More recently, the Audit Committee of the Vascular Surgical Society of Great Britain and Ireland has overseen a prospective study of 1304 patients [2]. The first half of this data base was assessed using Bayesian analysis to identify factors which were important in influencing outcome; the second half of the data base was used to validate the findings (Table 1). The age of the patient was extremely important in determining mortality. Smoking had little influence, although it is difficult to obtain the truth from patients regarding their smoking habits. Women fared worse than men, and patients with diabetes who were treated with diet or with insulin fared worse than those on oral medication. Aortic aneurysm surgery carried a worse outcome, particularly when compared with carotid surgery which carried a low risk of death. The most important factor was the degree of urgency of the admission, with emergency operations being associated

JVRG

Table 1. Bayes Probability Table.

Risk Factor		No	Odds Ratio	Weight
Age	0-60	262	2.9	10.7
(years)	61-70	388	1.38	3.2
	71-75	284	0.94	-0.6
	76-80	199	0.56	-5.8
	81-85	90	0.61	-4.9
	86-90	44	0.46	-7.7
	>90	12	0.21	-15.8
Sex	men	892	1.11	1.0
	women	409	0.81	-2.1
Smoking				
	current	459	0.97	-0.3
	ex	607	1.18	1.6
	never	204	0.9	-1.1
Diabetes				
	none	1073	1	0.0
	diet	42	0.76	-2.7
	tablet	98	1.92	6.5
	insulin	66	0.65	-4.3
Admission				
	elective	1051	2.07	7.3
	urgent	149	0.45	-8.1
	emergency	95	0.14	-19.5
Aortic aneurysm				
	yes	320	0.57	-5.6
	no	984	1.29	2.5
Carotid surgery				
	yes	226	4.56	15.2
	no	1078	0.85	-1.7

Weight refers to the importance of the factor. Negative marks are associated with poor outcome, positive with good outcome.

with a bad outcome. This was also shown to be very important in a prospective study of one single surgeon's arterial workload, with a mortality of 4.3% for 1149 elective operations, 10.6% for 376 urgent cases, and 23.9% for 188 emergency procedures [3]. The experience of the surgeon in assessing patients for particular operations may be helped, in future, by computer analysis of risk factors giving a numeric weight. This may enhance decision making about whether to operate on a particular individual.

Audit

Carotid endarterectomy is one of the most carefully analysed vascular operations, as the risk/benefit equation is particularly influenced by the operative mortality and morbidity. A recent survey showed that 20% of respondents did not audit their results, and retrospective analysis accounted for 62% of those who specified an audit technique [4]. Independent neurological assessment has a strong influence on the reported outcome of carotid surgery. An analysis of 50 studies showed an overall stroke and death rate of 5.6%, but this varied from 2.3% in reports by single surgeons to 5.5% for multiple surgical authors. If one or more authors was a physician, the rate was 6.4% and if the postoperative assessment was performed by a physician or neurologist it was 7.7% [5]. Case mix will also affect results, as the presenting symptom affects outcome. Patients who are asymptomatic have a better outcome than those who are symptomatic, and those with focal cerebral events do worse than those presenting with retinal symptoms [6,7].

The institution

The type of hospital in which vascular surgery is performed also affects outcome. Many studies have investigated the volume:outcome ratio of various institutions. An analysis of 678 Medicare patients showed that the overall stroke and death rate from carotid endarterectomy was 7% in low volume hospitals compared with 2.5% in the highest volume institutions [8]. The number of operations performed by any individual surgeon was not significant. This suggests that ancillary staff are important in the care of endarterectomy patients, and high numbers of cases may improve their expertise. A further analysis of 113,300 Medicare patients showed that those having carotid surgery in hospitals which participated in two major randomised clinical trials had a lower 30 day mortality than those from non-trial hospitals [9]. These clinical trials selected surgeons who had low complication rates for the operation. However, the minimum number of carotid endarterectomies that must be performed at any institution seems to be low. In a retrospective study of 48 hospitals in the state of Maryland over a 6 year period, 9918 carotid operations were identified; the threshold for acceptable results was eleven or more operations per hospital per year [10]. Another retrospective study on 1280 carotid endarterectomies from the eight University of Toronto-affiliated hospitals suggested that a surgeon volume of fewer than six cases per year was a significant predictor of poor outcome [11].

There is conflicting evidence about the outcome following aortic aneurysm surgery. In a study comprising 17,465 cases over a 4 year period of the Finnvasc national registry, hospital volume was not a significant factor in determining outcome. The surgeon's total vascular workload was important as was the number of elective aortic aneurysm repairs. The number of ruptured aneurysms had no significant influence [12]. However, a study of 9847 elective abdominal aortic aneurysm repairs has shown a significant inverse relationship between hospital volume and in-hospital death in New York State [13]. In another large series from the state of Florida, higher hospital volumes were associated with a better outcome for aortic aneurysm, carotid endarterectomy and lower limb arterial bypass operations [14]. There was no difference between teaching and non-teaching hospitals, which confirms findings from the UK [15].

The anaesthetist and adjunctive techniques used in theatre

Anaesthetists specialising in vascular procedures have recently formed a new society in the United Kingdom. However, there is very little evidence that anaesthetists concentrating on one surgical speciality affect outcome. Vascular surgeons know very quickly whether their colleague can cope with the demands of high risk patients having complex procedures, but objective data are hard to come by. One retrospective audit of 150 consecutive ruptured infrarenal abdominal aortic aneurysms suggested that anaesthetists specialising in vascular surgery resulted in a significantly better outcome at 30 days in patients over the age of 70, but there was no difference if patients of all ages were included [16].

Preoperative saline loading was shown in a non-randomised study to be beneficial in patients having aortic reconstructive procedures, with a reduction in pulmonary complications [17]. However, in a prospective randomised trial of pulmonary artery catheterisation with optimisation of haemodynamics in patients having elective vascular surgery, there was no significant difference in morbidity or mortality [18]. It was noted, however, that those with a pulmonary catheter received more fluid volume.

Two studies have shown a protective effect of normothermia during vascular procedures. In a randomised clinical trial, 300 patients having abdominal, thoracic or vascular surgical procedures with documented coronary disease or at high risk of a cardiac event, had either routine warming care or additional warming care to keep them normothermic [19]. Cardiac events and ventricular tachycardia were reduced in the normothermic group. The second study was a randomised trial of circulating water mattress compared with forced air blanket in 100 patients having infrarenal aortic aneurysm repair [20]. The forced air blanket was much more effective in keeping the core temperature normal both during and after surgery, and patients so treated had significantly less metabolic acidosis. Nevertheless, there was no difference in mortality, cardiac complications and length of stay. Patients who became hypothermic had lower cardiac output, thrombocytopenia, elevated prothrombin time and inferior APACHE II scores than those who remained normothermic.

There are several potential benefits from using autotransfusion during aortic surgery. These include reducing net blood loss, decreasing the risk of transmission of infection, preventing transfusion reactions, reducing the demands on blood transfusion services and, possibly, reducing cost. However, a randomised prospective trial of autotransfusion for aortic surgery failed to detect any significant difference in the number of allogeneic units transfused, the proportion of patients not receiving allogeneic blood, the postoperative haemoglobin and haematocrit, and complications [21].

Intensive care unit

Although many patients having arterial surgery can be nursed in a high dependency unit, there is still a role for intensive care, particularly for those undergoing thoracoabdominal aneurysm repair or emergency or urgent infrarenal aortic surgery. Intensive care unit protocols may affect the outcome. In a unique study, a consecutive series of patients having non-elective aortic aneurysm surgery were admitted to two different hospitals under the care of a single consultant surgeon. The intensive care units had different protocols for dealing with aneurysm patients. In one hospital, pulmonary artery catheters were placed in 96% of patients compared with 18% at the other; the former patients received much larger volumes of fluid and more inotropes, presumably to achieve set targets. In spite of this, more patients went into acute renal failure and the mortality rate was higher in the hospital with the increased use of pulmonary catheters [22]. This confirms the findings of studies on preoperative loading; pulmonary artery catheters increase the amount of fluid that patients are given [18]. When they are used incorrectly in order to achieve goals that are more suited to younger trauma victims, they may be harmful [23].

Conclusions

Factors other than the operative skill of the surgeon have been shown to affect outcome following arterial surgery. Randomised prospective trials have shown that good ideas in theory may not translate into better outcome in clinical practice, for instance the use of autotransfusion and preoperative saline loading. However, other factors such as warming blankets have been shown to be beneficial when assessed by rigorous trials. The role of intensive care units is much more difficult to assess, but there is evidence that goal-directed therapy may be harmful in elderly vascular patients having non-elective aortic aneurysm repair. Unfortunately virtually no randomised controlled trials exist on the role of nursing and physiotherapy in the care of vascular patients. However, a patient's physiology may be the most important determinant of outcome.

Non-surgical factors that affect surgical outcome

Sound evidence

- Patient age, type of operation and emergency operation are extremely important determinants of outcome from surgery.

- Pulmonary catheterisation for aortic surgery does not improve results.

- Warming during surgery reduces cardiac events and acidosis (but may not influence mortality or length of stay).

- High volume hospitals *almost* certainly produce better results than low volume hospitals; the influence of individual consultant operation volume is more difficult to assess.

Evidence needed

- The role of intensive care units and goal-directed therapy is not fully defined.

- The influence of nursing care and physiotherapy has never been assessed in any randomised trial.

References (randomised trials in bold)

1. Midwinter MJ, Tytherleigh M, Ashley S. Estimation of mortality and morbidity risk in vascular surgery using POSSUM and the Portsmouth predictor equation. *Br J Surg* 1999; 86: 471-4.

2. V-POSSUM. Personal communication. JJ Earnshaw.

3. Lagattolla NRF, McGuinness CL, Taylor PR. Influence of case mix and priority on outcome following arterial surgery. *Br J Surg* 1999; 86 Suppl 1; 110-111.

4. Chaturvedi S, Femino L. Are carotid endarterectomy complications rates being monitored? *Neurology* 1998; 50: 1927-8.

5. Rothwell PM, Warlow CP. Is self-audit reliable? *Lancet* 1995; 346: 1623.

6. Rothwell PM, Slattery J, Warlow CP. A systematic comparison of the risks of stroke and death due to carotid endarterectomy for symptomatic and asymptomatic stenosis. *Stroke* 1996; 27: 266-9.

7. Rothwell PM, Slattery J, Warlow CP. Clinical and angiographic predictors of stroke and death from carotid endarterectomy: systematic review. *BMJ* 1997; 315: 1571-7.

8. Cebul RD, Snow RJ, Pine R, Hertzer HR, Norris DG. Indications, outcomes and provider volumes for carotid endarterectomy. *JAMA* 1998; 279: 1282-7.

9. Wennberg DE, Lucas FL, Birkmayer JD, Brendenberg CE, Fisher ES. Variation in carotid endarterectomy mortality in the Medicare population: trial hospitals, volume and patient characteristics. *JAMA* 1998; 279: 1278-81.

10. Perler BA, Dardik AA, Burleyson GP, Gordon TA, Williams GM. Influence of age and hospital volume on the results of carotid endarterectomy: a statewide analysis of 9918 cases. *J Vasc Surg* 1998; 27: 25-33.

11. Kucey DS, Bowyer B, Iron K, Austin P, Anderson G, Tu JV. Determinants of outcome after carotid endarterectomy. *J Vasc Surg* 1998; 28: 1051-8.

12. Kantonenl, Lepantalo M, Salenius JP, Matzke S, Luther M, Ylonen K. Mortality in abdominal aortic aneurysm surgery: the effect of hospital volume, patient mix and surgeon's case load. *Eur J Vasc Endovasc Surg* 1997; 14: 375-9.

13. Sollano JA, Gelijns AC, Moskowitz AJ, et al. Volume-outcome relationships in cardiovascular operations: New York State, 1990-1995. *J Thorac Cardiovasc Surg* 1999; 117: 419-28.

14. Pearce WH, Parker MA, Feinglass J, Ujiki M, Manheim LM. The importance of surgeon volume and training in outcomes for vascular surgical procedures. *J Vasc Surg* 1999; 29: 768-78.

15. Galland RB, Wolfe JH. Mortality after elective aortic aneurysm repair: not where...but how many and by whom. *Ann R Coll Surg Eng* 1998; 80: 339-40.

16. Gibbs PJ, Darke SG, Parvin SD. Survival after repair of ruptured aortic aneurysm: an anaesthetic view. *Br J Surg.* 1998; 85: 554.

17. Garrison RN, Wilson MA, Matheson PJ, Spain DA. Preoperative saline loading improves outcome after elective, noncardiac surgical procedures. *Am Surg* 1996; 62: 223-31.

18. **Bender JS, Smith-Meek MA, Jones CE. Routine pulmonary artery catheterization does not reduce morbidity and mortality after elective vascular surgery: results of a prospective, randomised trial. *Ann Surg* 1997; 226: 229-36.**

19. **Frank SM, Fleisher LA, Breslow MJ, et al. Perioperative maintenance of normothermia reduces the incidence of morbid cardiac events. A randomised clinical trial. *JAMA* 1997; 277: 1127-34.**

20. **Elmore JR, Franklin DP, Youkey JR, Oren JW, Frey CM. Normothermia is protective during infrarenal aortic surgery. *J Vasc Surg* 1998; 28: 984-92.**

21. **Claggert GP, Valentine RJ, Jackson MR, Mathison C, Kakish HB, Bengtson TD. A randomized trial of intraoperative autotransfusion during aortic surgery. *J Vasc Surg* 1999; 29: 22-31.**

22. Sandison AJP, Wyncoll DLA, Edmondson RC, Van Heerden N, Beale RJ, Taylor PR. ICU protocol may affect the outcome of non-elective abdominal aortic aneurysm repair. *Eur J Vasc Endovasc Surg* 1998; 16: 356-361.

23. Hayes MA, Timmins AC, Yau EHS, Palazzo M, Hinds CJ, Watson D. Elevation of systemic oxygen delivery in the treatment of critically ill patients. *N Engl J Med* 1994; 33: 1717-22.

Non-surgical factors that affect
surgical outcome

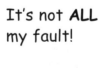

It's not **ALL**
my fault!

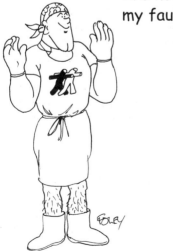

Chapter 31

Medico-legal implications associated with evidence based medicine

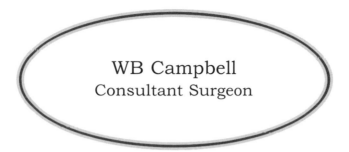

WB Campbell
Consultant Surgeon

DEPARTMENT OF SURGERY,
ROYAL DEVON AND EXETER HOSPITAL, EXETER

Introduction

'Evidence' is fundamental to the practice both of medicine and law, but the nature of evidence in medicine, and the way it is used, have become increasingly specific over recent years. 'Evidence based medicine' means practising in accordance with best current evidence [1,2], but many of the treatments doctors use are not well proven in a strictly scientific sense. This paradox has led to the concept of 'levels of evidence' (evidence from good randomised trials, from non-randomised trials, from cohort or case studies, from multiple time series, etc.) which are important in judging how effective or ineffective medical interventions may be. This gradation contrasts with the usual view of evidence in civil law, which is rather more black-and-white: evidence is generally considered to be true or false, and once a balance of probabilities exceeds 50%, then that probability is 'right'. It is worth recognising these rather different concepts of 'evidence' in the medical and legal worlds when addressing the medico-legal implications of evidence based medicine.

Any medico-legal action is based on the need to prove negligence. This involves two steps. First, liability must be proven, by showing that a practitioner failed to discharge his or her duty of care properly. Second, causation must be demonstrated, by establishing a link between the action (or lack of action) and harm to the patient. Both these steps may invoke the published evidence base. The 'Bolam test' is fundamental, requiring a standard of customary care and clinical judgement informed by scientific evidence and professional experience [3].

Medico-legal actions depend on expert opinions obtained by the lawyers for the plaintiff (or pursuer in Scotland) and by the defence. These experts advise, based on personal experience and opinion, citing selected areas of the literature as 'evidence'. Some may choose to present a convincing one-sided argument with highly selective citation, and a number of different experts may be enlisted in complex cases. Even for quite minor cases the process can be very protracted.

Two aspects are changing. First, the legal process in England and Wales is being altered to allow faster processing of apparently simple cases, with preference for a single expert who will be asked to provide a comprehensive report within a limited period of time [4]. Second, the drive towards 'evidence based medicine' with guidelines means that a judgement about what is 'right' or 'wrong' in medical practice appears to be more straightforward. This worries many doctors, who feel that they may be medico-legally vulnerable if they make thoughtful decisions which depart from the current 'evidence base' or guidelines.

Access to the evidence

The internet provides patients and any other interested parties with ready access to information, guidelines, and

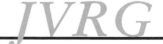

literature searches about medical conditions. While this has the obvious advantage of allowing them to be informed, it is also a treasure trove for those who are dissatisfied with their medical care and who want to sue doctors. If a doctor really has acted contrary to current best evidence, then the patient's internet findings may be proper exposure of poor practice. However, unhappy patients and others may latch on to information or publications which are controversial, not properly proven, or recognised as not cost effective.

When patients obtain information about a treatment which they feel they have been denied, there is usually some good and thoughtful reason for this in the individual case. It is to be hoped that a sympathetic explanation about the choice of treatment will resolve any concern, but doctors are likely to be both pressed and sued increasingly by patients who have interrogated the evidence base now available on the internet.

Systematic reviews

A few medical treatments become established or rejected on the basis of one or two big, landmark publications (eg. the indications for carotid endarterectomy since the European Carotid Surgery Trial[5] and the North American Symptomatic Carotid Endarterectomy Trial[6]). Much more often, however, the evidence for, or against the use of an intervention is scattered in various corners of the literature (perhaps in different languages) and may remain obscure until it is gathered together and appraised properly (for example aspirin prophylaxis in vascular disease[7]).

There are now well established principles for conducting systematic reviews[8]. Meta-analysis is the best recognised method and it is widely regarded as the closest we can approach to the current state of knowledge about the value of an intervention. When properly done, meta-analysis shows when the published evidence is sufficient to conclude that an intervention is effective or ineffective, or when the evidence is insufficient. If a meta-analysis bears the stamp of a respected organisation, such as the Cochrane Collaboration or the NHS Centre for Reviews and Dissemination, this adds to its authority[1].

Published meta-analyses are likely to be used in medico-legal proceedings and doctors failing to practise in accordance with their conclusions need to justify their actions. In general this is a reasonable and welcome trend but there are potential problems. First - when meta-analysis is used in a doctor's defence - lawyers and courts may not fully understand the significance and power of the meta-analysis data when a skilled expert counters them persuasively with selected excerpts from the literature. Second - when used against a doctor - some meta-analyses produce a conclusion which still leaves room for doubt, but may be presented as if it did not. Patching in carotid endarterectomy is a good example. Meta-analysis has shown an association

between patching and a reduction in the risk of ipsilateral stroke or death[9]: this might be used as evidence against a surgeon if a patient has a perioperative stroke when a patch was not used. However, the authors of the meta-analysis pointed out shortcomings of the available trials; there is no good evidence about the use of patches in arteries of different diameters and many vascular surgeons (even 'patchers') do not patch a wide internal carotid artery. Finally, there may be lack of understanding that while systematic reviews provide generalisable evidence, their findings need to be applied selectively to individual patients.

Guidelines

Guidelines are another product of the drive for evidence based medicine and they bother many doctors from a medico-legal point of view[3]. Guidelines represent a synthesis of the best available evidence and the opinions of the expert panels which have formulated them. On the whole, therefore, they are 'evidence based' but they also pronounce on areas for which the evidence is absent, poor, or extrapolated. This is a worry medico-legally, because guidelines produced by respected bodies could be used against a doctor who has contravened their advice on a matter which is not properly proven.

An example in vascular practice is the use of heparin prophylaxis in varicose vein surgery. Both the national THRIFT guidelines[10] and the European guidelines[11] on prophylaxis of venous thromboembolism place varicose veins high on the list of risk factors. However, the evidence for this relates only to patients having major abdominal or pelvic surgery: there is no evidence regarding patients having varicose vein operations. A surgeon who did not use prophylaxis might nevertheless be challenged medico-legally, using these influential guidelines, if a patient suffers thromboembolism after varicose vein surgery when prophylaxis was not used. In such circumstances, good evidence on the practice and opinions of the generality of other specialists may be valuable, and this is one area to which I have tried to contribute by publishing the results of questionnaires[12,13], happily supported by a great many colleagues.

Clinical guidelines might prove to be a two edged sword, because they need to be applied with discretion and a doctor who implements guidelines which are faulty, or who uses guidelines inappropriately, might perhaps be found negligent[3].

Practices with conflicting evidence

When there is limited evidence about a practice and that evidence is genuinely conflicting, uncertainty translates from clinical practice into the medico-legal arena because appraisal by different 'experts' may produce different yet forceful views. An example is the use of protamine for reversal of heparin in carotid endarterectomy. One large (non-randomised) study showed significant reduction in bleeding complications without significant adverse effects [14]: a subsequent non-randomised series [15] and a small randomised study [16] have shown an increased risk of stroke. Practice varies as a result and a surgeon who uses protamine could find him or herself threatened by expert opinions if a patient suffers a thrombotic stroke (quite possibly for other reasons).

Practices without good supporting evidence

These can pose problems medico-legally because doctors are vulnerable to the use of poor scientific evidence (because no good evidence exists) or the strongly held views of 'experts'. An example in vascular practice is the use of heparin, which is traditionally given during surgical and endovascular interventions, or as initial treatment in acute ischaemia; there is little specific evidence of benefit as a result. A surgeon might nevertheless be challenged medico-legally for failing to use heparin during intervention on the arteries of a limb, both on the grounds of published advice and common practice. In the absence of evidence which would withstand systematic review it is interesting to speculate on the conclusion of the arguments.

There are some interventions which are so obviously effective that no randomised trial has ever been required - for example balloon catheter embolectomy in the treatment of the bloodless limb caused by embolism. Arguing that this treatment might reasonably be witheld because there are no published trials would prevail neither in the clinical nor the medico-legal setting. However, one must be careful about using the concept 'it obviously works' inappropriately. From a radiological standpoint, balloon angioplasty of the superficial femoral artery for claudication quite clearly works when the artery is shown to be recanalised, the ankle pressure is restored to normal, and the patient walks unlimited distances the next day. But we now know that these results may not be longlasting and the benefit of femoropopliteal angioplasty for claudication has been called into question [17]. Based on the current evidence, how might a surgeon be judged who denied a patient access to angioplasty on the basis of dubious long-term results and uncertain cost effectiveness?

New treatments

These are always difficult, because the evidence is sparse when new treatments first become available; this is more of a problem with new surgical interventions than new drug therapies, which have a well developed system

of testing with huge commercial input. Endovascular treatment of aortic aneurysms is the obvious current example. Protection against medico-legal action depends on thorough patient information and consent, demonstrable levels of experience, and full participation in the recognised registries and trials. Compliance with the requirements of SERNIP (Safety and Efficacy Register for New Interventions and Products) in the United Kingdom ought to confer a degree of medico-legal protection - certainly departure from SERNIP principles would make a clinician medico-legally vulnerable.

Denying patients treatment which is not cost effective

Evidence based medicine is inextricably linked with cost effective medicine [2], particularly in the context of a cash limited health service. Advice about the cost effectiveness of treatments is already available in some regions from Development and Evaluation Committees (DECs) [18] and will soon be available nationally from the National Institute for Clinical Excellence (NICE) [19]. More often at present, cost-related decisions are made at local level and may be challenged medico-legally by patients. Occasionally these cases are given a high profile in the press; usually when they involve denial of potentially life-saving, but very expensive treatment.

In vascular practice the use of prostacyclin for advanced chronic ischaemia might fall into this category. There is some evidence of a beneficial effect [20], but the drug is expensive and local audit in my own hospital has failed to demonstrate sustained benefit in patients with critical ischaemia. It is therefore not funded for this indication. One could nevertheless envisage patients or their relatives attempting to press a medico-legal case because a limb was amputated without trying to prolong limb salvage by the use of prostacyclin.

Explaining and recording departures from the evidence base

All evidence of the effectiveness of interventions is generality, and there may be a great variety of reasons why the usual and proven treatment for a particular condition is not appropriate or best for an individual patient. While these reasons may be clear to the doctor, it is vital that they are explained properly to patients and their relatives, and that explicit records are kept. These records may be handwritten in the case notes, or included in typed letters or operation notes.

Inadequate communication remains a prime reason for complaints and medico-legal actions against doctors, and inadequate records pose a serious difficulty in providing a robust defence. At a time when evidence based medicine is burgeoning it is increasingly important for doctors to record thoroughly their reasons for advising interventions (or advising against them) when this advice apparently contravenes the current 'evidence base' or guidelines. Simply treating patients in the most thoughtful way - tempering the evidence with careful consideration of their individual circumstances - is no longer sufficient. We must be sure that our thoughts have been both well communicated and recorded, or we run the risk of needless medico-legal intrusion.

Acknowledgement

I thank Mr Stuart Bramley for his comments on the legal aspects of this chapter.

References (randomised trials in bold)

1. Grayson L. *Evidence-based medicine*. London. The British Library. 1997.

2. Lockett T. *Evidence-based and cost effective medicine for the uninitiated*. Oxford. Oxford Medical Press Ltd. 1997.

3. Hurwitz B. Legal and political considerations of clinical practice guidelines. *Br Med J* 1999; 318: 661-4.

4. Civil Procedure Rules 1998. Part 35.8.

5. **European Carotid Surgery Trialists' Collaborative Group. MRC European Carotid Surgery Trial; interim results for symptomatic patients with severe (70-99%) or with mild (0-29%) carotid stenoses.** *Lancet* **1991; 337: 1235-43.**

6. **North American Symptomatic Carotid Surgery Trial Collaborators. Beneficial effect of carotid endarterectomy in symptomatic patients with high-grade carotid stenosis.** *N Engl J Med* **1991; 325: 445-53.**

7. **Antiplatelet Trialists' Collaboration. Collaborative overview of randomised trials of antiplatelet therapy - II: Maintenance of vascular graft or arterial patency by antiplatelet therapy.** *Br Med J* **1994; 308: 159-168.**

8. Chalmers I, Altman DG. *Systematic reviews*. London. BMJ Publishing Group. 1995.

9. **Counsell CE, Salinas R, Naylor R, Warlow CP. A systematic review of the randomised trials of carotid patch angioplasty in carotid endarterectomy.** *Eur J Vasc Endovasc Surg* **1997; 13: 345-54.**

10. Thromboembolic Risk Factors (THRIFT) Consensus Group. Risk of and prophylaxis for venous thromboembolism in hospital patients. *Br Med J* 1992; 305: 567-74.

11. European Consensus Statement. *Prevention of venous thromboembolism*. London. Med-Orion. 1992.

12. Campbell WB, Ridler BMF. Varicose veins and deep vein thrombosis. *Br J Surg*. 1995; 82: 1494-7.

13. Hewin DF, Campbell WB. Ruptured aortic aneurysm: the decision not to operate. *Ann R Coll Surg Engl* 1998; 80: 221-5.

14. Treiman RL, Cossman DV, Foran RF, Levin PM, Cohen JL, Wagner WH. The influence of neutralising heparin after carotid endarterectomy on postoperative stroke and wound hematoma. *J Vasc Surg* 1990; 12: 440-6.

15. Mauney MC, Buchanan SA, Lawrence A, et al. Stroke rate is markedly reduced after carotid endarterectomy by avoidance of protamine. *J Vasc Surg* 1995; 22: 264-70.

16. **Fearn SJ, Parry AD, Picton AJ, Mortimer AJ, McCollum CN. Should heparin be reversed after carotid endarterectomy? A randomised prospective trial.** *Eur J Vasc Endovasc Surg* **1997; 13: 394-7.**

17. Fowkes FGR, Gillespie IN. Angioplasty (versus non-surgical management) for intermittent claudication. *Eur J Vasc Endovasc Surg* 1998, 16: 274.

18. Health Technology Evaluation. Research Reviews V. Eds. Milne R, Stein K, Best L. Southampton. Wessex Institute for Health Research and Development. 1998.

19. NHS Executive. *Faster access to modern treatment: how NICE appraisal will work*. Department of Health. 1999.

20. **U.K. Severe Ischaemia Study Group. Treatment of limb threatening ischaemia with intravenous iloprost: a randomised double-blind study placebo controlled study.** *Eur J Vasc Surg* **1991; 5: 511-6.**

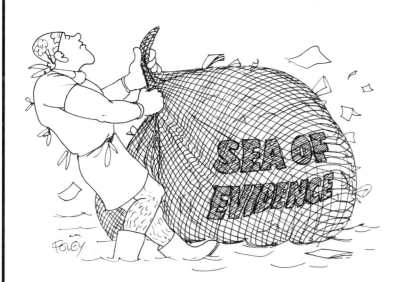

Appendix

THE JOINT VASCULAR RESEARCH GROUP

One of the main problems that bedevils vascular surgical research is that individual doctors do not manage a sufficient number of patients each year to achieve an adequate controlled trial within a limited period. This can be overcome by multicentre working, but the casual multicentre trial that runs on for several years only to be abandoned through a general waning of interest is well known to us all. It was to address these difficulties that on 25 March 1983, 13 British consultant vascular surgeons met in Southampton; the meeting was hosted by the local vascular surgeon, Tony Chant. This gathering gave life to a concept originally attributed to Simon Darke of Bournemouth; thus was the Joint Vascular Research Group (JVRG) born.

The prime objective of this collaborative group is to enter as many patients as possible into multicentre controlled trials of vascular procedures and to conduct studies of the natural history of vascular disease. The members agreed to meet twice a year (see below) to propose new trials and to assess the results of current work. Each trial becomes the responsibility of one member of the Group. Over time the JVRG has been responsible for many communications at scientific meetings and its members have contributed widely to textbooks and journals. A list of the original full papers produced by the JVRG is appended below; the present book is the second such publishing venture from the Group (the first was 'Vascular Surgery - Current Questions', edited by Aires Barros D'Sa, Peter Bell, Simon Darke and Peter Harris, and published in 1991).

The JVRG is a registered charity that is entirely self-supporting and relies on donations and profits from ventures such as this volume. The Group has grown since 1983 and membership is now by centre rather than individual. Twenty-two geographic centres now take part, including 25 hospitals (see below). The driving force is, however, very much the same as that which motivated the original Group 16 years ago; the original principles have served us well in expanding the evidence base of vascular surgery. Over the years the players have changed somewhat. Older and sometimes less productive members have drifted away to be replaced by younger more enthusiastic colleagues. In this way the JVRG has remained a vibrant organisation with an exciting role to play in a clinical future that will be increasingly evidence-based.

Original articles published by the JVRG

1. Darke SG, Lamont PM, Chant ADB, Barros D'Sa AAB, Clyne CAC, Harris PL, Ruckley CV, Bell PRF. Femoropopliteal versus femorodistal bypass grafting for limb salvage in patients with an isolated popliteal segment. *Eur J Vasc Surg* 1989; 3: 203-207.

2. Ruckley CV, Stonebridge PA, Prescott RJ for the Joint Vascular Research Group. Skewflap versus long posterior flap in below-knee amputations: multicentre trial. *J Vasc Surg* 1991; 13: 423-427.

3. Tyrell MR, Wolfe JH. Critical leg ischaemia: an appraisal of clinical definitions. Joint Vascular Research Group. *Br J Surg* 1993; 80: 177-180.

4. Ranaboldo CJ, Barros D'Sa AA, Bell PRF, Chant AD, Perry PM. Randomised controlled trial of patch angioplasty for carotid endarterectomy. The Joint Vascular Research Group. *Br J Surg* 1993; 80: 1528-1530.

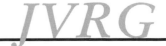

5. Varga ZA, Locke-Edmunds JC, Baird RN, Joint Vascular Research Group. A multicentre study of popliteal aneurysms. *J Vasc Surg* 1994; 20: 171-177.

6. Thompson JF, Mullee MA, Bell PRF, Campbell WB, Chant AD, Darke SG, Jamieson CW, Murie JA, Parvin SD, Perry M, Ruckley CV, Wolfe JH, Clyne CA. Intraoperative heparinisation, blood loss and myocardial infarction during aortic aneurysm surgery : a Joint Vascular Research Group Study. *Eur J Vasc Endovasc Surg* 1996; 12: 86-90.

7. Stonebridge PA, Prescott RJ, Ruckley CV. Randomised trial comparing infra-inguinal polytetrafluroroethylene bypass grafting with and without vein interposition cuff at the distal anastomosis. The Joint Vascular Research Group. *J Vasc Surg* 1997; 26: 543-550.

8. Galland RB on behalf of the Joint Vascular Research Group. Mortality following elective infrarenal aortic reconstruction. *Br J Surg* 1998; 85: 633-636.

9. Lambert AW, Wilkins DC on behalf of the Joint Vascular Research Group. Popliteal artery entrapment: collaborative experience. *Br J Surg* 1998; 85: 1367-1368.

10. Braithwaite BD, Davies B, Heather BP, Earnshaw JJ. Early results of a randomised trial of rifampicin-bonded Dacron grafts for extra-anatomic reconstruction. Joint Vascular Research Group. *Br J Surg* 1998; 85: 1378-1381.

Membership of the JVRG

Consultant Vascular Surgeons from the following Vascular Units currently contribute cases to JVRG studies :

Bath (Royal United Hospital)

Belfast (Royal Victoria Hospital)

Bournemouth (Royal Bournemouth General Hospital)

Bristol (Bristol Royal Infirmary)

Dundee (Ninewells Hospital)

Edinburgh (Edinburgh Royal Infirmary)

Exeter (Royal Devon and Exeter Hospital)

Gloucester/Cheltenham (Gloucestershire Royal and Cheltenham General Hospitals)

Hull (Hull Royal Infirmary)

Leeds (Leeds General Infirmary)

Leicester (Leicester Royal Infirmary)

Liverpool (Royal Liverpool Hospital)

London (Guys, Royal Free and St. Mary's Hospitals)

Newcastle (Freeman Hospital)

Northampton (Northampton General Hospital)

Nottingham (University Hospital)

Plymouth (Derriford Hospital)

Reading (Royal Berkshire Hospital)

Sheffield (Northern General Hospital)

Southampton (Southampton General Hospital)

Swansea (Morriston Hospital)

Torquay (Torbay Hospital)

JVRG Meeting Venues

1983	Southampton and London	**1992**	Torquay and London
1984	Lancaster and Birmingham	**1993**	Bournemouth and Manchester
1985	Edinburgh and London	**1994**	Torquay and Edinburgh
1986	Torquay and London	**1995**	Sheffield and London
1987	London and Newcastle	**1996**	Plymouth and Bournemouth
1988	Bristol and Leeds	**1997**	Bristol and London
1989	Leicester and Dundee	**1998**	Leeds and Hull
1990	Kirkby Lonsdale and London	**1999**	Gloucester and Leicester
1991	Belfast and Dublin	**2000**	Dovedale and London

Completed Trials

1. Critical ischaemia study.
2. In situ vein graft: proximal versus distal implantation.
3. Skew flap versus long posterior flap in below knee amputation.
4. Carotid endarterectomy patch versus no patch.
5. Polytetrafluoroethylene versus human umbilical vein in femoropopliteal bypass.
6. Heparin versus no heparin in aortic aneurysm surgery.
7. Popliteal artery aneurysm study.
8. Unilateral iliofemoral versus femorofemoral crossover bypass graft.
9. Unsealed versus collagen sealed aortic graft.
10. Vein interposition cuff versus no cuff in polytetrafluoroethylene femorodistal bypass grafts.
11. Randomised trial of aprotinin in ruptured abdominal aortic reconstruction.
12. Mortality following elective infrarenal aortic reconstruction.
13. Randomised trial of antibiotic bonding in extra-anatomic Dacron grafts.
14. Natural history of asymptomatic renal artery stenosis.
15. Prospective study of the incidence of renal failure after vascular surgery.
16. Multicentre study of wound and graft infection in vascular surgery: impact of methicillin-resistant *Staphylococcus aureus*.
17. Collaborative experience of popliteal entrapment syndrome.
18. Patterns of occlusive disease in patients with gangrenous toes.

Current Projects

1. Natural history of asymptomatic superficial femoral artery stenosis.
2. Register of rare diseases.
3. Sub-intimal angioplasty versus femoropopliteal grafting for long superficial femoral artery occlusion.
4. Prospective randomised trial of acute normovolaemic haemodilution in aortic surgery.

Appendix

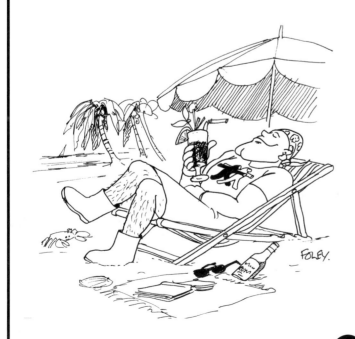